DEJA REVIEW™

USMLE Step 1

NOTICE

Medicine is an ever-changing science. As new research and clinical experience broaden our knowledge, changes in treatment and drug therapy are required. The authors and the publisher of this work have checked with sources believed to be reliable in their efforts to provide information that is complete and generally in accord with the standards accepted at the time of publication. However, in view of the possibility of human error or changes in medical sciences, neither the authors nor the publisher nor any other party who has been involved in the preparation or publication of this work warrants that the information contained herein is in every respect accurate or complete, and they disclaim all responsibility for any errors or omissions or for the results obtained from use of the information contained in this work. Readers are encouraged to confirm the information contained herein with other sources. For example and in particular, readers are advised to check the product information sheet included in the package of each drug they plan to administer to be certain that the information contained in this work is accurate and that changes have not been made in the recommended dose or in the contraindications for administration. This recommendation is of particular importance in connection with new or infrequently used drugs.

DEJA REVIEW™

USMLE Step 1

Third Edition

Mark K. Tuttle, MD

Interventional Cardiology Fellow
Beth Israel Deaconess Medical Center
Clinical and Research Fellow
Harvard Medical School
Boston, Massachusetts

John H. Naheedy, MD

Medical Director
Department of Radiology
Rady Children's Hospital San Diego
Assistant Professor
UC San Diego Medical Center
San Diego, California

Daniel A. Orringer, MD

Associate Professor
Department of Neurosurgery
NYU School of Medicine
New York, New York

New York   Chicago   San Francisco   Lisbon   London   Madrid   Mexico City
Milan   New Delhi   San Juan   Seoul   Singapore   Sydney   Toronto

Déjà Review™ USMLE Step 1, Third Edition

1 2 3 4 5 6 7 8 9   LCR   25 24 23 22 21 20

ISBN 978-1-260-44164-2
MHID 1-260-44164-4

This book was set in Palatino by MPS Limited.
The editors were Bob Boehringer and Christina M. Thomas.
The production supervisor was Catherine H. Saggese.
Project management was provided by Poonam Bisht, MPS Limited.
This book is printed on acid-free paper.

Library of Congress Cataloging-in-Publication Data

Names: Naheedy, John H., author. | Tuttle, Mark K., author. | Orringer, Daniel A., author.
Title: Deja review. USMLE step 1 / Mark K. Tuttle, John H. Naheedy, Daniel A. Orringer.
Other titles: USMLE step 1 | Deja review.
Description: Third edition. | New York : McGraw Hill, [2020] | Series: Deja review | John H. Naheedy's name appears first on previous edition. | Summary: "The Deja Review series provides a study guide to all core information. The high-yield "flashcard" format helps medical students recall the most important, must-know facts and concepts covered in their course work. This rapid-fire question & answer review book allows students to quickly navigate through the information needed for their success on USMLE Step 1 as well as their course exams. Mnemonics and keywords sprinkled throughout the text facilitate focus on core facts. An entire chapter at the end of book entitled "Make a Diagnosis" is devoted enirely to clinical vignettes, allowing students to reflect and recap on the topics they have just read in a clinical presentation"— Provided by publisher.
Identifiers: LCCN 2019055196 | ISBN 9781260441642 (paperback ; alk. paper) | ISBN 9781260441659 (ebook)
Subjects: MESH: Clinical Medicine—methods | Examination Question
Classification: LCC RC58 | NLM WB 18.2 | DDC 616.0076—dc23
LC record available at https://lccn.loc.gov/2019055196

In memory of John M. Stang, MD

To my wife Caroline, for her unwavering support and affection.
—Mark

To our families.
—John and Daniel

Contents

Student Editors

Blake Arthurs, MD
Family Medicine Resident
University of Michigan
Ann Arbor, Michigan
Chapters: Musculoskeletal, Pulmonary, and
    Reproductive and Endocrine, Make the
    Diagnosis

Ryoko Hamaguchi
MD Candidate
Class of 2020
Harvard Medical School
Boston, Massachusetts
Chapters: Gastroenterology,
    Hematology-Oncology, Neuroscience, and
    Make the Diagnosis

Cynthia Wang, MD/MPHS
Dermatology Resident
Washington University School of Medicine in
St. Louis
St. Louis, Missouri
Chapters: Skin and Connective Tissue, Renal
    and Genitourinary, Microbiology, Make the
    Diagnosis

Second Edition Contributing Authors

Alexander Choo
Medical Student
Class of 2010
University of California, San Diego
La Jolla, California
Chapters: Pulmonary, Skin and Connective Tissues, Musculoskeletal

Charlotte Gore
Medical Student
Class of 2010
University of California, San Diego
La Jolla, California
Chapters: Basic Principles, Neuroscience, Gastroenterology, Hematology and Oncology, Behavioral Science, Make the Diagnosis

Kristen A. Kipps
Medical Student
Class of 2010
University of California, San Diego
La Jolla, California
Chapters: Immunology, Microbiology and Infectious Diseases

Brian S. Pugmire
Medical Student
Class of 2010
University of California, San Diego
La Jolla, California
Chapter: Renal and Genitourinary

Krishna C. Ravi
Medical Student
Class of 2010
University of California, San Diego
La Jolla, California
Chapter: Cardiovascular

Omeed Saghafi
Medical Student
Class of 2010
University of California, San Diego
La Jolla, California
Chapter: Reproduction and Endocrinology

Preface

The main objective of a medical student preparing for Step 1 of the United States Medical Licensing Examination (USMLE) is to commit a vast body of knowledge to memory. We feel there are two main principles that will allow you to be successful in your preparations for Step 1: (1) repetition of key facts and (2) using review questions to gauge your comprehension and memory. The Déjà Review™ series is a unique resource that has been designed to allow you to review the essential facts and determine your level of knowledge on the subjects tested on Step 1. We also know, from experience, that building a solid foundation in the basic sciences will allow you to make a smooth transition into the clinical years of medical school and beyond.

ORGANIZATION

All concepts are presented in a question and answer format that covers the key facts on hundreds of commonly tested USMLE Step 1 topics. The material is divided into chapters organized by body systems. Special emphasis has been placed on the molecular and genetic basis of pathology, as this area has become increasingly emphasized in recent examinations.

This question and answer format has several important advantages:

- It provides a rapid, straightforward way for you to assess your strengths and weaknesses.
- It allows you to efficiently review and commit to memory a large body of information.
- It offers a break from tedious, convoluted multiple-choice questions.
- The "Make the Diagnosis" section exposes you to the prototypic presentation of diseases classically tested on the USMLE Step 1.
- It serves as a quick, last-minute review of high-yield facts.

The compact, condensed design of the book is conducive to studying on the go, especially during any downtime throughout your day.

HOW TO USE THIS BOOK

This text has been sampled by a number of medical students who found it to be an essential part of their preparation for Step 1, in addition to their course examinations. Remember, this text is not intended to replace comprehensive textbooks, course packs, or lectures. It is simply intended to serve as a supplement to your studies during your first 2 years of medical school and throughout your preparation for Step 1. We encourage you to begin using this book early in your first year to reinforce topics covered on your course examinations. We also recommend having the book spiral bound to make it more portable and easier to use outside of the library or classroom. You may cover up the answers and quiz yourself or even your classmates. For a greater challenge, try covering up the questions!

However you choose to study, we hope you find this resource helpful throughout your preclinical years and during your preparation for the USMLE Step 1. Best of luck!

Mark K. Tuttle, MD
John H. Naheedy, MD
Daniel A. Orringer, MD

CHAPTER 1

Basic Principles

MOLECULAR BIOLOGY, BIOCHEMISTRY, AND GENETICS

DNA, Genes, and Chromosomes

Which nucleotide bases are purines and which are pyrimidines?	"**CUT** the **PY**": Cytosine, Uracil, and Thymine = **PY**rimidines; "**PUR**e As Gold": **PUR**ines = adenine and guanine
Which proteins make up the core of a nucleosome?	Histones: H2A, H2B, H3, and H4
Which proteins are associated with DNA between nucleosomes?	Histone H1

Name the type of mutations described below:

Type of mutation that does not result in a change in amino acid sequence	Silent
Type of mutation that results in a change in amino acid sequence	Missense
Type of mutation that results in a stop codon	Nonsense: "NO sense"
Type of mutation that changes the reading frame	Frameshift
Type of mutation in which a portion of DNA is lost	Deletion
Type of mutation in which a single base is exchanged	Point

Name the type of cytogenetic disorders described below:

Failure of chromosomes to disjoin properly during cell division	Nondisjunction
Loss of a portion of a chromosome	Deletion
Two internal chromosomal breaks with inverted reincorporation of a portion of the chromosome	Inversion
Single breaks in two chromosomes resulting in the exchange of segments between chromosomes without loss of genetic material	Balanced reciprocal translocation
Single breaks in two acrocentric chromosomes resulting in one large chromosome and one small chromosome accompanied by the loss of some genetic information, hereditary form of Down syndrome	Robertsonian translocation
Mitotic error in early development leading to the development of two karyotypically distinct populations of cells in an organism	Mosaicism
What term is used to describe the AT-rich sequences in the genome where DNA replication begins?	Origin of replication

DNA Replication, Transcription, and Translation

Name the protein(s) involved in replication or DNA repair with the functions listed below:

Stabilize single-stranded DNA	Single-stranded DNA-binding proteins
Recognition of AT-rich sequences at the origin of replication and separation of DNA strands in bacteria (prokaryotes)	DnaA protein
Unwinding DNA double helix	DNA helicases
Prevention of supercoiling during replication	DNA topoisomerases
Placement of RNA primer at site where replication is initiated	Primase, and a RNA polymerase
Removal of RNA primers from DNA synthesized discontinuously	DNA polymerase I (specifically, the 5′-3′ exonuclease activity)

DNA chain elongation in prokaryotes	DNA polymerase III
Proofreading of newly synthesized DNA strand	DNA polymerase III (specifically, the 3′-5′ exonuclease activity)
Repair UV damage to DNA	UV-specific endonuclease, exonuclease, and DNA ligase
Removal of damaged bases from DNA	Apurinic or apyrimidinic endonuclease, exonuclease, and DNA ligase
What term is used to describe the DNA strand synthesized continuously toward the replication fork?	Leading strand
What term is used to describe the DNA strand synthesized discontinuously away from the replication fork?	Lagging strand
What are the three stop codons?	UGA, UAA, UAG (**U** Go **A**way, **U** Are **A**way, **U** Are Gone)
In which direction are DNA and RNA synthesized?	5′ → 3′
What is the start codon?	AUG
Name the type of RNA responsible for each of the following functions:	
Largest RNA molecule	mRNA (messenger RNA)
Most abundant type of RNA	rRNA (ribosomal RNA)
Smallest RNA molecule	tRNA (transfer RNA)
Portion of RNA transcript encoding information for protein synthesis	Exons ("exons are expressed")
Portion of RNA transcript that is found between sequences of RNA encoding information for protein synthesis	Introns
Type of RNA covalently bound to a single amino acid	tRNA
Name the term used to describe the region of genomic DNA where RNA polymerase and transcription factors bind to regulate transcription	Promoter
Name the term used to describe the region of genomic DNA where transcription factors activators bind to enhance transcription	Enhancer

Name the term used to describe the region of genomic DNA where repressors bind

Silencer

Name the enzyme responsible for each of the following functions:

Synthesis of rRNA

RNA polymerase I

Synthesis of mRNA

RNA polymerase II

Synthesis of tRNA

RNA polymerase III

Name three major regulatory mechanisms of transcription in eukaryotes

1. Regulation by transcription factors at the level of the promoter
2. Regulation by histones binding to specific genomic regions
3. Regulation of DNA structure (including methylation, gene rearrangement, and amplification)

What genetic structure regulates transcription in prokaryotes?

An operon

Name the elements of an operon responsible for each of the following functions:

Region where proteins bind to enable transcription

Promoter region

Molecule that binds at the promoter

Activator or repressor

Sequence in DNA where regulatory proteins bind

Operator

Molecule that binds the operator to regulate transcription

Repressor

What are three modifications made to an RNA transcript before it leaves the nucleus?

1. 5′ Capping with 7-methylguanosine
2. 3′ Polyadenylation
3. Splicing of introns

Which small molecule provides the energy for charging a tRNA with its amino acid?

Adenosine triphosphate (ATP)

Which small molecule provides the energy for binding tRNA to the ribosome and for translocation?

Guanosine triphosphate (GTP)

Which molecules, central to the discipline of molecular biology, recognize and cleave specific sequences of a DNA molecule?

Restriction enzymes

Microbiology Techniques

Name the molecular biology
techniques described below:

Method of separating molecules based on movement through a gel placed in an electric field	Gel electrophoresis
Technique for detecting specific DNA sequences using restriction enzymes and a radiolabeled DNA probe	Southern blot
Technique for detecting specific RNA sequences using restriction enzymes and a radiolabeled DNA probe	Northern blot
Technique for detecting specific protein sequences using radiolabeled antibodies	Western blot
A rapid technique for amplifying a specific DNA sequence in vitro	Polymerase chain reaction (PCR)
Technique for detecting different alleles at a gene of interest using restriction enzymes	Restriction fragment length polymorphism analysis
Technique for detecting the presence of antigen or antibody using radiolabeled antibodies	Radioimmunoassay (RIA)
Technique for detecting the presence of antigen or antibody using antibodies linked to enzymes with detectable activity	Enzyme-linked immunosorbent assay (ELISA)

Inherited Diseases

Name inheritance patterns described
below:

Twenty-five percent of offspring from two carrier parents affected	Autosomal recessive (AR)
Commonly cause defects in structural genes	Autosomal dominant (AD)
Commonly cause defects in enzymes	AR
Defect seen in multiple generations in both sexes	AD
Defects not typically seen in consecutive generations	AR

Disease is not observed in females	X-linked (XL) recessive
Disease is transmitted by mother	Mitochondrial inheritance
Half of male offspring from affected mother will manifest disease	XL recessive
Disease manifestations commonly present after puberty	AD (since mutation exists in gene pool, must be able to survive to reproduce)

What are the conditions for a population to be in Hardy-Weinberg equilibrium?

1. No mutation at locus of interest
2. No selection for allele at locus of interest
3. Random mating
4. Closed population (no migration)

What are the two Hardy-Weinberg equations?

1. $p^2 + 2pq + q^2 = 1$
2. $p + q = 1$ (p and q are separate alleles and pq is the heterozygote frequency)

Name the disease or condition associated with each of the following statements:

Lack of UV-specific endonuclease causing dry skin and malignant melanoma	Xeroderma pigmentosum
Lack of aldolase B causing hypoglycemia, jaundice, and cirrhosis	Fructose intolerance
Lack of fructokinase causing fructosemia and fructosuria	Essential fructosuria
Lack of galactose-1-phosphate uridyltransferase causing cataracts, hepatosplenomegaly (HSM), and mental retardation	Galactosemia
Deficiency of lactase causing bloating, flatulence, and diarrhea on consumption of dairy products	Lactose intolerance
Lactic acidosis and neurologic deficits in an alcoholic	Pyruvate dehydrogenase deficiency
Hemolytic anemia in patients of Mediterranean descent after eating fava beans or taking antimalarial medication	Glucose-6-phosphate dehydrogenase deficiency
Hemolytic anemia due to deficiency in glycolysis	Hexokinase, glucose-phosphate isomerase, aldolase, triose-phosphate isomerase, phosphoglycerate kinase, enolase, or pyruvate kinase deficiency

Inappropriate hepatocellular accumulation of glycogen caused by a deficiency of glucose-6-phosphatase, associated with severe fasting, hypoglycemia, lactic acidosis, hyperlipidemia, and impaired fructose metabolism	von Gierke disease/type I glycogen storage disease
Inappropriate accumulation of glycogen in the liver, heart, and muscle caused by a deficiency of lysosomal α-1,4-glucosidase, resulting in cardiomegaly	Pompe disease/type II glycogen storage disease
Inappropriate accumulation of glycogen in liver and heart due to deficiency of α-1,6-glucosidase, a debranching enzyme often leading to muscular hypotonia	Cori disease/type III glycogen storage disease
Inappropriate accumulation of glycogen in skeletal muscle fibers due to deficiency of glycogen phosphorylase, leading to myalgia and myoglobinuria with exercise	McArdle disease/type V glycogen storage disease
Defect in cystathionine synthase leading to the presence of homocysteine in the urine	Homocystinuria
Defect of renal tubular amino acid transporter for cysteine, ornithine, lysine, and arginine	Cystinuria
Inadequate catabolism of branched-chain amino acids (Ile, Val, and Leu) due to lack of α-ketoacid dehydrogenase leading to mental retardation	Maple syrup urine disease
Lack of phenylalanine hydroxylase (PAH) leading to a buildup of phenylalanine resulting in mental retardation, hypopigmentation, eczema, and a mousy odor	Phenylketonuria (can also get Phe buildup due to deficiency of tetrahydrobiopterin, BH4, cofactor of PAH)
Lack of homogentisic acid oxidase leading to a buildup of homogentisate, causing darkening of the urine and connective tissues	Alkaptonuria
Lack of tyrosinase leading to a lack of melanin	Albinism

Lack of adenosine deaminase inhibits DNA synthesis by causing the accumulation of metabolites in the purine salvage pathway; one of the causes of severe combined immunodeficiency syndrome	Adenosine deaminase deficiency
Lack of hypoxanthine-guanine phosphoryltransferase (HGPRTase) causing an overproduction of uric acid leading to neurologic deficits, hyperuricemia, and behavioral abnormalities, including self-mutilation	Lesch-Nyhan Syndrome (Lacks Nucleotide Salvage)
Trisomy 21 → mental retardation, slanted palpebral fissures, hypertelorism, macroglossia, atrial septal defect (ASD), duodenal atresia, early-onset Alzheimer disease, and multiple visceral anomalies	Down syndrome
Expansion of unstable region of X chromosome (abnormal *FMR1* gene with CGG expansion) leading to mental retardation, enlarged testes, and craniofacial anomalies	Fragile X syndrome
XL recessive deficiency of α-galactosidase A → buildup of ceramide trihexoside which causes pain in the extremities, ocular abnormalities, angiokeratomas, cardiovascular disease, and renal failure	Fabry disease
AR deficiency of galactosylceramide β-galactosidase leading to cerebral accumulation of galactocerebroside, which causes progressive neurologic degeneration	Krabbe disease (aka globoid cell leukodystrophy)
AR deficiency of β-glucocerebrosidase leading to the accumulation of glucocerebroside in the brain, bone marrow, liver, spleen → HSM, aseptic necrosis of femur, and neurologic dysfunction	Gaucher disease

AR deficiency of sphingomyelinase on chromosome 11 leading to buildup of sphinogmyelin and cholesterol in histiocytes of the liver, spleen, and lymphatic system, resulting in cortical atrophy, cherry red spot on macula, HSM	Niemann-Pick disease
AR deficiency of hexosaminidase A on chromosome 18, leading to the accumulation of GM_2 ganglioside within lysosomes resulting in neurologic degeneration and developmental delay, and cherry red spot on macula	Tay-Sachs disease
AR deficiency of arylsulfatase A, leading to an accumulation of cerebroside sulfate and dysfunction and demyelination of the central and peripheral nervous systems resulting in ataxia and dementia	Metachromatic leukodystrophy
XL recessive deficiency of iduronate sulfatase, leading to an accumulation of heparan and dermatan sulfate resulting in mental retardation, coarse facial features, and short stature	Hunter syndrome

Name the genetic disease associated with each of the following clinical or pathologic findings:

Cherry red spot of the macula	Tay-Sachs disease and Niemann-Pick disease
Cells containing "crinkled paper" cytoplasm and glycolipid-laden macrophages	Gaucher disease

Carbohydrate, Protein, and Lipid Metabolism

Describe the effect of insulin on the following metabolic processes:

Glycogen synthesis in muscle and liver	Increase
Gluconeogenesis in the liver	Decrease
Glycogenolysis in the liver	Decrease
Glucose uptake in muscle and adipose tissue	Increase

Triacylglycerol degradation	Decrease
Triacylglycerol synthesis	Increase
Protein synthesis	Increase

Describe the effect of glucagon on the following metabolic processes:

Glycogenolysis in the liver	Increase
Gluconeogenesis in the liver	Increase
β-Oxidation of fatty acids in the liver	Increase
Amino acid uptake by liver	Increase

Which small molecule accepts reducing equivalents and is typically involved in catabolic processes?	NAD$^+$
Which small molecule donates reducing equivalents and is typically involved in anabolic processes?	Nicotinamide adenine dinucleotide phosphate (NADPH)

Name the cellular compartment (cytosol, mitochondria, or both) where each of the following processes occur:

Citric acid cycle	Mitochondria
Fatty acid oxidation	Mitochondria
Fatty acid synthesis	Cytosol
Gluconeogenesis	Both
Glycolysis	Cytosol
Heme synthesis	Both
Hexose monophosphate (HMP) shunt	Cytosol
Protein synthesis	Cytosol (rough ER)
Steroid synthesis	Cytosol (smooth ER)
Urea cycle	Both

Name the molecule(s) that serve as the primary source of energy for the following organs:

Liver	Amino acids, lipids, glucose, fructose, and lactate

Central nervous system (CNS)	Glucose
Heart	Lipids, ketone bodies, lactate, and glucose
Adipose tissue	Glucose and lipids
Type I skeletal muscle fibers (slow twitch, "red")	Lipids and ketone bodies
Type II skeletal muscle fibers (fast twitch, "white")	Glucose

What are the four major enzymes that function in gluconeogenesis?

1. Pyruvate carboxylase
2. PEP carboxykinase
3. Fructose-1,6-bisphosphatase
4. Glucose-6-phosphatase
   (Pathway Produces Fresh Glucose)

Name four important cellular processes that require reducing equivalents supplied primarily by the pentose phosphate pathway

1. Fatty acid and steroid biosynthesis
2. Glutathione-mediated reduction of H_2O_2
3. Cytochrome P-450 system
4. Respiratory burst in phagocytes

Which molecule serves as donor of methyl groups in many metabolic processes?

S-adenosylmethionine

Which metabolic process is responsible for transferring reducing equivalents from RBCs and muscle tissue to the liver?

Cori cycle

Which two amino acids play key roles in the transport of nitrogen from the periphery to the liver?

1. Alanine
2. Glutamine

Name the eight intermediates of the citric acid cycle

1. Citrate (**Cindy**)
2. Isocitrate (**Is**)
3. α-Ketoglutarate (**Kinky**)
4. Succinyl-CoA (**So**)
5. Succinate (**She**)
6. Fumarate (**Fornicates**)
7. Malate (**More**)
8. Oxaloacetate (**Often**)

Name a toxin that directly blocks the flow of electrons through the electron transport chain

Cyanide

Cyanide is a by-product of the metabolism of which antihypertensive?

Nitroprusside

Name a toxin that directly inhibits mitochondrial ATPase	Oligomycin
What are the primary metabolic substrates released by the liver in the fed state and the fasting state?	Very low-density lipoprotein (VLDL) (fed); glucose and ketone bodies (fasting)

Name the apolipoprotein or lipoprotein responsible for each of the following functions:

Activates lecithin-cholesterol acyltransferase	Apolipoprotein A-I
Binds to low-density lipoprotein (LDL) receptor, mediates VLDL secretion	Apolipoprotein B-100
Delivery of cholesterol from the tissues to the liver	High-density lipoprotein (HDL)
Delivery of cholesterol produced by the liver to the tissues	LDL
Delivery of triglycerol absorbed in the small intestine to tissues	Chylomicron
Delivery of triglycerol produced by the liver to tissues	VLDL
Mediates chylomicron remnant uptake	Apolipoprotein E
Serves as a cofactor for lipoprotein lipase	Apolipoprotein C-II
Which enzyme, found in the liver and bone marrow, catalyzes the rate-limiting step of heme synthesis?	Aminolevulinate synthase
What are the major intermediates in the degradation of heme?	Heme → biliverdin → bilirubin → bilirubin diglucuronide (conjugated bilirubin)
Conjugated bilirubin is excreted in which bodily fluid?	Bile
Which compound produced by intestinal bacterial degradation of conjugated bilirubin gives urine its yellow color?	Urobilinogen
Which common physical finding in severe liver disease results from the accumulation of bilirubin (hyperbilirubinemia)?	Jaundice

Name the essential amino acids	"PriVaTe **TIM HALL**": Phe, Val, Trp, Thr, Ile, Met, His, Arg, Leu, Lys
Which amino acids (AAs) are exclusively ketogenic?	Leu and Lys
Which AAs can be ketogenic or glucogenic?	Tyr, Ile, Phe, and Trp
Which AAs are exclusively glucogenic?	All the amino acids not listed in the above two items
Which AAs are negatively charged at physiologic pH (7.4)?	Asp, Glu (the two acidic AAs)
Which AAs are positively charged at physiologic pH (7.4)?	Arg, Lys (the two basic AAs), His also basic but weakly charged at pH 7.4
Which AA is used to carry ammonium from the muscles to the liver?	Alanine
Which small molecule, essential to the excretion of ammonium, is derived from the removal of ammonium from glutamine?	α-Ketoglutarate
What are the intermediates of the urea cycle?	1. Ornithine (**Ordinarily**) 2. Carbamoyl phosphate (**Careless**) 3. Citrulline (**Crappers**) 4. Aspartate (**Are**) 5. Arginosuccinate (**Also**) 6. Fumarate (**Frivolous**) 7. Arginine (**About**) 8. Urea (**Urination**)
What is the limiting reagent for hepatic ethanol (EtOH) catabolism?	NAD^+
Which metabolic abnormality in chronic alcoholics results from depletion of NAD^+ in the liver?	Hypoglycemia (due to inhibition of gluconeogenesis)
Depletion of NAD^+ inhibits which two major metabolic processes?	1. The conversion of pyruvate to lactate 2. Oxaloacetate to malate
In what metabolic state does the liver commonly produce ketone bodies?	During starvation (or diabetic ketoacidosis)

G-Proteins

Which two second messengers are increased by the activation of a Gq protein?	1. IP3 2. Diacylglycerol (DAG)
Which enzyme is induced by the activation of a Gq protein?	Protein kinase C
Which enzyme is induced by the activation of a Gs protein?	Protein kinase A
Which second messenger is increased by the activation of a Gs protein?	cAMP
Which enzyme is inhibited by the activation of a Gi protein?	Protein kinase A
Which second messenger is decreased by the activation of a Gi protein?	cAMP

Enzymes

What is the shape of the plot of reaction velocity against substrate concentration for enzymes following Michaelis-Menten kinetics?	Hyperbolic
For an enzyme following Michaelis-Menten kinetics, how does halving enzyme concentration affect V_{max}?	V_{max} will be halved; (V_{max} is directly proportional to enzyme concentration for all substrate concentrations)
What is the shape of a plot of reaction velocity against substrate concentration for enzyme with a single allosteric regulator?	Sigmoid or "S" shaped
Name two important parameters of the cellular environment that directly affect enzyme kinetics	1. pH 2. Temperature
The inverse of V_{max} (the maximum reaction velocity) for a given enzyme is represented by what point on a Lineweaver-Burk plot?	The y intercept
The inverse of K_m (the Michaelis-Menten constant) for a given enzyme is represented by what point on a Lineweaver-Burk plot?	The x intercept

An enzyme with a small K_m will have a high or low affinity for its substrate?	High affinity ($K_m = 1/2V_{max}$)
How does a competitive inhibitor affect K_m?	Increases
How does a noncompetitive inhibitor affect K_m?	No effect
How does a competitive inhibitor affect V_m?	No effect
How does a noncompetitive inhibitor affect K_m?	Decreases

Cell Cycle

Name the phase of the cell cycle associated with each of the following cellular events:

Quiescence	G_0
Centrosome duplication	S
RNA, protein, organelle synthesis	G_0
DNA, RNA, histone synthesis	S
Release of E2F from Rb	G_1/S transition
Cyclin-dependent kinase (Cdk)-cyclin A and Cdk-cyclin B are active	G_2/M transition
Cdk-cyclin D and Cdk-cyclin E are active	G_1/S transition
Chromatin condensation, mitotic spindle formation	M: prophase
Kinetochore assembly	M: prometaphase
Centrosomes move to opposite poles	M: prophase
Nuclear envelope and nucleolar disappearance	M: prometaphase
Chromosome alignment at metaphase plate	M: metaphase
Kinetochore separation	M: anaphase
Nuclear envelope and nucleolar formation	M: telophase
Cytoplasmic division (cytokinesis)	M: cytokinesis
Most variable phase of cell cycle	G_1

Which two important molecules are involved in the G_1 to S checkpoint?	Rb, p53
What is the significance of p53?	Allows cell to detect DNA defects and repair them before proceeding with replication

Cell Membranes

What are the major categories of molecules that make up the cell membrane?	Cholesterol, phospholipids, sphingolipids, glycolipids, and proteins
Where in the cell membrane are glycoproteins found?	Exclusively in the noncytoplasmic side
What is the effect of increasing the cholesterol content of a cell membrane?	Membrane fluidity is decreased

NUTRITION

Name the fat-soluble vitamins	Vitamins A, D, E, and K
Where are these vitamins absorbed?	Ileum
What conditions cause fat-soluble vitamin deficiencies?	Malabsorption syndromes (eg, cystic fibrosis, celiac disease, ileal disease [eg, Crohn's], ileal resection)
Why do toxicities occur more commonly with fat-soluble vitamins?	Fat-soluble vitamins can accumulate in fatty tissues; varying fat content with age leads to different thresholds of toxicity for children versus elderly; and water-soluble vitamins are more easily excreted in the urine
Which prolonged dietary deficiency of protein and calories is characterized by retarded growth and cachexia in children?	Marasmus
Which disease, characterized by protein deficiency with adequate caloric intake, results in retarded growth, anemia, and severe edema?	Kwashiorkor
Name the vitamin(s) associated with each of the following statements:	
Composes NAD^+ and $NADP^+$	Vitamin B_3 (niacin)
Remains in the body with stores lasting up to 3–5 years	Vitamin B_{12} (cobalamin)

Important in purine/pyrimidine synthesis	Folate
Important part of visual pigments and epithelial cell differentiation	Vitamin A (retinol)
Antioxidant that delays cataracts and atherosclerosis	Vitamin E (α-tocopherol)
Component of CoA and fatty acid synthase	Vitamin B_5 (pantothenic acid)
Cofactors for pyruvate-dehydrogenase complex	Vitamins B_1 (thiamine), B_2 (riboflavin), B_3 (niacin), and B_5 (pantothenic acid)
Found only in animal products; Schilling test used to detect deficiency	Vitamin B_{12} (cobalamin)
Cofactor for norepinephrine (NE) synthesis and collagen cross-linkage; Fe absorption	Vitamin C (ascorbic acid)
Cofactor in transamination reactions	Vitamin B_6 (pyridoxine)
Toxicity causes nausea, stupor, and hypercalcemia	Vitamin D
Important in methionine synthesis and isomerization of methylmalonyl-CoA	Vitamin B_{12} (cobalamin)
Toxicity causes skin changes, arthralgias, and premature epiphyseal closure; CNS manifestations include increased intracranial pressure (pseudotumor ceribri)	Vitamin A (retinol)
Catalyzes γ-carboxylation of coagulation factors, synthesized by GI flora	Vitamin K
The most toxic vitamin in overdose	Vitamin D
The most common vitamin deficiency in the United States	Folate
Name the vitamin deficiency associated with each of the following findings:	
Wernicke-Korsakoff syndrome, beriberi	Vitamin B_1 (thiamine); B_1 = Ber1Ber1
Rickets, osteomalacia, and hypocalcemic tetany	Vitamin D
Neonatal hemorrhage and ↑ prothrombin time (PT)	Vitamin K

Megaloblastic anemia with neurologic dysfunction	Vitamin B_{12} (cobalamin)
Dermatitis, diarrhea, and dementia (pellagra)	Vitamin B_3 (niacin)
Deficiency caused by long-term raw egg ingestion	Biotin (avidin in egg whites binds biotin)
Megaloblastic anemia without neurologic dysfunction	Folate
Dry skin, dry eyes, and night blindness	Vitamin A (retinol)
Hemolysis (from RBC fragility) and ataxia	Vitamin E (-tocopherol)
EEG abnormalities and peripheral neuropathy; caused by isoniazid (INH) and oral contraceptives	Vitamin B_6 (pyridoxine)
Cheilosis, corneal vascularization, and angular stomatitis	Vitamin B_2 (riboflavin)
Neural tube defects during pregnancy	Folate
Scurvy, hemorrhages, and impaired wound healing	Vitamin C (ascorbic acid)
Deficiency caused by *Diphyllobothrium latum* infection, sprue, pernicious anemia, and Crohn's disease	Vitamin B_{12} (cobalamin)

Name the trace element associated with each of the following statements:

Important in protein synthesis; deficiency causes acrodermatitis and ↑ sense of taste/smell	Zinc
Involved in hemoglobin synthesis; excess caused by ceruloplasmin deficiency	Copper
Cofactor for glutathione peroxidase; deficiency causes cardiomyopathy	Selenium
Involved in collagen cross-linkage; excess causes pulmonary fibrosis	Silicon
Involved in methionine metabolism; deficiency mimics vitamin B_{12} deficiency	Cobalt (constituent of cobalamin)
Reduces insulin resistance, glucose tolerance factor	Chromium

EMBRYOLOGY

Name the embryonic structure
described below:

Border between future mouth and pharynx; formed by both hypoblast and epiblast cells	Buccopharyngeal membrane
Produces β-human chorionic gonadotropin (hCG)	Syncytiotrophoblast
Forms the lining of the cytotrophoblast	Extraembryonic somatic mesoderm
Consists of the syncytiotrophoblast, cytotrophoblast, and extra embryonic somatic mesoderm	Chorion
Forms the covering of the yolk sac	Extraembryonic visceral mesoderm

The following developmental
milestones occur how long after
contraception?

Implantation	Within 1 week
Bilaminar disc	Within 2 weeks
Gastrulation	Within 3 weeks
Formation of the primitive streak and neural plate	Within 3 weeks
Organogenesis, peak of susceptibility to teratogens	Weeks 3–8
Limb formation	Week 4
Cardiac contractions begin	Week 4
Male and female genitals can be distinguished	Week 10

Name the abnormality/abnormalities
caused by the following teratogens:

Angiotensin-converting enzyme (ACE) inhibitors	Renal dysgenesis → oligohydramnios, pulmonary hypoplasia, and limb contractures
Tetracycline	Yellow teeth and enamel hypoplasia
Aminoglycosides	Eighth cranial nerve damage → deafness
Oral hypoglycemics	Neonatal hypoglycemia
Warfarin	Craniofacial (nasal hypoplasia) and CNS defects, stillbirth

Phenytoin	Fetal hydantoin syndrome: craniofacial and limb defects, mental deficiencies
Valproic acid	Spina bifida
Lithium	Cardiac (Ebstein) anomaly
Isotretinoin	Craniofacial (small ears), CNS, cardiac, and thymus defects
Indomethacin	Constriction of ductus arteriosus
Diethylstilbestrol (DES)	Clear cell vaginal cancer and cervical/uterine malformations in female offspring
Thalidomide	Limb reduction defects
Alcohol	Fetal alcohol syndrome: craniofacial defects (absent philtrum, flattened nasal bridge, and microphthalmia), growth restriction, and brain, cardiac, and spinal defects
Tobacco	Growth restriction, prematurity, low birth weight
Radiation	Growth restriction, CNS defects, and leukemia

Name the embryonic layer that gives rise to each of the following tissues:

Adrenal cortex	Mesoderm
Anterior pituitary	Ectoderm (oral ectoderm/Rathke pouch)
Aorticopulmonary septum	Ectoderm (neural crest)
Autonomic nerves	Ectoderm (neural crest)
Long bones and vertebrae	Mesoderm
Facial bones	Ectoderm (neural crest)
CNS neurons and astrocytes	Ectoderm (neural tube)
Connective tissue	Mesoderm
Epidermis	Ectoderm (surface ectoderm)
Epithelial lining of the GI tract	Endoderm
Myocardium	Mesoderm
Kidneys	Mesoderm
Lens of eye	Ectoderm (surface ectoderm)
Liver parenchyma	Endoderm
Mammary glands	Ectoderm (surface ectoderm)
Melanocytes	Ectoderm (neural crest)

Striated muscle	Mesoderm
Nucleus pulposus	Mesoderm (notochord)
Pancreas	Endoderm
Parafollicular cells of the thyroid	Ectoderm (neural crest)
Retina	Ectoderm (neural tube)
Schwann cells	Ectoderm (neural crest)
Spleen	Mesoderm
Parathyroid	Endoderm
Posterior pituitary	Ectoderm (neural tube)
Thymus	Endoderm
Thyroid	Endoderm
Kidneys, ureters, and gonads	Mesoderm

BASIC PATHOLOGY

Cellular Adaptation

Give the appropriate term for each of the following definitions:

Complete failure of cell production	Aplasia
Relative decrease in cell production	Hypoplasia
Increase in cell size	Hypertrophy
Replacement of one adult (differentiated) cell (epithelial or mesenchymal) type with another adult cell type	Metaplasia
Uncontrolled proliferation of cells	Neoplasia
Decrease in cell substance results in a decrease in cell size; may result in decreased tissue/organ size	Atrophy
Increase of organ/tissue size due to an increase in the number of cells	Hyperplasia

Cell Injury

Name the mechanism of cell injury
characterized by each of the following
statements:

Mitochondrial dysfunction $\rightarrow\downarrow$ | Ischemic/hypoxic cell injury
cellular ATP $\rightarrow$ failure of Na^+/K^+
ATPase, failure of protein synthesis

Causes lipid peroxidation of | Reactive oxygen species (O_2-free
membranes | radicals)

Associated with ionizing radiation, | Reactive oxygen species (O_2-free
UV light, and reperfusion after | radicals)
ischemic injury

Prevented by enzymes such as | Generation of reactive oxygen species
glutathione peroxidase, catalase, | (O_2-free radicals)
and superoxide dismutase

Which molecules are released in | Cytochrome c and H^+
response to mitochondrial damage?

Cytoskeletal abnormalities, ATP deple- | Defective membrane permeability
tion, and cell swelling are associated
with which key event in cell injury?

What is the effect of increased cyto- | Activation of ATPase, endonuclease,
plasmic calcium ions in a cell undergo- | phospholipase, and proteases
ing apoptosis or necrosis?

Necrosis/Apoptosis

Classify the following as features of
apoptosis or necrosis:

Cellular blebbing and cell | Apoptosis
shrinkage

Involves many contiguous cells | Necrosis

Physiologic, programmed cell | Apoptosis
removal

Active form of cell death (requires | Apoptosis
energy consumption)

Gross, irreversible cellular injury | Necrosis

Involves single cells or groups of | Apoptosis
cells

Involution and shrinkage of | Apoptosis
affected cells and fragments

Marked inflammatory reaction | Necrosis

State the function of each of the
following molecules during apoptosis:

Caspases (cysteine protease)	Protein cleavage
Endonucleases	DNA cleavage
Phosphatidylserine and thrombospondin	Cell surface molecules recognized by phagocytes
Tumor necrosis factor (TNF)-α receptor and FAS (CD95)	Death receptors
Bcl-2 and Bcl-x	Major antiapoptotic proteins
Cytochrome c	Activation of procaspase 9
Apoptosis-activating factor-1 (Apaf-1)	Cytoplasmic receptor for cytochrome c
TNF-α	Bindings of this ligand to its receptor induce association with a death domain
Granzyme B	Activation of the caspase cascade (released by cytotoxic T cells)

Name the type of necrosis
characterized by each of the following
features:

Enzymatic degradation of tissue seen in abscesses	Liquefactive necrosis
Commonly seen in tuberculous granulomas	Caseous necrosis
Fibrin-like, proteinaceous deposition in arterial walls	Fibrinoid necrosis
Lipase-induced autodigestion of adipose tissue $\rightarrow$ saponification	Fat necrosis
Interruption of blood supply to organs supplied by end arteries; architecture well preserved	Coagulative necrosis
Results from vascular occlusion; most commonly affects lower extremities or bowel	Gangrenous necrosis

Cell Changes/Accumulations

What type of cellular change is characterized by excess accumulation of intracellular triglycerides?	Fatty change (steatosis)
What type of calcification is caused by hypercalcemia?	Metastatic calcification

What type of calcification occurs in previously damaged tissues?	Dystrophic calcification
Name four endogenous pigments that accumulate in cells	1. Melanin 2. Bilirubin 3. Hemosiderin 4. Lipofuscin
Name four diseases associated with protein misfolding	1. Alzheimer disease 2. α-1-Antitrypsin deficiency 3. Cystic fibrosis 4. Amyloidosis

Name the cellular pigment described below:

Identified with Prussian blue dye; can result in organ damage or simple deposition	Hemosiderin
Yellowish, fat-soluble "wear-and-tear" pigment	Lipofuscin
Formed in the epidermis from tyrosine	Melanin

Inflammation

Which three classes of adhesion molecules are involved in inflammation?	1. Selectins (E, P, and L) 2. Immunoglobulin (Ig) family (intercellular adhesion molecule [ICAM], platelet cell adhesion molecule [PCAM]) 3. Integrins
What are the five steps in the extravasation of inflammatory leukocytes?	1. Margination 2. Pavementing 3. Tumbling (rolling) 4. Adhesion 5. Transmigration
Which two groups of cell adhesion molecules pair mediate tumbling?	1. Selectins on endothelial cells 2. Sialylated glycoproteins (eg, sialyl-Lewis-X) on leukocytes
Which two groups of cell adhesion molecules pair mediate leukocyte adhesion to endothelial cells?	1. ICAM and vascular cell adhesion molecule (VCAM) (Ig superfamily) on endothelial cells 2. Integrins on leukocytes
Which factors induce endothelial expression of P-selectin?	Platelet activation factor (PAF), histamine, and thrombin

Which factors induce endothelial expression of ICAM and VCAM?	Interleukin (IL)-1 and TNF

Name five chemotactic factors for neutrophils

1. Bacterial products
2. C5a
3. LTB4
4. Chemokines (IL-8)
5. Fibrin split (degradation) products

Name six functional responses of leukocytes following their activation

1. Eicosanoid production
2. Cytokine secretion
3. Generation of reactive oxygen species
4. Degranulation
5. Altered cell adhesion molecule expression
6. Upregulation of receptors (toll-like, G protein-coupled, opsonin, cytokines)

What term is used to describe the process of coating substances (with Ig or C3b) to facilitate phagocytosis?

Opsonization

Which neutrophil intracellular micro-bicidal mechanism uses the HMP shunt to generate an oxidative burst?

H_2O_2-myeloperoxidase (MPO)-halide system of bacterial killing

Name two processes associated with impaired leukocyte adhesion

1. Recurrent bacterial infections
2. Altered wound healing

Decide whether each of the following substances causes vasoconstriction or vasodilation:

Bradykinin	Vasodilation
Thromboxane (TXA)	Vasoconstriction
Prostacyclin (PGI$_2$)	Vasodilation
Leukotrienes (LTC$_4$, LTD$_4$, and LTE$_4$)	Vasoconstriction
Prostaglandins (PGD$_2$, PGE$_2$, and PGF$_2$)	Vasodilation

Remember: most substances also cause analogous effects on bronchial tone

Name seven substances that increase vascular permeability

1. Histamine
2. Serotonin
3. C3a and C5a
4. Leukotrienes (LTC4, LTD4, and LTE4)
5. Bradykinin
6. Nitric oxide (NO)
7. PAF (low concentration)

Which two enzymes stimulate the release of arachidonic acid from membrane phospholipids?	1. Phospholipase A_2 2. Phospholipase C
What are the two major pathways in arachidonic acid metabolism?	1. Cyclooxygenase (COX) 2. Lipoxygenase
What signaling molecules are produced by the COX pathway?	TXA_2 (in platelets), PGI_2 (in endothelial cells), and other prostaglandins (in other tissues)
What are the two major enzymes involved in prostaglandin production?	1. COX-1 2. COX-2
Which COX enzyme serves in homeostatic functions?	COX-1
What products does the lipoxygenase pathway produce?	HPETEs and leukotrienes
Which arachidonic acid metabolite is thought to sensitize nerve endings to pain mediators?	PGE_2 ($\downarrow PGE_2 \rightarrow$ analgesic effects)
Name four acute-phase responses of inflammation:	1. Systemic effects (fever and leukocytosis) 2. Hepatic synthesis of acute-phase reactants (C-reactive protein [CRP], ferritin, complement, and prothrombin) 3. Synthesis of adhesion molecules 4. Neutrophil degranulation
Which substance links the kinin, coagulation, plasminogen, and complement systems?	Factor XIIa (Hageman factor)
Which group of plasma proteins participates in immune-mediated lysis of cells?	Complement system
Which substance produced by endothelial cells relaxes smooth muscle and inhibits platelet aggregation?	NO
Which factor is a pyrogen and causes fever?	IL-1 $\rightarrow PGE_2$
Name four possible outcomes of acute inflammation:	1. Complete resolution 2. Abscess/ulcer/fistula formation 3. Healing by fibrosis and scarring 4. Progression to chronic inflammation

Which pattern of chronic inflammation is characterized by nodular collections of epithelioid histiocytes and multinucleated giant cells?

Granulomatous inflammation

Name three etiologies of granulomatous inflammation:

1. Infectious (*Mycobacterium tuberculosis*, *Histoplasma*, cat scratch disease, leprosy, syphilis)
2. Foreign bodies
3. Idiopathic (eg, sarcoidosis, Crohn's disease)

Tissue Repair

What are the four factors determining the size of a cell population?

1. Proliferation
2. Cell death
3. Cell differentiation
4. Replacement by stem cells

What are the three categories of cells based on their inherent proliferative activity?

1. Permanent (cardiac myocytes, neurons)
2. Quiescent (hepatocytes, endothelial cells, lymphocytes)
3. Labile (epidermis, GI, and respiratory tract epithelial cells; bone marrow; hair follicles)

Name five factors that mediate cellular proliferation during the process of tissue repair:

1. Platelet-derived growth factor (PDGF)
2. Epidermal growth factor (EGF) and transforming growth factor-alpha (TGF-α)
3. Fibroblast growth factors (FGFs)
4. Hepatocyte growth factor
5. Vascular endothelial growth factor (VEGF)

What highly vascular, newly formed connective tissue fills defects left by removal of cellular debris?

Granulation tissue

What are the four key components to the orderly formation of a scar?

1. Angiogenesis and granulation tissue formation
2. Fibroblast emigration and proliferation
3. Deposition of extracellular matrix
4. Maturation and remodeling → scar

Name five factors that delay or impede tissue repair:	1. Impaired circulation 2. Persistent infection 3. Retention of debris or foreign body 4. Nutritional deficiency (eg, protein and vitamin C) 5. Metabolic disorders (eg, diabetes mellitus)

Hemodynamic Dysfunction

Name five causes of edema:	1. ↑Hydrostatic pressure 2. ↑Capillary permeability 3. ↓Oncotic pressure 4. ↑Na+ retention (renal disorders or congestive heart failure [CHF]) 5. Lymphatic obstruction
Describe the contents of a transudate	Low-protein content (SG <1.012), few cells, and little protein
What type of fluid accumulation forms as a result of increased vascular permeability due to endothelial cell destruction?	Exudate
What is the composition of exudate?	High protein (SG >1.020), ↑inflammatory leukocytes, and ↑protein
Name two organs commonly affected by chronic passive congestion and their related pathologic findings:	1. **Lungs:** hemosiderin-laden macrophages or "heart-failure cells" (from left heart failure) 2. **Liver:** nutmeg liver (from right heart failure)
Name the two types of infarcts and several examples of each:	1. Anemic (white) infarcts: heart, spleen, and kidneys 2. Hemorrhagic (red) infarcts: lungs, testes, and GI tract (occurs in areas with collateral circulation)

Thrombosis

What is Virchow triad?	The three primary influences on thrombus formation: 1. Endothelial injury 2. Stasis 3. Hypercoagulability
Name the three components necessary for hemostasis:	1. Vascular endothelium 2. Platelets 3. Coagulation cascade

Name five factors that promote platelet aggregation:	1. ADP 2. Thrombin 3. TXA_2 4. Collagen 5. Platelet-activating factor
Which product of the COX pathway limits further platelet aggregation?	PGI_2
Where are proteins C and S made?	Endothelial cells
Classify the following as features of the extrinsic or the intrinsic pathway:	
Involves activation of factor VII	Extrinsic pathway
Clinically monitored by the PT	Extrinsic pathway
Initiated by activation of factor XII	Intrinsic pathway
Monitored by partial thromboplastin time (PTT)	Intrinsic pathway
Name the component(s) of the coagulation cascade associated with each of the following features:	
Vitamin K-dependent coagulation factors	Factors II, VII, IX, X, proteins C and S
Ion necessary for proper function of the coagulation cascade	Calcium
Factors inhibited by antithrombin III (AT III)	Thrombin, factors IX, X, XI, and XII
Complex that activates proteins C and S	Thrombomodulin-thrombin complex
The most important fibrinolytic protease	Plasmin
Converts plasminogen to plasmin	Tissue plasminogen activator (t-PA), also urokinase plasminogen activator
Cleaved by activated protein C (APC) → inhibition of coagulation	Factors Va and VIIIa
Which molecule dramatically enhances the activity of AT III?	Heparin
What is the most frequent cause of hereditary thrombophilia?	Factor V (Leiden) mutation (2%–15% of white population)
Hereditary thrombophilia can also be caused by deficiency of what major antithrombotic proteins?	AT III, protein C, and protein S

How does the Leiden mutation confer hypercoagulability?	Renders mutant factor V resistant to cleavage by APC
Which prothrombotic disorder is characterized by autoantibodies that induce platelet activation?	Antiphospholipid antibody syndrome

Name the type of thrombus associated with each of the following:

Sterile vegetations of heart valves in patients with hypercoagulable states	Nonbacterial thrombotic endocarditis
Noninfective heart valve vegetations from circulating immune complexes	Libman-Sacks endocarditis

Embolism

Name the type of embolism described by each of the following statements:

Venous thrombus that gains access to arterial circulation through a right-to-left shunt	Paradoxical embolus
Associated with decompression sickness	Air embolus
Occurs at parturition; can lead to disseminated intravascular coagulation (DIC) and death	Amniotic fluid embolus
Embolus obstructing the bifurcation of the pulmonary artery	Saddle embolus
Important cause of death in immobilized, post-op patients	Pulmonary embolus
Occur after severe, multiple long bone fractures	Fat emboli

Shock

Name the type of shock described by each of the following statements:

Associated with gram-negative endotoxemia	Septic shock
Circulatory collapse from pump failure of left ventricle (LV)	Cardiogenic shock
IgE-mediated systemic vasodilation with ↑ vascular permeability	Anaphylactic shock

Caused by severe hemorrhage or fluid loss	Hypovolemic shock
Associated with severe trauma causing reactive peripheral vasodilation	Neurogenic shock
Which two mediators are associated with systemic vasodilation in septic shock?	1. NO 2. PAF

Name the characteristic manifestations of shock on each of the following organs:

Lungs	Pulmonary edema
Liver	Steatosis and centrilobular necrosis
Colon	Patchy mucosal hemorrhages
Adrenals	Lipid depletion of cortex
Kidneys	Acute tubular necrosis

BASIC PHARMACOLOGY

Absorption/Distribution

In which part of the GI tract are most oral drugs absorbed?	Duodenum
Name three factors that influence absorption of drugs:	1. Chemical properties (active transport vs. passive diffusion) 2. pH (percent of drug in the uncharged state determines rate of absorption) 3. Physical factors (blood flow, surface area, and contact time with absorptive surfaces)
What is first-pass metabolism?	Hepatic degradation/alteration of an oral drug after absorption, before it enters the general circulation

Complete the following formulas:

(Rate of drug elimination)/(plasma drug concentration) =	Clearance (CL)
(Amount of drug in body)/(plasma drug concentration) =	Volume of distribution (V_d)
$(C_p \times V_d)/F$ =	Loading dose (also defined as the amount of drug necessary to rapidly raise a desired plasma concentration of the drug)

$(C_p \times CL)/F =$

Maintenance dose (also defined as the amount of drug necessary to maintain a desired plasma concentration of the drug)

$(0.693 \times V_d)/CL =$

Half-life $(t_{1/2})$

C_p = target plasma concentration, F = bioavailability

If a patient was known to be a rapid metabolizer, would the loading dose or maintenance dose have to be adjusted to maintain a desired plasma concentration of the drug?

The loading dose would be unchanged; the maintenance dose would need to be increased

How do dosage calculations change for patients with impaired renal/hepatic function?

Loading dose stays the same, maintenance dose decreases

List four conditions that alter drug distribution

1. Edematous state (eg, CHF and nephrotic syndrome)
2. Pregnancy ($\uparrow$ intravascular volume)
3. Obesity (accumulation of lipophilic agents in fat cells)
4. Hypoalbuminemia (no albumin to bind drugs $\rightarrow \uparrow$ availability)

Metabolism/Elimination

Name four clinical situations that would result in increased drug half-life

1. Prerenal state ($\downarrow$ renal plasma flow)
2. Renal disease $\rightarrow$ decreased extraction ratio
3. Adding a second drug that displaces the first from albumin, thus $\uparrow V_d$
4. $\downarrow$ Metabolism (hepatic insufficiency or drug interaction)

Classify each of the following statements as characteristic of phase I or phase II metabolism:

Produces slightly polar, water-soluble metabolites

Phase I

Involves mixed-function oxidase (P-450)

Phase I

Involves conjugation reactions (acetylation, glucuronidation, and sulfation)

Phase II

Produces very polar, inactive metabolites that are excreted by the kidneys

Phase II

Reduction, oxidation, and hydrolysis	Phase I
Phase that may be compromised first in geriatric patients	Phase I
Phase that may be compromised in neonates	Phase I

Classify each of the following statements as characteristic of first- or zero-order drug elimination:

Constant *fraction* of drug eliminated per unit of time	First-order elimination
Constant *amount* of drug eliminated per unit of time	Zero-order elimination
Plasma concentration decreases linearly with time	Zero-order elimination
Plasma concentration decreases exponentially with time	First-order elimination
Elimination rate is independent of concentration	Zero-order elimination

Pharmacodynamics

What term describes the maximum effect a drug can produce?	Efficacy
What term describes the measure of the amount of drug needed to produce a given result?	Potency
What term describes the dose of a drug that produces the desired effect?	Effective dose (ED)
What term describes the dose of a drug that produces death?	Lethal dose (LD)
What term describes the measure of the safety of a drug?	Therapeutic index
How is therapeutic index calculated?	LD_{50}/ED_{50} (LD_{50} = dose lethal in 50% of the population, ED_{50} = dose effective in 50% of the population)
How does a competitive antagonist affect the dose-response curve?	Shifts it to the right ($\uparrow ED_{50}$)

How does a noncompetitive antagonist affect the dose-response curve?	Shifts it downward ($\downarrow$ maximal response)
How does a partial agonist differ from a full agonist?	Acts like an agonist when an agonist is not present; acts like an antagonist if an agonist is present

Toxicology

Name the antidote for each of the following toxins:

Iron	Deferoxamine
Copper/gold/arsenic	Penicillamine
Lead	CaEDTA, succimer, dimercaprol (BAL in oil), and oral penicillamine
Arsenic/mercury	Dimercaprol
Carbon monoxide	100% O_2 and hyperbaric O_2
Cyanide	Nitrite, vitamin B_{12}, and thiosulfate
Methemoglobin	Methylene blue
Methanol/ethylene glycol	EtOH, fomepizole, and dialysis
Acetaminophen (Tylenol)	N-acetylcysteine
Aspirin (salicylates)	Alkalinize urine (promotes excretion) and dialysis
Opioids	Naloxone (IV, IM, and inhaled) or naltrexone (PO)
Benzodiazepines	Flumazenil
Organophosphates, anticholinesterases	Atropine and pralidoxime (PAM)
Heparin	Protamine sulfate
Warfarin	Vitamin K, fresh frozen plasma (FFP), prothrombin complex concentrate (PCC) for acute reversal
Factor Xa inhibitors (enoxaparin, apixaban, rivaroxaban)	Andexanet alfa
tPA	Aminocaproic acid
Digoxin	Antidig Fab fragments (first stop drug and stabilize K^+, Mg^{2+}, and lidocaine)

P-450

Classify each of the following drugs as inhibitors or inducers of P-450:

Inducers: "Queen Barb takes Phen-phen and Refuses Greasy Carbs"

Inhibitors: "Inhibitors Stop Cyber-Kids from Eating Grapefruits"

Barbiturates	Inducer
INH	Inhibitor
Spironolactone	Inhibitor
Rifampin	Inducer
Cimetidine	Inhibitor
Ketoconazole	Inhibitor
Phenytoin and carbamazepine	Inducer
Quinidine	Inducer
Disulfiram	Inhibitor
Sulfonamides	Inhibitor
Steroids	Inhibitor
Macrolides (erythromycin)	Inhibitor
Chloramphenicol	Inhibitor
Griseofulvin	Inducer
Grapefruit	Inhibitor
Verapamil	Inhibitor
Chronic EtOH use	Inducer
Acute EtOH use	Inhibitor

CHAPTER 2

Immunology

IMMUNOLOGY BASICS

Cells of the Immune System

Name the type of immune cell that fits each description given below:

Major cells involved in innate immunity	Monocytes, macrophages, neutrophils, natural killer (NK) cells
Cell-mediated immune response	T lymphocyte
Humoral immunity	B lymphocyte
Primary phagocytic cell in acute inflammation	Neutrophil
Type of cell necessary for transplant rejection	T lymphocyte
Contains myeloperoxidase and lysozyme	Neutrophil
Major mediator of a type 1 hypersensitivity reaction	Mast cell
Major mediator of the antiparasitic response	Eosinophil
Granules contain histamine and heparin	Basophil and mast cells
Major antigen-presenting cells in tissues	Macrophages and B cells
Demonstrates a multilobed ("hypersegmented") nucleus in vitamin B_{12} or folate deficiency	Neutrophil
Secretes interleukin (IL)-1 to promote T cell activity	Macrophage
Expresses IgE receptors on its cell membrane to mediate the allergic response	Basophil

Expresses high levels of major histocompatibility complex (MHC) class II on its cell membrane	Macrophage
Macrophage precursor	Monocyte
Cell type increased in atopic asthma	Eosinophil
Recognizes antigen presented in the context of MHC class II molecules	T-helper cell
Antibody-producing cell with abundant rough endoplasmic reticulum	Plasma cell
Major source of IL-2 production	T-helper cell (specifically T_H1 cells)
Major cell of the humoral immune response	B lymphocyte

Immunoglobulins

Name the type of immunoglobulin (Ig) associated with the following features:

Most abundant type of Ig	IgG
First class of Ig produced in an immune response upon exposure to antigen	IgM
Able to fix complement	IgG and IgM
Found on the lining of mucous membranes and in secretions, including breast milk and saliva	IgA
Able to cross placenta	IgG
Type of Ig commonly occurring as a dimer	IgA
Type of Ig commonly occurring as a pentamer	IgM
Ig elevated in patients with asthma and allergies	IgE
Responsible for long-term immunity	IgG
Causes mast cells and basophils to release histamine when triggered by antigen	IgE
Type of Ig found embedded in the cell membrane of developing B cells	IgD

Total levels and concentration of this antibody can be estimated using radioimmunosorbent test (RIST) and radioallergosorbent test (RAST)	IgE
What term is used to describe the portion of a molecule that serves as an antigenic determinant?	Epitope
What term is used to describe a small molecule that can serve as an antigenic determinant only if it is attached to a larger carrier molecule?	Hapten
What type of chemical bonds are critical in linking the heavy and light chains of Igs?	Disulfide bonds
What term is used to describe the region in an antibody that determines antigen specificity?	The hypervariable region or complementarity determining region (CDR)
Name five mechanisms by which antibody diversity is created:	1. Mutations in the genes encoding the CDR region 2. Random VJ recombination in light chains 3. Random VDJ recombination in heavy chains 4. Random assembly of light and heavy chains 5. Imperfect recombination of VDJ genes

T-Cells

Name the T-lymphocyte cell surface protein associated with the following features:	
Antigen-specific receptor on 95% of T cells	$\alpha\beta$ T-cell receptor ($\alpha\beta$ TCR)
Antigen-specific receptor on 5% (or less) of T cells	$\gamma\delta$ T-cell receptor ($\gamma\delta$ TCR)
Signal transduction protein always associated with TCR	CD3
T-cell marker expressed in immature T cells	CD2

Responds to MHC class II molecule expressed by antigen-presenting cells	CD4
Responds to MHC class I molecule expressed on all cells	CD8
Found specifically on T-helper cells	CD4
Found specifically on cytotoxic T cells	CD8
Cells with this surface marker ↓ in HIV/AIDS	CD4
Type of T cell that destroys virally infected cells	CD8

HLA Subtypes

Name the HLA haplotype(s) associated with the following diseases:

Ankylosing spondylitis	HLA-B27
Type 1 diabetes mellitus	HLA-DR3/DR4
Multiple sclerosis	HLA-DR2
Rheumatoid arthritis	HLA-DR4

Cytokines

Name the cytokine described below:

Endogenous pyrogen	IL-1 (produced by macrophages)
Promotes IgA synthesis	IL-5
Induces IL-2 production by T cells	IL-1
High concentrations induce cell death in some tumors and cause cachexia	Tumor necrosis factor (TNF)-α
Induces T- and B-cell activity during the initial stages of an immune response	IL-1
Induces production of IgE and IgG	IL-4 (produced by T-helper cells)
Induces differentiation of eosinophils and promotes growth in B cells	IL-5 (produced by T-helper cells)
Chemotactic factor for neutrophils	IL-8 (produced by monocytes and endothelial cells)

Secreted by activated T cells and induces maturation of bone marrow stem cells	IL-3
Inhibits production of interferon-gamma (IFN-γ) by T-helper cells	IL-10 (produced by T_H2 cells)
Inhibits production of IFN-γ	IL-4
Inhibits differentiation of TH1 cells	IL-10
Stimulates TH1 differentiation	IL-12 (produced by macrophages and B cells)
Activates T-helper, T-cytotoxic, natural killer, and B cells	IL-2 (produced by T-helper cells)
Promotes production of IFN-γ T-helper cells	IL-12
Low concentrations promote neutrophil activity and IL-2 receptor expression	TNF-α
Inhibits growth and function of T and B cells and promotes collagen secretion during tissue repair	Transforming growth factor-beta (TGF-β)

Gel and Coombs Hypersensitivity Reactions

Name the Gel and Coombs hypersensitivity reaction described below:

Mediated by IgE bound to mast cells and basophils	Type 1 (immediate or anaphylactic hypersensitivity)
Antibody-mediated cytotoxic reaction	Type 2 (cytotoxic reaction)
Occurs in response to environmental allergies	Type 1
Antigen-sensitized T cells release cytokines, which induce an inflammatory response up to 48 hours after initial contact with antigen	Type 4 (delayed-type hypersensitivity)
Associated with the release of histamine, platelet-activating factor, leukotrienes, prostaglandins, and thromboxanes	Type 1

Binding of cytotoxic T cells or complement to F_c portion of antibody causes target cell lysis	Type 2
Immune complex deposition in tissues results in an inflammatory response	Type 3 (immune complex reaction)

Name the type of hypersensitivity reaction responsible for the following diseases or conditions:

Arthus reaction	Type 3
Asthma	Type 1
Chronic transplant rejection	Type 4
Contact dermatitis, reaction to poison ivy	Type 4
Drug allergies	Type 1
Environmental allergies	Type 1
Erythroblastosis fetalis	Type 2
Goodpasture syndrome	Type 2
Graves' disease	Type 2
Hemolytic anemia	Type 2
Immune complex-mediated glomerulonephritis	Type 3
Lambert-Eaton	Type 2
Myasthenia gravis	Type 2
Multiple sclerosis	Type 4
Pernicious anemia	Type 2
Purified protein derivative (PPD)/tuberculin skin test	Type 4
Rheumatic fever	Type 2
Rheumatoid arthritis	Type 3
Systemic anaphylaxis	Type 1
Serum sickness	Type 3
Systemic lupus erythematosus (SLE)	Type 3
Transfusion reaction due to ABO incompatibility	Type 2

Complement

Which class of bacteria is particularly susceptible to complement-mediated lysis?	Gram-negative organisms
Which antibody isotypes activate the classic pathway of the complement cascade?	IgG and IgM
Which molecules activate the alternative pathway of the complement cascade?	Aggregated IgA, endotoxin, and other components of the bacterial cell wall

Name the component(s) of the complement cascade responsible for the following functions:

Neutralization of viruses	C1 to C4
Opsonization	C3b
Neutrophil and macrophage chemotaxis	C5a
Synthesis of membrane attack complex (MAC)	C5b to C9
Formation of C3 convertase	C3b, Bb (alternative pathway) or C4b, C2b (classic pathway)

Name the disease or condition caused by a deficiency of the following complement components:

C1 esterase inhibitor	Hereditary angioedema
C3	Sinus and upper respiratory tract infections
C5b to C9	Recurrent Neisseria infections
Decay accelerating factor	Paroxysmal nocturnal hemoglobinuria

Transplant Rejection and MHC Basics

For each of the following descriptions, name the type of transplant rejection:

Preformed antibodies in host react against graft antigens	Hyperacute rejection (minutes to hours)
Activation of previously sensitized T cells	Accelerated rejection (hours to days)

Involves T-cell activation, differentiation, and antibody production	Acute rejection (days to weeks)
Immune complex deposition combined with subacute cell cytotoxicity	Chronic rejection (months to years)
What are the four different classes of grafts?	1. Autograft (from self) 2. Syngeneic (from identical twin or clone) 3. Allograft (from same species) 4. Xenograft (from different species)
The activity of cytotoxic T cells against tumor or virally infected cells requires which cell surface receptor for antigen presentation?	MHC class I
The activity of cytotoxic T cells against pathogens phagocytosed by macrophages requires which cell surface receptor for antigen presentation?	MHC class II

PATHOLOGY OF THE IMMUNE SYSTEM

Autoantibodies

Describe the disease associated with the following autoantibodies:

Antinuclear antibodies (ANA)	SLE (sensitive but not specific for SLE)
Antiacetylcholine esterase (ACh)	Myasthenia gravis
Antibasement membrane	Anti-GBM disease (Goodpasture)
Anticentromere	**CREST** syndrome (**C**alcinosis, **R**aynaud, **E**sophageal dysmotility, **S**clerodactyly, **T**elangiectasias)
Anti-dsDNA	SLE (highly specific for SLE)
Antiepithelial cell	Pemphigus vulgaris
Antigliadin	Celiac sprue
Antihistone	Drug-induced lupus
Anti-IgG F$_c$ (rheumatoid factor)	Rheumatoid arthritis
Anti-Jo1	Myositis
Antimicrosomal	Hashimoto thyroiditis

Antimitochondrial	Primary biliary cirrhosis
Antinuclear ribonucleoprotein (nRNP)	Mixed connective tissue disease
Antiplatelet	Idiopathic thrombocytopenic purpura
Anti-Scl-70 (DNA topoisomerase 1)	Systemic sclerosis
Anti-Smith	SLE (highly specific for SLE)
Anti-SS-A (Ro) and anti-SS-B (La)	Sjögren syndrome
Antithyroglobulin	Hashimoto thyroiditis
Anti-thyroid-stimulating hormone receptor (TSHr)	Graves' disease
Anti-voltage-gated calcium channel	Lambert-Eaton syndrome
Cytoplasmic pattern of antineutrophil cytoplasmic antibodies (c-ANCA)	Granulomatosis with polyangiitis (GPA)
Perinuclear pattern of antineutrophil cytoplasmic antibodies (p-ANCA)	Microscopic PolyANgiitis, Polyarteritis Nodosa (PAN), and Churg-Strauss syndrome
List the four types of nuclear antigens against which ANAs are directed:	1. DNA 2. Histones 3. Nonhistone proteins 4. Nucleolar antigens

Systemic Lupus Erythematosus

What pathologic finding is common to all tissues affected by SLE?	Acute necrotizing vasculitis of small arteries and arterioles caused by immune complex deposition
Describe the effect of SLE on each of the following organs:	
Skin	Malar rash, discoid rash, photosensitivity
Joints	Arthritis and arthralgias
Brain	Neuropsychiatric changes or seizures (2° to cerebral vasculitis), cognitive dysfunction
Eyes	Cotton-wool spots, retinal hemorrhages
Heart	Pericarditis, Libman-Sacks Endocarditis (SLE → LSE)
Lungs	Pleuritis, pulmonary fibrosis
Gastrointestinal (GI)	Oral and nasopharyngeal ulcers

Spleen	Splenomegaly and onion skinning of splenic vessels
Kidneys	Wire-loop glomerular lesions and mesangial immune complex deposits → glomerulonephritis
Hematology	Hemolytic anemia, leukopenia, thrombocytopenia, antiphospholipid antibody syndrome
Blood vessels	Raynaud phenomenon

Libman-Sacks endocarditis causes sterile vegetations to form on both sides of which cardiac valve most often?	Mitral valve

Name five medications capable of inducing a lupus-like syndrome:	1. Hydralazine 2. Isoniazid 3. Phenytoin 4. Procainamide 5. Penicillamine

Name the disease related to SLE that is characterized by immune complex deposition at the dermal-epidermal junction	Discoid lupus erythematosus

Immunodeficiencies

Name the immunodeficiency associated with the following clinical and pathologic features:

B-cell deficiency causing recurrent respiratory tract bacterial infections in boys >6 months of age	X-linked (XL) agammaglobulinemia
T-cell deficiency due to failure of development of the third and fourth pharyngeal pouches	Thymic aplasia (DiGeorge syndrome)
Defective B and T cells, most cases caused by XL recessive mutation in γ-chain of cytokine receptors or autosomal recessive (AR) mutation in adenosine deaminase	Severe combined immunodeficiency
AR disease characterized by IgA deficiency, cerebellar dysfunction, and conjunctival telangiectasias	Ataxia-telangiectasia

XL deficiency of nicotinamide adenine dinucleotide phosphate (NADPH) oxidase activity, resulting in an impaired neutrophil respiratory burst and leading to increased bacterial and fungal infections	Chronic granulomatous disease
Recurrent bacterial infections early in life due to a defect in CD40 ligand that prevents B-cell class switching	Hyper-IgM syndrome
AR microtubule defect resulting in decreased phagocytosis, partial albinism, and neuropathy	Chediak-Higashi disease
AR syndrome characterized by failure of neutrophil chemotaxis-associated eczema, elevated IgE, noninflamed staphylococcal abscesses	Job (hyper-IgE) syndrome
XL recessive disease characterized by recurrent infections, thrombocytopenia, eczema	Wiskott-Aldrich syndrome
Mutation of the Btk tyrosine kinase gene resulting in the underproduction of all classes of antibodies	XL agammaglobulinemia
Defect in the receptor for IL-7	Severe combined immunodeficiency
Associated with *Staphylococcus aureus*, *Streptococcus pneumoniae*, and *Haemophilus influenzae* respiratory infections and persistent *Giardia lamblia* infections	XL agammaglobulinemia
Associated with recurrent GI and pulmonary infections	Isolated IgA deficiency
Frequent viral and fungal infections in a patient with hypocalcemia due to low PTH levels	Thymic aplasia (DiGeorge syndrome)
Associated with tetany and congenital defects of the heart and aorta	Thymic aplasia (DiGeorge syndrome)
Small thymus devoid of lymphocytes, hypoplastic lymph nodes, and splenic white pulp	Severe combined immunodeficiency
↑ IgA, normal IgE, and ↓ IgM levels	Wiskott-Aldrich syndrome
Hypogammaglobulinemia commonly due to failure of T-cell-mediated B-cell maturation	Common variable immunodeficiency

Autoimmune and Connective Tissue Disorders

Name the autoimmune disease of
connective tissue associated with the
following clinical and pathologic
findings:

Keratoconjunctivitis sicca or   Sjögren syndrome
xerophthalmia, xerostomia, and
evidence of other connective tissue
disease

Autoimmune inflammatory disorder   Polymyositis
associated with malignancy;
frequently caused muscle weakness

Heliotrope rash   Dermatomyositis

Rapidly progressive diffuse fibrosis   Systemic sclerosis
of skin and involved organs
including the heart, GI tract, kidney,
lung, muscle, and skin

CREST syndrome of calcinosis,   Localized scleroderma
Raynaud phenomenon, esophageal
dysfunction, sclerodactyly,
telangiectasias

↑ Serum creatine kinase (CK) levels   Polymyositis

What is the most common cause of   Renal crisis (accounts for 50% of deaths
death due to systemic sclerosis?   related to systemic sclerosis)

Which autoimmune disease of   Mixed connective tissue disease
connective tissue lacks renal
involvement?

Amyloidoses

Name the group of disorders   Amyloidoses
characterized by extracellular
deposition of protein in a β-pleated
sheet conformation

Which stain is used to identify the   Congo red
presence of amyloid in tissue that
exhibits apple green birefringence
under polarized light?

Which molecular configuration is   Cross-β-pleated sheet
common to all forms of amyloid?

CHAPTER 3

Microbiology

BACTERIOLOGY

Taxonomy Basics

Name two genera of gram-positive cocci:	1. *Streptococcus* 2. *Staphylococcus*
Name four genera of gram-positive bacilli:	1. *Clostridium* 2. *Listeria* 3. *Bacillus* 4. *Corynebacterium*
Which of these gram-positive bacilli are spore forming?	*Clostridium* and *Bacillus*
Which gram-positive cocci are catalase positive (+)?	*Staphylococcus*
Which of these is also coagulase (+)?	*Staphylococcus aureus*
Which coagulase-negative *Staphylococcus* is novobiocin resistant?	*Staphylococcus saprophyticus* (*Staphylococcus epidermidis* is novobiocin-sensitive)
Name the streptococci that typically show the following pattern of hemolysis:	
α **(green/partial hemolysis) "α*lmost hemolytic*"**	*Streptococcus pneumoniae* and viridians group (eg, *Streptococcus mutans*)
β **(clear hemolysis) "β*etter hemolysis*"**	Group A (*Streptococcus pyogenes*) and group B (*Streptococcus agalactiae*)

Laboratory Evaluation of Bacteria

How are *S. pneumoniae* and viridans streptococci differentiated in the laboratory?

S. pneumoniae is bile soluble and optochin sensitive

How can capsulated *S. pneumoniae* bugs be detected in the laboratory?

Quellung positive (capsule swells when antisera is added)

What determines the Lancefield grouping of streptococci?

C-carbohydrate in the bacterial cell wall

How are groups A and B differentiated in the laboratory?

Group A is sensitive to bacitracin

How are spores from gram-positive rods killed?

Autoclave (spores are resistant to heat and most chemicals)

Name the gram-negative organisms associated with each of the following statements:

Three pathogenic gram-negative cocci

1. *Neisseria meningitidis*
2. *Neisseria gonorrhoeae*
3. *Moraxella catarrhalis*

Six gram-negative coccobacilli

1. *Haemophilus influenzae*
2. *Pasteurella*
3. *Brucella*
4. *Bordetella pertussis*
5. *Francisella*
6. *Legionella*

Three clinically important gram-negative rods that are typically lactose fermenting

1. *Enterobacter*
2. *Escherichia coli*
3. *Klebsiella* (all implicated in urinary tract infections [UTIs])

Two obligate intracellular organisms

1. *Chlamydia* (steals adenosine triphosphate [ATP] from host)
2. *Rickettsia* (lacks coenzyme A [CoA] and nicotinamide adenine dinucleotide [NAD] → cannot produce own ATP)

Four obligate aerobes

1. *Nocardia*
2. *Pseudomonas*
3. *Mycobacterium tuberculosis*
4. *Bacillus*

Three obligate anaerobes	1. *Clostridium* 2. *Bacteroides* 3. *Actinomyces* (no catalase and/or superoxide dismutase → susceptible to oxidative damage)
How are the pathogenic *Neisseria* species differentiated in the laboratory?	*N. meningitidis* ferments maltose
How can *Pseudomonas* be rapidly differentiated from many lactose nonfermenters in the laboratory?	*Pseudomonas* is oxidase positive

Bacteriology Basics

Which cell membrane structure is unique to gram-positive organisms?	Teichoic acid
Which molecule, unique to the bacterial cell wall, provides rigid support and resistance against osmotic pressure?	Peptidoglycan
Which heat-stable lipopolysaccharide (LPS) is found in the cell wall of gram-negative bacteria?	Endotoxin
Which is the only gram-positive organism with LPS-lipid A?	*Listeria monocytogenes*
Name five important systemic effects of endotoxin (particularly, lipid A):	1. ↑ Interleukin (IL)-1 → fever 2. ↑ Tissue necrosis factor (TNF) → hemorrhagic tissue death 3. ↑ Nitric oxide → hypotension and shock 4. Activation of alternate complement pathway →↑ C3a (edema) and C5a (polymorphonuclear [PMN] chemotaxis) 5. Activation of factor XII → coagulation cascade → DIC
Which has a higher toxicity, endotoxins or exotoxins?	Exotoxins: fatal dose on the order of 1 mg (vs. hundreds of micrograms for endotoxins)

Name the mechanism of DNA transfer characterized by the following statements:

DNA is taken up directly from the environment by competent cells	Transformation (can occur in eukaryotic cells, too)
	Medically important natural transformers: **HHSNG**: "Here, Have Some New Genes": *H. pylori, H. influenzae, S. pneumoniae, N. gonorrhoeae*
Plasmid or chromosomal DNA transferred from one bacterium to another via cell-to-cell contact	Conjugation
DNA transferred by a virus from one cell to another; can be generalized or specialized	Transduction
DNA segments able to excise and reincorporate into different locations	Transposons

Name the bacterium whose exotoxin has the following effects:

Superantigen that induces IL-1 and IL-2 synthesis in toxic shock syndrome; also leads to food poisoning	*S. aureus*
α-Toxin is a lecithinase → gas gangrene	*Clostridium perfringens*
Prevents the release of the neurotransmitter (NT) glycine from Renshaw cells in spinal cord → paralysis	*Clostridium tetani*
↑ Adenylate cyclase by adenosine diphosphate (ADP) ribosylation → whooping cough	*B. pertussis*
Exotoxin encoded by β-prophage; α subunit → inactivates elongation factor 2 (EF-2) halting protein synthesis; β subunit → permits entry into cardiac and neural tissue	*Corynebacterium diphtheriae*
Erythrogenic superantigen → rash in scarlet fever	*S. pyogenes*

Prevents release of acetylcholine (ACh) at nerve terminals → paralysis; spores in canned food and honey, construction sites	*Clostridium botulinum*
Heat-stable toxin ↑ guanylate cyclase; heat-labile toxin ↑ adenylate cyclase by ADP ribosylation of G protein → watery diarrhea	*E. coli*
Inactivates the 60S ribosome → kills intestinal cells	*Shigella dysenteriae*
Irreversible ADP ribosylation of G protein →↑ adenylate cyclase →↑ Cl⁻ and H₂O in gut → voluminous stools	*Vibrio cholerae*
Exotoxin A inhibits protein synthesis by blocking EF-2	*Pseudomonas*
Which virulence factor allows organisms to colonize mucosal surfaces?	IgA protease (eg, *S. pneumoniae* and *H. influenzae*)

Name the bacterial structure associated with each antigenic classification given below:

K-antigen	Capsule (related to virulence of the bacteria) **K = Kapsule**
O-antigen	Outer portion of the polysaccharide of endotoxin **O = Outer**
H-antigen	Flagella (seen in motile species)

Name the key virulence factor(s) associated with each of the following organisms:

Group A streptococcus	M-protein (antiphagocytic), streptokinase (thrombolytic, dissolves blood clot), and hyaluronidase (dissolves hyaluronan cell-cell bonds, allowing spread through tissue)

S. aureus	Protein A (prevents complement fixation and phagocytosis), penicillinase (inactivates penicillin), and hyaluronidase (dissolves hyaluronan cell-cell bonds, allowing spread through tissue), TSST-1 (causes toxic shock syndrome)
Streptococcus viridans	Extracellular dextran → helps bind to heart valves, causing endocarditis
Yersinia pestis	F1 capsular antigen (antiphagocytic) and protease (degrades clots)
V. cholerae	Ctx A (irreversibly ADP ribosylates cAMP leading to constitutive secretory diarrhea), Ctx B (binds gangliosides on cell surface)
Vibrio vulnificus	Metalloproteinase (tissue damage), capsule (antiphagocytic), RtxA (cytotoxin)
Enterotoxigenic E. coli	Heat-labile toxin (ADP ribosylates cAMP, similar to cholera toxin)
Enterohemorrhagic E. coli	Shiga-like toxin (Stx 1+2, irreversibly inactivates mammalian 60S ribosome, halting protein synthesis)
S. dysenteriae	Shiga toxin (irreversibly inactivates mammalian 60S ribosome, halting protein synthesis)
Bartonella henselae	Hypoxia-inducible factor-1 (HIF-1) (angiogenic factor which can lead to bacillary angiomatosis in immunocompromised)
N. gonorrhoeae	IgA protease (cleaves IgA), adhesin (promotes cell invasion), pilus (allows binding to non-ciliated epithelium)
H. influenzae	Capsule: six types (A–F) and IgA protease
Borrelia	Antigenic variation
M. tuberculosis	Mycosides (cord factor, wax D, and sulfatides)

Infectious Diseases

Name the organism(s) associated with
each of the following characteristics:

Gram-positive rods with metachromatic granules	*C. diphtheriae*
Three urease (+)	*Helicobacter pylori, Proteus,* and *Ureaplasma urealyticum*
Aerosol transmission from environmental water source (eg, air conditioner)	*Legionella pneumophila*
Contain mycolic acid in membranes	*Mycobacterium* and *Nocardia*
Peptidoglycan wall lacks muramic acid	*Chlamydiae*
Produces pyocyanin (blue-green) pigment	*Pseudomonas aeruginosa*
Produces yellow-gold pigment	*S. aureus*
Only bacterial membrane containing cholesterol	*Mycoplasma pneumoniae*
Filamentous, branching rods in a cervicofacial infection	*Actinomyces israelii*
Two forms: elementary and reticulate bodies	*Chlamydiae*
Pleomorphic gram-negative rods in "school of fish" pattern	*Haemophilus ducreyi*
Clue cells on wet mount	*Gardnerella vaginalis*
High titer of cold agglutinins (IgM)	*M. pneumoniae*
Two fungi-like bacteria	*A. israelii* and *Nocardia asteroides*

Name the organism(s) associated with
the following pathology:

Fitz-Hugh and Curtis syndrome	*Chlamydia trachomatis* or *N. gonorrhoeae*

Invades gastrointestinal (GI) mucosa → diarrhea; motile; can disseminate hematogenously	*Salmonella*
Infected dog or cat bites (or scratches)	*Pasteurella multocida*
Ghon complex	*M. tuberculosis* (1° tuberculosis [TB]) **Note:** hilar nodes plus Ghon focus usually in lower lobe
Meningitis and pneumonia in neonates	*H. influenzae*
Atypical pneumonia with avian reservoir	*Chlamydia psittaci*
Gas gangrene in traumatic open wounds	*C. perfringens*
Infects skin and superficial nerves	*Mycobacterium leprae*
Fibrocaseous cavitary lung lesion	*M. tuberculosis* (2° TB) **Note:** usually at apex because ↑ affinity for ↑ O2 environments
Mycobacterium causing disseminated disease in acquired immunodeficiency syndrome (AIDS) patients and pneumonia classically in elderly, well-mannered women who suppress their cough (Lady Windermere syndrome)	*Mycobacterium avium-intracellulare*
Mycobacterium causing cervical lymphadenitis in kids	*Mycobacterium scrofulaceum* (ie, scrofula)

For each of the following clinical findings, name the organism responsible and the drug(s) of choice:

Oral/facial abscesses with sulfur granules in sinus tracts	*A. israelii*—penicillin G (IV)
Currant jelly sputum	*Klebsiella*—first- or second-generation cephalosporins
Woolsorter's disease	*Bacillus anthracis*—penicillin G or ciprofloxacin

Food poisoning from reheated rice	*Bacillus cereus*—antibiotic treatment generally not required (illness due to enterotoxin not bacteria)
Scarlet fever, impetigo, and pharyngitis	*S. pyogenes*—penicillin
Pontiac fever	*L. pneumophila*—macrolide (erythromycin and azithromycin)
Gram-positive coccus causing sepsis/meningitis in a newborn	*S. agalactiae*—ampicillin **Note:** group **B**, think **B**abies
Pneumonia in elderly, thin, well-mannered women who suppress their cough (Lady Windermere syndrome)	*M. avium-intracellulare*
Acute epiglottitis, meningitis, otitis, and pneumonia	*H. influenzae*—second-generation cephalosporins (treat meningitis with ceftriaxone, plus rifampin for contacts)
Gastritis and majority of duodenal ulcers	*H. pylori*—triple therapy
Waterhouse-Friderichsen syndrome	*N. meningitidis*—ceftriaxone
Pneumonia in cystic fibrosis and burn patients	*Pseudomonas cepacia*—bactrim or ciprofloxacin
Bacterial vaginosis with discharge and fishy odor	*G. vaginalis*—metronidazole
Burn and wound infections with fruity odor	*P. aeruginosa*—aminoglycoside plus antipseudomonal (eg, piperacillin and tazobactam)
Acute postinfectious glomerulonephritis	*S. pyogenes*—penicillin G
Pseudomembranous enterocolitis	*Clostridium difficile*—metronidazole or oral vancomycin
Community-acquired-pneumonia (most common cause) with rust-colored sputum	*S. pneumoniae*—beta-lactam + macrolide (cover for atypical pathogens) or respiratory fluoroquinolone
Atypical "walking" pneumonia in young adult	*M. pneumoniae*—erythromycin or doxycycline

Urethritis/pelvic inflammatory disease (PID), neonatal conjunctivitis, and pneumonia	*C. trachomatis* types D to K—erythromycin eye drops in neonates, azithromycin for urethritis, pneumonia
Lyme disease	*Borrelia burgdorferi*—doxycycline
Malignant, vesicular papules covered with black eschar → bacteremia and death	*B. anthracis*—penicillin G or ciprofloxacin
Pneumonia, sepsis, otitis externa, UTIs, hot-tub folliculitis, osteomyelitis	*P. aeruginosa*—aminoglycoside plus antipseudomonal piperacillin and tazobactam
Undulant fever, Bang's disease	*Brucella* sp.—doxycycline plus gentamicin or rifampin (pasteurize milk to prevent)
Bubonic plague	*Y. pestis*—gentamicin
Rocky Mountain spotted fever	*Rickettsia rickettsii*—tetracycline/doxycycline
Trench fever (lasts 5 days; recurs in 5-day cycles)	*Bartonella quintana*—gentamicin/doxycycline
Tabes dorsalis, aortitis, and gummas	*Treponema pallidum* (3° syphilis)—penicillin G
Q fever (acute)	*Coxiella burnetii*—doxycycline
Weil disease	*Leptospira interrogans*—penicillin G
Yaws	*Treponema pertenue*—penicillin G
Pott disease	*M. tuberculosis* (disseminated)—four-drug anti-tuberculous therapy, including rifampin plus isoniazid (INH)
Dental caries	*S. mutans*—amoxicillin or amoxicillin/clavulanic acid (prevention with topical fluoride/chlorhexidine)
Rheumatic fever	*S. pyogenes* (prodrome of pharyngitis only, not cellulitis)—penicillin G
Scalded skin syndrome and toxic shock syndrome	*S. aureus*—penicillin agent (vancomycin if methicillin-resistant *S. aureus* [MRSA])

Hansen disease	*M. leprae*—dapsone plus clofazimine or rifampin
Lymphogranuloma venereum	*C. trachomatis* types L1, L2, L3—doxycycline
What is the infectious differential for a rash affecting the palms and soles?	Rocky Mountain spotted fever, 2° syphilis, hand-foot-and-mouth disease (coxsackie A), and Kawasaki syndrome

Name the mode of transmission and reservoir(s) for each of the following bacteria:

Brucella sp.	Contact with animals or dairy products; cows
Francisella tularensis	Tick or deerfly bite; rabbits and deer
P. multocida	Animal bite/scratch; cats and dogs
B. burgdorferi	Ixodes tick bite; lives on deer and mice
Y. pestis	Flea bite; rodents (eg, prairie dogs)
R. rickettsii	Tick bite; dogs, rabbits, and rodents (endemic to eastern United States)
Rickettsia prowazekii	Human body louse; humans and flying squirrels

Name the laboratory test described below:

Detects antirickettsial antibodies	Weil-Felix reaction (cross-reacts with proteus)
Sensitive for treponemes	Fluorescent treponemal antibody-absorption test (FTA-ABS) (+) (earliest and longest, used as confirmatory test for syphilis if RPR is reactive)
Useful in screening for TB	Purified protein derivative (PPD) test
Screening for TB in persons with prior BCG (Bacillus Calmette-Guérin) vaccine	Interferon gamma-release assay (IGRA)

Name the screening test for syphilis and four biological false positives:	VDRL test 1. Viruses (mononucleosis and hepatitis) 2. Drugs (narcotics) 3. Rheumatoid arthritis/fever 4. Leprosy and lupus

Name the normal, dominant flora for each of the following locations:

Nose	*S. aureus*
Oropharynx	Group D streptococci (viridans)
Dental plaques	*S. mutans*
Colon	*Bacteroides fragilis* > *E. coli*
Vagina	*Lactobacillus*; colonized by *E. coli* and group B streptococcus
Skin	*S. epidermidis*

Name the nosocomial pathogen(s) associated with each of the following:

Urinary catheter	*E. coli* and *Proteus mirabilis*
Respiratory therapy equipment, ventilators	*P. aeruginosa*
Wound infections	*S. aureus*
Water aerosols	*Legionella* sp.

Tuberculosis

Decide whether each of the following statements is more closely associated with 1° or 2° TB:

Radiographic finding = Ghon complex; classically affects lower lobes	1° TB
Miliary TB	2° TB
Fibrocaseous cavitary lung lesion; classically affects apical lungs (↑ affinity for ↑ O2 environment)	2° TB

Symptoms of cough/hemoptysis, fever, night sweats, and weight loss	2° TB
What type of hypersensitivity reaction is seen after infection with *M. tuberculosis*?	Type IV or delayed-type hypersensitivity (basis for PPD test)
How does the interferon gamma-release assay (IGRA) work in the diagnosis of latent TB?	A blood sample is incubated with mycobacterial antigens and then tested for release of interferon-γ, indicating a previous exposure
What phenomenon leads to a false-negative PPD in patients with active TB?	Anergy; chronic TB infection (or HIV) leads to immune suppression and inhibition of the type IV hypersensitivity reaction that causes a positive tuberculin skin test
What unique type of cell is seen in association with caseating granulomas in TB?	Langerhans giant cell
What is the mode of transmission of *M. tuberculosis*?	Airborne (droplet nuclei)
What term describes the lymphatic and hematogenous spread of TB, causing numerous small foci of infection in extrapulmonary sites?	Miliary TB
Name five common sites of extrapulmonary TB:	1. CNS (tuberculous meningitis) 2. Vertebral bodies (Pott disease) 3. Psoas major muscle → abscess 4. GI tract (liver and cecum) 5. Cervical lymph nodes → scrofuloderma
What is an effective screening tool for latent TB?	Tuberculin skin test (eg, PPD) or IGRA
Testing for latent TB in persons with prior BCG (Bacillus Calmette-Guérin) vaccine	IGRA
How is active TB infection diagnosed?	Clinical and radiologic signs of 2° TB and demonstration of presence of mycobacteria; PPD and IGRA may yield false-negative results and should not be used in this setting

What assays are used to diagnose active TB infection? — Acid-fast stain, nucleic acid amplification, culture

What is the management of latent TB? — INH and rifapentine once weekly? 3 months OR rifampin daily for 4 months OR INH daily for 6 to 9 months

What is the treatment for active TB? — Respiratory isolation and initial four-drug therapy (**RIPE: R**ifampin, **I**NH, **P**yrazinamide, **E**thambutol)

What is the major toxicity of most TB drugs? — Hepatotoxicity; INH → vitamin B6 deficiency (always supplement treated patients); ethambutol → optic neuritis

ANTIBIOTICS

Name the drug(s) whose mechanism of action is described below:

Binds penicillin-binding proteins → inhibits transpeptidase → blocks cell wall synthesis; also releases autolytic enzymes (bactericidal) — α-Lactam antibiotics (penicillin, cephalosporins, cephalomycins, carbapenems, and monobactams)

Forms reactive cytotoxic metabolites inside cell — Metronidazole

Binds and inactivate β-lactamase → protects antibiotic — β-Lactamase inhibitors

Inhibits 50S peptidyl transferase
Blocks entry of aa-tRNA to 30S ribosomal complex — Chloramphenicol
Tetracyclines

Blocks transpeptidation of D-ala — Vancomycin

Inhibits dihydrofolate reductase — Trimethoprim (TMP)

Para-aminobenzoic acid (PABA) antimetabolites →↑ dihydropteroate synthase — Sulfonamides

Binds to 30S subunit → block formation of 70S initiation complex → misreading of mRNA — Aminoglycosides

Binds to 50S subunit → inhibit translocase	Macrolides (erythromycin and azithromycin)
Blocks DNA topoisomerase (gyrase)	Quinolones (ciprofloxacin and levofloxacin)
Blocks 50S peptide bond formation	Clindamycin
Inhibits DNA-dependent RNA polymerase	Rifampin
Interferes with mycolic acid synthesis	INH
Bind to bacterial/fungal cell membranes → disrupt osmotic properties	Polymyxins
PABA antagonist → blocks purine synthesis	Sulfones (dapsone and sulfoxone)

Name the antibacterial drug(s) associated with each of the following unique toxicities:

Kernicterus in infants	Sulfonamides and ceftriaxone
Interstitial nephritis	Penicillins
Disulfiram-like reactions	Metronidazole, second-generation cephalosporins
Photosensitivity rash	Doxycycline
Gray baby syndrome	Chloramphenicol
Megaloblastic anemia	TMP
Hemolytic anemia in G6PD-deficient patient	Sulfonamides, chloramphenicol, nitrofurantoin, and INH
Hepatotoxicity, vitamin B_6 deficiency, lupus-like syndrome	INH **Note:** ↑ $t_{1/2}$ in slow acetylators
Pseudomembranous colitis	Any antibiotic, leading to *C. difficile* infection
Fanconi syndrome	Tetracycline (ingestion of expired drug)
Ototoxicity and nephrotoxicity	Aminoglycosides

Red, pruritic rash on torso with rapid IV infusion (red man syndrome)	Vancomycin
Reversible cholestatic hepatitis; ↑ GI motility	Erythromycin
Achilles tendonitis; cartilage damage in laboratory animals	Fluoroquinolones
Red-orange discoloration of bodily secretions	Rifampin
Discolors teeth; suppresses bone growth in kids	Tetracycline
Aplastic anemia (dose independent)	Chloramphenicol
Neurotoxicity and nephrotoxicity	Polymyxins

Name six uses for metronidazole:

1. *Giardia*
2. *Entamoeba*
3. *Trichomonas*
4. *G. vaginalis*
5. Anaerobes (*C. difficile, Bacteroides*)
6. *H. pylori* (part of triple therapy)

Which drug is used as solo prophylaxis for TB?

INH

How do organisms develop resistance against vancomycin?

d-lac (or d-ser) replaces terminal d-ala in cell wall → ↑ affinity of vancomycin for cell wall

VIROLOGY

Taxonomy/Basics

Name six medically important DNA viral families:

HHAPPPy:
1. Hepadnaviridae
2. Herpesviridae
3. Adenoviridae
4. Poxviridae
5. Parvoviridae
6. Papovaviridae

Name two families of circular DNA viruses:	1. Papovaviridae 2. Hepadnaviridae
Name the only ssDNA viral genome:	Parvovirus
Name the only DNA virus that replicates in the cytoplasm:	Poxviridae (carries its own DNA-dependent RNA polymerase)
Name three naked DNA viruses:	**PAP:** 1. Parvo 2. Adeno 3. Papov
Name the only dsRNA viral genome:	Reoviruses (eg, rotavirus)
Name the family of the smallest RNA viruses:	Picornaviruses
Name four families of naked RNA viruses:	**CRAP:** 1. Calicivirus 2. Reovirus 3. Astrovirus 4. Picornavirus
Name two families of RNA viruses that do not replicate solely in the cytoplasm:	1. Influenza viruses 2. Retroviruses
Where do most enveloped viruses acquire their membranes?	From plasma membrane (except herpesviruses—nuclear membrane)
Name four families of segmented viruses:	**BOAR** (all RNA viruses) 1. Bunyaviridae 2. Orthomyxoviridae (influenza viruses) 3. Arenaviridae 4. Reoviridae
Name the only diploid viruses:	Retroviruses
What types of nucleic acids do not require special enzymes to be infectious?	Those with same structure as host nucleic acids (eg, positive-stranded ssRNA and most naked dsDNA)
Name the type of viral genetic strategy described below:	
The virus contains its own genetic material but is coated with surface proteins from another virus, which determine its infectivity	Phenotypic mixing

Occurs when viruses exchange segments of their genomes	Reassortment
Occurs when a nonmutated virus assists a mutated one by making a functional gene product that serves both itself and the mutated virus	Complementation
Exchanging oligonucleotides by crossing-over within base sequences	Recombination
What type of antigenic change in the influenza virus causes *epidemics*?	Antigenic drift (minor changes from random mutation)
What type of antigenic change in the influenza virus causes *pandemics*?	Antigenic shift (reassortment of genome, including animal acquisition) (**D**rifting is a **S**low Process, **S**hifting is a **R**apid Process)

For each of the following vaccines, state whether it is live attenuated or killed:

Sabin polio	Live attenuated
Salk polio	Killed (Sal**K** = **K**illed)
May revert to virulence	Live attenuated (very rare)
For whom is it dangerous to receive live vaccines?	Immunocompromised hosts (ie, transplant recipients, AIDS patients, and pregnant women)

Infectious Diseases

Name the virus(es) associated with each of the following statements:

Tzanck prep shows multinucleated giant cells	Herpes simplex virus (HSV)-1, HSV-2, and varicella-zoster virus (VZV)
Viral culture with buffy coat	Cytomegalovirus (CMV)
Transmitted by bat, raccoon, and skunk bites	Rabies virus
Transmitted by arthropods	Arboviruses

Cowdry type A inclusion bodies	Herpesviruses (HSV-1, CMV, and VZV)
Number 1 cause of diarrhea in kids <3 years old (y/o)	Rotavirus
Number 1 cause of viral pneumonia in infants <6 months old	Respiratory syncytial virus (RSV)
Severe (but rare) sequelae include giant cell pneumonia and subacute sclerosing panencephalitis (SSPE)	Measles virus (rubeola)
Councilman bodies in liver	Yellow fever virus
Reactivation of virus in brain of AIDS patient → demyelination, death	JC virus → progressive multifocal leuko-encephalopathy (PML)
Bullet-shaped, helical nucleocapsid; travels up nerve axons to CNS in retrograde fashion	Rabies virus
Koplik spots	Measles virus (rubeola)
Atypical lymphocytes	Epstein-Barr virus (EBV) and CMV
Nosocomial infection associated with the newborn nursery	CMV and RSV
Negri bodies in neurons	Rabies virus
Incomplete RNA virus → requires envelope	Hepatitis D virus
Positive heterophile antibody test	EBV
Necrosis of large motor neurons in anterior horn spinal cord → flaccid paralysis	Poliovirus

For each of the following clinical findings, name the associated virus:

Shingles	VZV
Suboccipital lymphadenopathy	Rubella virus
Herpangina, hand-foot-and-mouth disease	Coxsackie A virus

Gingivostomatitis, keratitis, and temporal lobe encephalitis	HSV-1
Genital and neonatal infections	HSV-2
Fever, hepatosplenomegaly pharyngitis, and posterior auricular lymphadenopathy; "kissing disease"	EBV (mononucleosis)
Common cold	Rhinoviruses (>100 serotypes; associated with 85% of cases)
PML	JC polyomavirus
Chickenpox	Varicella
Small, pearly, umbilicated papular epidermal growths near genitals	Molluscum contagiosum virus
German measles and congenital infections	Rubella virus
Explosive gastroenteritis; recent epidemics on cruise ships and schools	Norwalk virus
Exanthem subitum (roseola)	Human herpesvirus (HHV)-6
Contains hemagglutinin and neuraminidase virulence factor; undergoes antigenic shift and responsible for pandemics	Influenza A
Fever, black vomitus, and jaundice; transmitted by *Aedes* mosquito	Yellow fever virus
Pericarditis, myocarditis, and pleurodynia	Coxsackie B virus
Acute viral hepatitis	Hepatitis A and B
Mononucleosis, congenital infection, and pneumonia	CMV
Subacute sclerosing panencephalitis	Measles (rubeola) virus
Intussusception from hyperplasia of Peyer patches	Adenoviruses
Kaposi sarcoma	HHV-8

Aseptic meningitis, orchitis, and parotitis	Mumps virus
Barking cough and laryngeal swelling	Parainfluenza viruses (croup)
Hepatitis from IV drug abuse or blood transfusion	Hepatitis C virus
Hydrophobia, seizures, and fatal encephalitis	Rabies virus
Cause of common and genital warts	Human papillomavirus (HPV)
Hepatitis with high mortality rate in pregnant women	Hepatitis E virus
Reye syndrome	Influenza viruses (occurs with aspirin [ASA] ingestion)
Epidemic keratoconjunctivitis; childhood URIs	Adenoviruses
Cough, coryza, and conjunctivitis	Measles (rubeola) virus
Erythema infectiosum (fifth disease); transient aplastic anemic crisis	Parvovirus B19

Name the oncogenic virus associated with the following cancers:

Burkitt lymphoma	EBV
Hepatocellular carcinoma	Hepatitis B and C viruses
Hairy cell leukemia	HTLV-2
Adult T-cell lymphoma	HTLV-1
Nasopharyngeal carcinoma	EBV
Kaposi sarcoma	HHV-8
Cervical, penile, and anal carcinoma	HPV types: 16, 18, 31, 33, and 45

Name the family of viruses characterized by the following:

Smallpox, molluscum contagiosum, and vaccinia	Poxviridae
Hantavirus and California encephalitis	Bunyaviridae
Marburg and Ebola hemor-rhagic fever	Filoviridae
Lassa fever and lymphocytic choriomeningitis	Arenaviridae

Human Immunodeficiency Virus

What are the three major routes of HIV transmission?	1. Sexual contact 2. Vertical (mother to newborn) transmission 3. Parenteral
What is the most common mode of HIV transmission on a global basis?	Heterosexual contact
What type of virus is HIV?	Human retrovirus of the lentivirus family
What test is used to screen for HIV infection?	Enzyme-linked immunosorbent assay (ELISA) looks for AB to viral proteins; ↑ sensitivity
What test is used to confirm HIV(+) screening results?	Western blot assay (high false nega-tive within 2 months of infection); ↑ specificity
Which enzyme creates dsDNA from RNA for integration into host genome?	Reverse transcriptase (RT)
What test is used to monitor the effects of antiretroviral therapy?	HIV RT-polymerase chain reaction (RT-PCR) (measures viral load)
What is the strongest measure of dis-ease progression in an HIV(+) patient?	CD4+ T-cell count
Name two key glycoproteins on the surface of the HIV viral envelope:	1. gp41 (fusion) 2. gp120 (attachment) proteins; together = gp160
Name two key HIV viral core proteins:	1. p24 (nucleocapsid) 2. p17 (matrix protein)

Name three key HIV retroviral enzymes contained in the core:	1. RT 2. Integrase 3. Protease (all encoded by *pol* gene)
Which viral antigen peaks within 2 months of infection, then rises again years later?	p24
What are the two cell surface molecules to which gp120 must bind?	1. CD42; a chemokine receptor (CCR5 or CXCR4)
HIV infects which three cell types?	1. CD4+ T cells 2. Monocytes/macrophages 3. Dendritic cells
The induction of what cellular transcription factor during an immune response leads to activation of transcription of HIV proviral DNA?	Nuclear factor-kappa B (NF-?B)
Protease inhibitors of HIV prevent cleavage of the protein product of what viral genes?	*Gag* and *pol* genes
What are the three mechanisms by which HIV-infected CD4+ T cells are lost?	1. HIV cytopathic effect 2. Apoptosis 3. HIV-specific cytotoxic T-cell killing
What are the three stages of HIV infection?	1. Acute retroviral infection 2. Chronic phase 3. AIDS
What is the surrogate measure of viral load in an HIV(+) patient?	HIV-1 RNA
What is the strongest measure of disease progression in AIDS?	CD4+ T-cell count
Which tissues are the major reservoirs of HIV-infected T cells and macrophages in patients?	1. Lymph nodes 2. Spleen 3. Tonsils
Which cell type in the brain is infected by HIV?	Microglial cells
List the major immune abnormalities in AIDS:	1. Decreased number of CD4+ T cells 2. Decreased T-cell function 3. Polyclonal activation of B cells 4. Altered macrophage function

What is the clinical picture of direct viral disease from HIV?

Constitutional symptoms (weight loss, fever, fatigue, and night sweats) and/or neurologic symptoms (encephalopathy with dementia and aseptic meningitis)

How is AIDS defined?

CD4+ <200 or AIDS-defining illness, regardless of CD4+ count

Name the common AIDS opportunistic organisms or infections/diseases associated with the following:

    Four fungal infections

1. Candidiasis (GI tract)
2. Cryptococcosis (meningitis)
3. Histoplasmosis (disseminated)
4. Coccidioidomycosis (disseminated)

    Five bacterial infections

1. *M. tuberculosis* (lung/disseminated)
2. *M. avium-intracellulare* (lung)
3. *Nocardia* (lung/CNS/disseminated)
4. *Salmonella* (disseminated)
5. Encapsulated organisms

    Four viral infections

1. HSV
2. VZV (shingles)
3. CMV (retinitis or colitis)
4. JC virus (PML)

    Three protozoal infections

1. *Pneumocystis* (lung or disseminated)
2. *Toxoplasma* (lung/CNS)
3. *Cryptosporidium* (GI)

State the typical CD4+ count associated with each of the following HIV complications:

    Opportunistic infections are typically seen, especially *Pneumocystis jirovecii* pneumonia

<200 cells/mL

    ***Mycobacterium avium* complex (MAC), CMV, and cryptosporidiosis**

<50 cells/mL

    Toxoplasmosis

<100 cells/mL

    TB becomes more common

<400 cells/mL

List four common neoplasms in patients with AIDS:	1. Kaposi sarcoma 2. Non-Hodgkin B-cell lymphoma 3. CNS lymphoma 4. Squamous cell carcinoma of the cervix or anus
What has been shown to minimize the risk of perinatal HIV transmission?	Zidovudine (AZT) given to pregnant women, cesarean delivery, and avoiding breast feeding

Prions

Which infectious agents lack both DNA and RNA?	Prions (made of proteins only)
What are symptoms of prion diseases?	Rapidly progressing dementia, psychiatric disturbances, and cerebellar symptoms (ataxia, myoclonus); all prion diseases are fatal
Name four prion diseases:	1. Creutzfeldt-Jakob disease (rapidly progressive dementia) 2. Mad cow disease 3. Kuru 4. Fatal familial insomnia
What type of histopathologic change is seen in these diseases?	Spongiform encephalopathy

Antiviral Agents

For each of the following drugs, provide: 1. The mechanism of action (MOA) 2. Indication(s) (IND) 3. Significant side effects and unique toxicity (TOX) (if any):	
Acyclovir and valacyclovir	**MOA:** guanosine analog; activated by herpes thymidine kinase → inhibits viral DNA polymerase **IND:** HSV (treatment and prophylaxis for oral, genital, and ocular herpes), VZV (chickenpox and shingles) **TOX:** neurotoxic (delirium and tremors) and nephrotoxic

Ganciclovir	**MOA:** guanosine analog; activated by human thymidine kinase → inhibits CMV DNA polymerase **IND:** CMV (retinitis, pneumonia, colitis), especially in immunocompromised people **TOX:** bone marrow suppression, nephrotoxic, and → spermatogenesis (toxicity > acyclovir because activated by human enzyme)
Foscarnet	**MOA:** pyrophosphate analog; inhibits viral DNA polymerase (no activation required) **IND:** CMV, HSV (refractory infections) **TOX:** reversible nephrotoxicity and anemia
Nucleoside RT inhibitors (zidovudine—azidothymidine [AZT], didanosine—ddI, zalcitabine—ddC, lamivudine—3TC, and stavudine—d4T)	**MOA:** nucleoside analogs; activated by phosphorylation → inhibits RT → prevents incorporation of viral genome into host DNA **IND:** part of combination therapy for HIV **TOX:** bone marrow suppression, peripheral neuropathy, pancreatitis (especially ddI), lactic acidosis, and macrocytic anemia (AZT)
Nonnucleoside RT inhibitors (nevirapine, delavirdine, and efavirenz)	**MOA:** binds directly to and inhibits HIV RT → prevents incorporation of viral genome into host DNA **IND:** part of combination therapy for HIV **TOX:** rash (including Stevens-Johnson), ↑ liver enzymes, inhibits P-450, vivid dreams/CNS changes (with efavirenz)
Protease inhibitors (saquinavir, ritonavir, indinavir, nelfinavir, and amprenavir)	**MOA:** blocks protease enzyme → inhibits assembly of viral core and new viruses **IND:** part of combination therapy for HIV **TOX:** GI upset, insulin resistance, ↑ lipids, fat redistribution syndromes, interstitial nephritis, and thrombocytopenia (indinavir)

Integrase inhibitors (raltegravir)	**MOA:** blocks HIV integration into host cell DNA by reversibly inhibiting HIV integrase **IND:** part of combination therapy for HIV **TOX:** headache, nausea, diarrhea, rash
Fusion inhibitors (enfuvirtide, maraviroc)	**MOA:** binds gp41, preventing viral entry (enfuvirtide); binds CCR-5 on T-cell/monocyte surface, preventing association with HIV protein gp120 (maraviroc) **IND:** part of combination therapy for HIV **TOX:** injection site reactions
Amantadine and rimantadine	**MOA:** inhibits viral penetration and uncoating; releases dopamine (DA) from intact nerve terminals **IND:** influenza A treatment/prophylaxis, Parkinson disease **TOX:** CNS effects: confusion, ataxia, and slurred speech (less with rimantadine); teratogenesis
Zanamivir and oseltamivir	**MOA:** neuraminidase inhibitor ↑ alters virion aggregation and release **IND:** influenza A and B treatment and prophylaxis (oseltamivir) **TOX:** bronchospasm in patients with asthma/COPD (zanamivir)
Ribavirin	**MOA**: guanosine analog; activated by phosphorylation ↑ inhibits inosine-5′-monophosphate (IMP) dehydrogenase **IND**: RSV, hantavirus, and chronic hepatitis C **TOX**: hemolysis (when given IV), teratogen
Sofosbuvir	**MOA:** NS5B inhibitor **IND:** hepatitis C **TOX:** fatigue, headache
Glecaprevir	**MOA:** NS3/4a protease inhibitor **IND:** hepatitis C **TOX:** headache, diarrhea, abnormal LFTs

Interferon-α	**MOA:** human glycoproteins that interfere with ability of viruses to replicate (block protein synthesis and degrade mRNA) **IND:** chronic hepatitis B and C, genital warts, Kaposi sarcoma, and hairy cell leukemia **TOX:** bone marrow suppression
What constitutes highly active antiretroviral therapy (HAART)?	Two nucleoside RT inhibitors and a protease inhibitor, nonnucleoside RT inhibitor, or integrase inhibitor **Note:** no patient should ever be on monotherapy as resistance is common
When is HAART typically initiated?	CD4+ <500 cells/mL or very high viral load
Which drug is used to prevent vertical transmission during pregnancy?	Zidovudine (AZT)

MYCOLOGY

Which four endemic mycoses can mimic TB?	1. Histoplasmosis 2. Coccidioidomycosis 3. Paracoccidioidomycosis 4. Blastomycosis
What is a dimorphic fungus?	Lives in two forms: cold = mold (<37°C), heat = yeast
Name the fungus associated with each of the following statements:	
"Spaghetti and meatball" appearance on KOH prep	*Malassezia furfur*
Contains cancer-causing aflatoxins	*Aspergillus flavus*
Dimorphic fungus living on rose thorns and splinters	*Sporothrix schenckii*
Urease (+), stains with India ink, and latex agglutination (+)	*Cryptococcus neoformans*

Organism found inside macrophages; spread in pigeon and bat droppings	*Histoplasma capsulatum*
Budding yeast, pseudohyphae; germ tubes at 37°C	*Candida albicans*
Wide angle (>90°) branching of irregular nonseptated hyphae	*Mucor* and *Rhizopus* sp.
Big, broad-based budding dimorphic fungus	*Blastomycosis* **B-B-B-B-B** (**B**ig, **B**road-**B**ased **B**udding **B**lasto)
45° angle branching and septated hyphae; fruiting bodies	*Aspergillus* sp.
Narrow-based unequal budding yeasts with capsular halo	*C. neoformans*
Endemic to Ohio and Mississippi river valleys	*H. capsulatum*
"Flying-saucer" appearance of silver stain	*P. jirovecii*
"Captain's wheel" appearance; endemic to rural Latin America	*Paracoccidioidomycosis*

For each of the following diseases, name the fungus/yeast responsible and the drug of choice:

Rose gardener disease with ascending lymphangitis	*S. schenckii*—potassium iodide
Tinea nigra	*Phaeoannellomyces werneckii*—topical salicylic acid
Thrush in an immunocompromised patient	*C. albicans*—nystatin (swish and swallow) and amphotericin B if systemic infection
San Joaquin (desert valley) fever; endemic to southwest United States, California	*Coccidioides immitis*—fluconazole and amphotericin B

Interstitial pneumonia of the immunocompromised	*P. carinii* (or *P. jirovecii*)—TMP-sulfamethoxazole (SMX) or pentamidine (prophylaxis when CD4+ <200 cells/mL)
Tinea (pityriasis) versicolor	*M. furfur*—topical miconazole or selenium sulfide
Meningitis from pigeon droppings	*C. neoformans*—amphotericin + flucytosine for 2 weeks followed by fluconazole
Tinea cruris/capitis/corporis/unguium/pedis	*Trichophyton, Epidermophyton,* or *Microsporum* sp.—topical miconazole, oral griseofulvin for capitis and unguium
Fungus ball in lungs or invasive disease	*Aspergillus fumigatus*—voriconazole

Antifungals

Name the drug whose mechanism of action is described below:

Blocks ergosterol (unique to fungi) synthesis by inhibiting P-450	Azole family (ketoconazole, fluconazole, miconazole, voriconazole, and posaconazole)
Binds ergosterol → produces membrane pores	Amphotericin B and nystatin
Blocks ergosterol synthesis by blocking squalene epoxidase	Terbinafine
Interferes with microtubule formation → inhibits mitosis	Griseofulvin
Converted to 5-fluorouracil (5-FU) → blocks formation of purines	Flucytosine

Name the antifungal drug(s) associated with each of the following unique toxicities:

Rigors, acute febrile reaction, nephrotoxicity, and arrhythmias	Amphotericin B—follow BUN/creatinine daily **Note:** newer lipid formulations (ie, AmBisome less nephrotoxic)

Photosensitivity, mental confusion, bone marrow suppression, and induces P-450	Griseofulvin
Antiandrogenic effects, adrenal suppression, and liver dysfunction	Azole family (especially ketoconazole)
Bone marrow suppression and alopecia	Flucytosine

PARASITOLOGY

Protozoa

Name the protozoan associated with each of the following statements:

Transmitted by Tsetse fly; shows antigenic variation	*Trypanosoma brucei* (*gambiense* and *rhodesiense*)
Transmitted by *Anopheles* mosquito	*Plasmodium*
Transmitted by Reduviid bug	*Trypanosoma cruzi*
Transmitted by cysts in meat or cat feces	*Toxoplasma*
Transmitted by sandfly	*Leishmania*
Primary amoebic encephalitis; enters through cribriform plate	*Naegleria fowleri*
Obligate intracellular parasite; cysts on acid-fast stain	*Cryptosporidium*
Maltese "X" cross shape	*Babesia*
Pear-shaped, binucleate, flagellated trophozoite	*Giardia lamblia*
Blood smear shows trophozoites and schizonts	*Plasmodium*
Macrophages containing amastigotes	*Leishmania donovani*

For each of the following clinical findings, name the associated protozoan and the treatment:

Megacolon, megaesophagus, and cardiomegaly (with apical atrophy)	*T. cruzii* (Chagas disease)—nifurtimox
Cyclic fever, headache, anemia, and splenomegaly	*Plasmodium*—chloroquine for erythrocyte forms and primaquine for latent forms (*Plasmodium vivax* and *Plasmodium ovale*)
Chloroquine-resistant malaria	*Plasmodium falciparum*—mefloquine or quinine and pyramethamine/sulfadoxine
Bloody diarrhea with "flask-shaped" ulcers, liver abscesses, and trophozoites in stool	*Entamoeba histolytica*—metronidazole and iodoquinol
Black fever or "kala-azar"	*L. donovani*—sodium stibogluconate (pentavalent antimony)
Severe, watery diarrhea in AIDS patient	*Cryptosporidium*—supportive (hydration, improve immune status)
Flatulence, bloating, and foul-smelling diarrhea	*G. lamblia*—metronidazole
African sleeping sickness	*T. brucei* (*gambiense* and *rhodesiense*)—suramin (acutely) or melarsoprol (for CNS symptoms)
Encephalitis with brain abscesses in immunocompromised host; congenital defects	*Toxoplasma gondii*—pyrimethamine and sulfadoxine or clindamycin
Vaginitis with foul-smelling, frothy discharge	*Trichomonas vaginalis*—metronidazole
Fever and hemolytic anemia after *Ixodes* tick bite	*Babesia* sp.—quinine and clindamycin
Why are many Africans resistant to *P. vivax* infection?	They carry sickle cell trait and/or they lack antigens Duffy a and b on RBCs
What causes the cyclic symptoms in malaria?	Immune response to burst RBCs that release merozoites

Helminths

For each of the following clinical findings, name the associated helminth and the treatment:

Larvae penetrate skin of feet; GI infection → anemia	*Ancylostoma duodenale* or *Necator americanus* (hookworms)—mebendazole or pyrantel pamoate
Worms visibly crawling in conjunctiva; spread by deerfly	*Loa loa*—diethylcarbamazine
Fever, periorbital edema, and myositis after ingesting raw pork	*Trichinella spiralis*—thiabendazole
River blindness; spread by female blackflies	*Onchocerca volvulus*—ivermectin (**rIV**ERmectin for RIVER blindness)
Elephantiasis from lymphatic blockage	*Wuchereria bancrofti*—diethylcarbamazine
Larvae penetrate skin → autoinfection; GI infection	*Strongyloides stercoralis* (threadworm)—thiabendazole or ivermectin
Intestinal infection and anal pruritis; ↑ incidence in children; positive "tape test"	*Enterobius vermicularis* (pinworms)—mebendazole or pyrantel pamoate
Fluke associated with squamous cell carcinoma of the urinary tract	*Schistosoma haematobium*—praziquantel
Granulomatous hepatitis and chorioretinitis	*Toxocara canis*—diethylcarbamazine
GI infection; competes for food → malnutrition in children; eggs visible in feces	*Ascaris lumbricoides*—mebendazole or pyrantel pamoate
Inflammation and 2° bacterial infection of lungs from undercooked crab meat	*Paragonimus westermani*—praziquantel
Biliary tract inflammation from undercooked fish	*Opisthorchis* (*Clonorchis*) *sinensis*—praziquantel
Undercooked pork larval worm → mass lesions in brain; cysticercosis	*Taenia solium*—praziquantel or niclosamide, albendazole for cysticercosis

Hydatid liver cysts from eggs in dog feces → anaphylaxis if antigens released from cysts	*Echinococcus granulosus*—albendazole, careful surgical removal of cysts (pre-injected with EtOH)
Fish tapeworm causing vitamin B12 deficiency	*Diphyllobothrium latum*—praziquantel
Cercariae penetrate skin → granulomas and inflammation of liver and spleen; snails are hosts	*Schistosoma sp.*—praziquantel
Which cell count is elevated during many helminth infections and can be detected by routine CBC?	*Eosinophils*
Which is the most common helminth infection in the United States?	*E. vermicularis*

Name the antiparasitic drug(s) associated with each of the following unique toxicities:

Cinchonism (flushing, tinnitus, blurry vision, confusion, rash)	Quinine
Hemolytic anemia in G6PD-deficient person	Chloroquine, primaquine, quinine, and TMP-SMX
Mazzotti reaction (pyrexia, hypotension, and respiratory distress caused by death of parasites)	Diethylcarbamazine (with *Onchocerca*)

CHAPTER 4

Neuroscience

EMBRYOLOGY

Name the structure(s) in the adult nervous system that arise from the following embryonic components:

Telencephalon	Cerebral hemispheres and lateral ventricles
Diencephalon	Thalamus, optic nerves, and third ventricle
Mesencephalon	Midbrain and aqueduct
Metencephalon	Pons, cerebellum, and superior fourth ventricle
Myelencephalon	Medulla and inferior fourth ventricle
Neural crest cells	Peripheral sensory and autonomic nerves and sensory ganglia

What is the level of the conus medullaris in a newborn and in an adult?

L2 or L3 (newborn), L1-2 (adult)

NEUROANATOMY AND NEUROPHYSIOLOGY

Organization of the Nervous System

What are the divisions of the autonomic nervous system?

Sympathetic, parasympathetic

Where are the preganglionic cell bodies of the sympathetic nervous system?

Intermediolateral horn of the spinal cord from T1 to L3

Where are the preganglionic cell bodies of the parasympathetic nervous system located?

Brainstem (cranial nerve nuclei) and spinal cord from S2 to S4

Which is the primary neurotransmitter (NT) of both sympathetic and parasympathetic ganglia?	Acetylcholine (ACh)
Which is the primary type of cholinergic receptor of both sympathetic and parasympathetic ganglia?	Nicotinic
Which NT mediates the transmission of impulses from sympathetic neurons to effector organs?	Norepinephrine (NE)
Which NT mediates the transmission of impulses from parasympathetic neurons to effector organs?	ACh
Which NT mediates the transmission of impulses from somatic neurons to skeletal muscle?	ACh
What types of receptors are present on the effector organs innervated by the sympathetic nervous system?	$\alpha1$, $\alpha2$, $\beta1$, and $\beta2$
What type of receptor is present on the effector organs innervated by the parasympathetic nervous system?	Muscarinic
What type of receptor is present on muscle innervated by the somatic nervous system?	Nicotinic

Sympathetic Nervous System

Name the effect of the sympathetic nervous system on the following organ systems and the type of receptor which mediates each effect:	
Eyes	Pupillary dilation ($\alpha1$)
Salivary glands	Increased thick, viscous secretions
Bronchioles	Bronchodilation (β_2), ↑ secretions
Heart	Tachycardia (β_1), ↑ contractility (β_1), ↑ AV nodal conduction (β_1)
Vascular smooth muscle	Vasoconstriction of cutaneous mucous membrane and splanchnic vessels (α_1); vasodilation in skeletal muscle (β_2)

Gastrointestinal (GI) tract	↓ Muscle motility and tone (β_2), contraction of sphincters (α_1)
Male sex organs	Ejaculation (α_2)
Uterus	Relaxation (β_2), contraction (α_1)
Bladder and ureters	Relaxation of detrusor (β_2), contraction of trigone and sphincter (α_1)
Sweat glands	↑ Secretions (muscarinic)
Kidneys	↑ Renin secretion (β_1)
Adipocytes	↑ Lipolysis (β_1)
Pancreas	↓ Insulin secretion ($\alpha2$), ↑ insulin secretion (β_2)

Parasympathetic Nervous System

What is the effect of the parasympathetic nervous system on the following organ systems:	
Eyes	Pupillary constriction
Bronchioles	Bronchoconstriction
Heart	Bradycardia, ↓ contractility, ↓ AV nodal conduction
GI tract	↑ Motility, relaxation of sphincters
Male sex organs	Erection via vasodilation
Bladder and ureters	Contraction of detrusor, relaxation of sphincters and trigone
What type of cholinergic receptor mediates all of the effects on the organs above?	Muscarinic

Motor and Sensory Fibers

Name the function of each of the following types of sensory fibers:	
Ia (A-α)	Proprioception, muscle spindles
Ib	Proprioception, Golgi tendon organs
II (A-β)	Touch, pressure, and vibration; secondary afferents of muscle spindles
III (A-δ)	Touch, pressure, fast pain, and temperature

| IV (c) | Slow pain and temperature (unmyelinated) |

What is the electrochemical effect of an inward Na⁺ current on a sensory fiber? — Depolarization

What is the electrochemical effect of an inward Na^+ current on a sensory fiber? — Depolarization

Name the function of each of the following components of a sensory pathway:

Sensory receptor	Translates environmental stimulus into an electrical impulse
First-order neuron	Carries impulse from sensory receptor into central nervous system (CNS)
Second-order neuron	Carries impulse from primary neuron to the thalamus
Third-order neuron	Carries impulse from second-order neuron to the cerebral cortex
Fourth-order neuron	Carries impulses from third-order neurons to appropriate somatosensory area of cerebral cortex

Name the type of mechanoreceptor described below:

Onion-like subcutaneous receptors that respond to vibration and tapping	Pacinian corpuscle
Primary receptors of the dermal papillae that mediate two-point tactile discrimination	Meissner corpuscle
Encapsulated receptor that responds to pressure	Ruffini corpuscle
Disc-shaped touch receptor of the deep dermis	Merkel tactile disc

Rods or cones?

Sensitive to low-intensity light	Rods
Sensitive to high-intensity light	Cones
Receptor used primarily for night vision	Rods
Receptor used primarily for day vision	Cones
Present in fovea	Cones
High visual acuity	Cones

Receptor which adjusts to low light conditions most rapidly	Cones
Receptor capable of color vision	Cones

Name the type of muscle sensor for each of the following functions:

Detection of static and dynamic changes in muscle length	Muscle spindles
Detection of muscle tension	Golgi tendon organs
Detection of vibration	Pacinian corpuscles
Detection of pain	Free nerve endings

What type of motoneuron is responsible for ensuring that a muscle will respond appropriately throughout contraction, despite changes in tension?	γ-Motoneurons
What type of muscle reflex, mediated by type Ia afferent fibers, causes muscle contraction in response to muscle stretch?	Stretch or myotatic reflex
What type of muscle reflex, mediated by type Ib afferent fibers, causes muscle relaxation in response to muscle contraction?	Golgi tendon reflex
What type of muscle reflex, mediated by types II, III, and IV afferent fibers, causes ipsilateral flexion and contralateral extension?	Flexor withdrawal reflex
What are the components of the afferent limb of a myotatic reflex arc?	Muscle spindle receptor $\rightarrow$ Ia fiber $\rightarrow$ dorsal root ganglion
What comprises the efferent limb of a myotatic reflex arc?	Ventral motor neuron

For each of the following muscle stretch reflexes, name the muscle group and spinal level tested:

Ankle jerk	Gastrocnemius (S1)
Knee jerk	Quadriceps (L3-L4)
Biceps jerk	Biceps (C5-C6)

Forearm jerk	Brachioradialis (C5-C6)
Triceps jerk	Triceps (C7-C8)

What type of posturing is caused by a transecting lesion above the level of the medulla but below the midbrain?

Decerebrate rigidity (abnormal extension posture)

What type of posturing is caused by a transecting lesion above the level of the red nucleus (midbrain)?

Decorticate rigidity (abnormal flexion posture)

Which is the major NT of cerebellar Purkinje cells?

γ-Aminobutyric acid (GABA)

Note: the output of Purkinje cells is always inhibitory

Meninges

What are the three layers of the meninges?

"The meninges **PAD** the CNS"
1. Pia
2. Arachnoid
3. Dura

What meningeal space, which lies between the pia and arachnoid, contains the cerebrospinal fluid (CSF)?

Subarachnoid space

What structure produces CSF?

The choroid plexus of the lateral, third, and fourth ventricles

What structures reabsorb CSF into venous circulation?

The arachnoid granulations

Trace the flow of CSF from the choroid plexus into venous circulation

Choroid plexus → lateral ventricles → interventricular foramina (of Monro) → third ventricle → cerebral aqueduct → fourth ventricle → lateral foramina (of Luschka) or median foramen (of Magendie) → subarachnoid space → arachnoid granulations → superior sagittal sinus

What are the three major functions of CSF?

1. To provide support and protection to the CNS
2. To remove metabolic waste products
3. To transport hormones and cytokines throughout the CSF and to the systemic circulation

Vasculature of the Central Nervous System

Name the blood vessel that supplies
each of the following structures:

Anterior two-thirds of the spinal cord, the medullary pyramids, medial lemniscus, and root fibers of cranial nerve (CN) XII	Anterior spinal artery
Retina	Central artery of the retina (a branch of the ophthalmic artery)
Lateral geniculate body, globus pallidus, posterior limb of internal capsule	Anterior choroidal artery (an important branch of internal carotid artery)
Hypothalamus and ventral thalamus	Posterior communicating artery
Leg-foot area of motor and sensory cortices	Anterior cerebral artery (ACA)
Anterior putamen, caudate nucleus, and anteroinferior internal capsule	Medial striate arteries (branches of the ACA)
Broca (expressive) and Wernicke (receptive) speech areas, face and arm areas of motor cortices, frontal eye field	Middle cerebral artery (MCA)
Internal capsule, caudate nucleus, putamen, globus pallidus	Lateral striate arteries (branches of the MCA)
Nucleus ambiguus and the inferior surface of the cerebellum	Posterior inferior cerebellar artery
Caudal lateral pontine tegmentum (including portions of the nuclei of CN V, VII) and the inferior cerebellar surface	Anterior inferior cerebellar artery
Superior surface of cerebellum, cerebellar nuclei, and the cochlear nuclei	Superior cerebellar artery
Majority of midbrain, portions of the thalamus, lateral and medial geniculate bodies, occipital lobe, inferior aspect of the temporal lobes, and the hippocampus	Posterior cerebral artery (PCA)
Majority of the dura	Middle meningeal artery

Name the cerebral veins that drain
directly into the superior sagittal sinus: Bridging veins

Name the cerebral vein that drains deep cerebral veins into the straight sinus:

Vein of Galen

CN III, CN V_1, CN V_2, CN VI, post-ganglionic sympathetic fibers, and both internal carotid arteries all pass through which structure?

Cavernous sinus

Axonal Transport

Name the cytoplasmic structure in the nerve cell body and dendrites that are involved in protein synthesis:

Nissl substance

Name the type of axonal transport described below:

Transport responsible for delivery of synthesized NTs away from the cell body

Fast anterograde axonal transport

Transport responsible for delivery of cytoskeletal and cytoplasmic components away from the cell body

Slow anterograde transport

Transport responsible for returning growth factor, viruses, and toxins to the cell body for degradation

Fast retrograde transport

Kinesin-dependent transport

Fast anterograde axonal transport

Dynein-dependent transport

Fast retrograde transport

Name the process of anterograde axonal and myelin degeneration accompanied by Schwann cell proliferation:

Wallerian degeneration

Supporting Cells of the Nervous System

Name the type of cell described below:

Primary supportive cell type of the CNS

Astrocyte

Myelin-producing cell type of the CNS

Oligodendrocyte

CNS scavenger cell type, derived from mesoderm

Microglia

CSF-producing cell type

Ependymal cell

Myelin-producing cell type of the peripheral nervous system (PNS)

Schwann cells

What type of intercellular connections is responsible for maintaining the integrity of the blood-brain barrier?

Tight junctions

What proteins are commonly used to identify astrocytes?

Glial fibrillary acidic protein (GFAP) and glutamine synthetase

Pigments and Inclusions

Name the process or disease associated with the following neuronal histopathologic findings:

    Lipofuscin granules

Aging

    Depletion of neuromelanin in substantia nigra and Lewy bodies

Parkinson disease

    Negri bodies

Rabies

    Amyloid plaques and neurofibrillary tangles

Alzheimer disease

    Cowdry type A inclusion bodies

Herpes simplex encephalitis

Spinal Tracts

Name the spinal tract responsible for each of the following functions:

    Voluntary control of skeletal muscle

Lateral corticospinal/pyramidal tract

    Sensation of pain and temperature

Lateral spinothalamic tract

    Two-point discrimination and vibratory sensation

Dorsal column-medial lemniscus tract

    Control of facial muscles

Corticobulbar tract

    Coordination of muscle tone, posture, balance, and motor activity

Dentothalamic tract

Describe the major difference between the innervation of the lower and upper facial muscles

Corticobulbar fibers innervate the lower facial muscles unilaterally, while upper facial muscles are innervated bilaterally

Name the structure in the spinal cord composed of ascending fibers of the dorsal column-medial lemniscus pathway originating in the upper extremities:

Cuneate fasciculus

Name the structure in the spinal cord composed of ascending fibers of the dorsal column-medial lemniscus pathway originating in the lower extremities:

Gracile fasciculus (medial to cuneate fasciculus)

At what level of the brainstem do fibers of the dorsal column-medial lemniscus pathway cross?

Caudal medulla

What type of receptors provides input to the lateral spinothalamic tract?

Free nerve endings

At what level do fibers of the spinothalamic tract cross?

At the same level or 1 to 2 levels above/below where they enter the spinal cord

Name the structure where fibers of the lateral spinothalamic tract cross the midline:

Ventral white commissure/anterior commissure

Where do fibers of the dorsal column-medial lemniscus pathway, the trigeminothalamic, and lateral spinothalamic tract all terminate?

The sensory cortex

What part of the cortex gives rise to the fibers of the lateral corticospinal and corticobulbar tracts?

The motor, premotor, and sensory areas of the cortex (Brodmann areas 6, 4, and 3, 1, 2)

Fibers of the lateral corticospinal tract pass through which limb of the internal capsule?

Posterior limb

Name the structure where fibers of the lateral corticospinal tract cross the midline:

Medullary pyramids

Classify each of the following clinical findings as upper motor neuron (UMN) or lower motor neuron (LMN) signs:

Spastic paresis	UMN
Flaccid paralysis	LMN
Babinski sign (upgoing toes)	UMN
Fasciculations and fibrillations	LMN
Areflexia	LMN
Atrophy	LMN
Hyperreflexia	UMN

Cranial Nerves

Name the cranial foramen that each of the CNs below pass through:

I	Cribriform plate
II	Optic canal
III, IV, V$_1$, VI	Superior orbital fissure
	Note: all of these nerves pass through the cavernous sinus as well
V$_2$	Foramen **R**otundum
V$_3$	Foramen **O**vale (for divisions of the trigeminal nerve think "**S**tanding **R**oom **O**nly")
VII, VIII	Internal acoustic meatus
IX, X, XI	Jugular foramen
XII	Hypoglossal canal
Middle meningeal artery	Foramen spinosum

Name the function(s) for each CN listed below:

I: olfactory	Smell
II: optic	Vision
III: oculomotor	1. Eye movement 2. "Parasympathetic" ciliary and pupillary sphincter mm **Note:** mm is used as the abbreviation for "muscles"
IV: trochlear	Contraction of superior oblique muscle
V$_1$: trigeminal—ophthalmic branch	Sensation from nose to forehead
V$_2$: trigeminal—maxillary branch	Sensation from lateral nose, upper lip, superior buccal area
V$_3$: trigeminal—mandibular branch	1. Sensation from areas of the lower face not covered by V$_1$ and V$_2$ 2. Movement of the **M**uscles of **M**astication (**M**asseter, te**M**poralis, **M**edial, and lateral pterygoids), tensor veli palatini, and tensor tympani
VI: abducens	Contraction of lateral rectus muscle

VII: facial	1. Parasympathetic—lacrimal, submandibular, and sublingual glands 2. Mm of facial expression, stapedius, stylohyoid, and the posterior belly of the digastric muscle 3. Taste—anterior two-thirds of tongue 4. Sensation—skin of external ear
VIII: vestibulocochlear	Hearing and sense of balance
IX: glossopharyngeal	1. Parasympathetic—parotid gland 2. Motor—stylopharyngeus mm 3. Taste—posterior one-third tongue 4. Sensation—parotid gland, carotid body and sinus, pharynx, and middle ear 5. Cutaneous sensation—external ear canal
X: vagus	1. Parasympathetic—trachea, bronchi, heart, GI tract 2. Contraction of laryngeal, pharyngeal, and esophageal striated mm 3. Taste—epiglottis and palate 4. Sensation—trachea, GI tract 5. Cutaneous sensation—external ear
XI: accessory	Movement of sternocleidomastoid and trapezius muscles
XII: hypoglossal	Contraction of muscles of tongue
Which three CNs are purely sensory nerves?	1. CN I 2. CN II 3. CN VIII
Which five CNs are purely motor nerves?	1. CN III 2. CN IV 3. CN VI 4. CN XI 5. CN XII
Which four CNs have both motor and sensory components?	1. CN V 2. CN VII 3. CN IX 4. CN X
Which two CNs are rostral to the midbrain?	1. CN I 2. CN II
Which two CNs nuclei are located in the midbrain?	1. CN III 2. CN IV

Which four CNs have at least a portion of their nuclei in the pons?	1. CN V 2. CN VI 3. CN VII 4. CN VIII
Which seven CNs have at least a portion of their nuclei in the medulla?	1. CN V 2. CN VI 3. CN VII 4. CN VIII 5. CN IX 6. CN X 7. CN XII
Name the only CN that crosses the midline and exits the brainstem posterior to the ventricular system:	CN IV—exits the brainstem posteriorly and crosses the midline after exiting the caudal midbrain
What nucleus serves as the origin of preganglionic parasympathetic fibers projecting to the ciliary ganglion?	Edinger-Westphal nucleus of CN III
What visceral sensory nucleus, located in the medulla, is a relay center for taste, sensory input from the carotid sinus, carotid body, and the vagus nerve?	Nucleus Solitarius
What visceral motor nucleus, located in the medulla, is involved in coordinating swallowing and speech?	Nucleus aMbiguus
Which are the afferent and efferent limbs of the corneal reflex?	CN V_1 and CN VII
Which are the afferent and efferent limbs of the pupillary light reflex?	CN II and CN III
Which are the afferent and efferent limbs of the gag reflex?	CN IX and CN X
Name the site of a lesion, within the visual tract, capable of causing each of the following deficits:	
Ipsilateral blindness	Transection of the optic nerve
Binasal hemianopia	Bilateral lateral compression of optic chiasm
Bitemporal hemianopia	Midsagittal transection or midline pressure on the optic chiasm (often caused by a pituitary tumor)

Right hemianopia *without* macular sparing	Transection of the left optic radiation
Right upper quadrantanopia	Transection of the lower division of the left optic radiation
Right lower quadrantanopia	Transection of the upper division of the left optic radiation
Right hemianopia *with* macular sparing	Destruction of the left visual cortex

What are five key structures of the pupillary light reflex pathway?

1. Ganglion cells of the retina
2. Pretectal nucleus of the midbrain
3. Edinger-Westphal nucleus
4. Ciliary ganglion
5. Postganglionic parasympathetic fibers of CN III

What are four key structures of the pupillary dilation pathway?

1. Paraventricular nucleus of the hypothalamus
2. Ciliospinal center of Budge at the level of T1 to T2
3. Superior cervical ganglion
4. Postganglionic sympathetic fibers traveling along the internal carotid artery and its branches to the eye

What part of the cortex is responsible for voluntary eye movements?

Frontal eye field (Brodmann area 8)

What side will a patient's eyes deviate toward if there is a lesion of the right frontal eye field?

Right side ("Look toward the lesion of frontal eye fields")

What structure connects the nucleus of CN VI and the nucleus of CN III?

Medial longitudinal fasciculus (MLF)

What type of lesion will result in medial rectus palsy (inability to adduct the eye) on attempted lateral gaze but normal adduction on accommodation?

Intranuclear ophthalmoplegia (a lesion of the MLF)

What classic idiopathic lesion is characterized by ptosis, miosis, and anhydrosis?

Horner syndrome

Name the condition characterized by a pupil that will accommodate but cannot react to light:

Argyll-Robertson pupil (associated with tertiary syphilis, lupus, and diabetes mellitus)

Name the condition caused by a lesion in the afferent fibers of the light reflex pathway:

Marcus Gunn pupil

What are the primary sensory receptors of the auditory pathway?

Inner hair cells of the organ of Corti

Where does the auditory pathway terminate?

Bilateral input from both auditory tracts terminates in primary auditory cortex in superior temporal gyrus (Brodmann areas 41 and 42)

What type of cells is responsible for relaying auditory stimuli from the organ of Corti to the cochlear nuclei?

Bipolar cells of the spiral or cochlear ganglion

What pontine nucleus plays a key role in sound localization?

Superior olivary nucleus

Conduction deafness is caused by a lesion of which components of the auditory system?

External auditory canal, tympanic membrane, or the middle ear

Sensorineural deafness is caused by a lesion of which components of the auditory system?

Cochlea, cochlear nerve, or the cochlear nuclei

Patients with presbycusis have trouble hearing what types of sounds?

High-frequency sounds

Which cells of the vestibular system respond to angular acceleration and deceleration?

The hair cells of the three semicircular canals

What structures of the vestibular system respond to linear acceleration and deceleration?

The hair cells of the utricle

What type of cells is responsible for relaying vestibular stimuli from the hair cells to the vestibular nuclei?

Bipolar cells of the vestibular ganglion

What structures provide input to the vestibular nuclei?

Hair cells of the semicircular canal, hair cells of the utricle, and the flocculonodular lobe of the cerebellum

What structures receive signals from the vestibular nuclei?

The thalamus, spinal cord, cerebellum, and CNs III, IV, and VI

Cerebellum, Thalamus, Hypothalamus

What are the three primary functions of the cerebellum?

1. Maintenance of posture and equilibrium
2. Control of muscle tone
3. Coordination of voluntary muscle activity

What type of tremor may result from a cerebellar lesion?

Intention tremor

A positive Romberg sign (loss of balance when the eyes are closed) suggests a lesion to which tract of the CNS?

Dentothalamic tract (the main cerebellar pathway) or dorsal column (tabes dorsalis in neurosyphilis)

Name the thalamic nucleus/nuclei responsible for the relay of impulses for each modality listed below:

Vision

Lateral geniculate nucleus ("Lateral to Look")

Hearing

Medial geniculate nucleus ("Medial for Music")

Proprioception, pain, pressure, touch, vibration

Lateral portion of ventral posterior nucleus (VPL, "Posterior for Proprioception, Pain")

Facial sensation

Medial portion of ventral posterior nucleus (VML)

Motor

Ventral anterior/lateral nuclei

Limbic function

Dorsomedial, anterior nuclei

Which portion of the internal capsule contains fibers of the corticobulbar tract?

The genu

Which portion of the internal capsule contains fibers of the corticospinal, spinothalamic, visual, and auditory tracts?

The posterior limb

Which arteries supply the posterior limb of the internal capsule?

Perforating branches of the anterior choroidal artery and lenticulostriate arteries

Name the major hypothalamic nucleus (or nuclei) responsible for each function listed below:

Regulation of the release of gonadotropic hormones	Medial preoptic nucleus (which contains the sexually dimorphic nucleus)
Regulation of circadian rhythms	Suprachiasmatic nucleus
Regulation of body temperature	Anterior nucleus (lesion results in hyperthermia) and posterior nucleus (lesion results in poikilothermia)
Regulation of water balance, synthesis of antidiuretic hormone, oxytocin, and corticotropin-releasing factor	Paraventricular and supraoptic nuclei
Regulation of appetite	VentroMedial nucleus (lesion resulting from eating Very Much [hyperphagia, obesity]) and lateral hypothalamic nucleus (lesions cause anorexia and starvation)
Regulation of hypothalamus	Arcuate or infundibular nucleus
Regulation of emotional expression	Mammillary nucleus (a component of the limbic system)
What is the most epileptogenic part of the cerebrum?	The hippocampus
What system within the CNS plays a central role in the initiation and coordination of somatic motor activity?	The striatal or extrapyramidal motor system
What are the major components of the striatal motor system?	Neocortex, basal ganglia (striatum [caudate + putamen], globus pallidus, subthalamic nucleus, substantia nigra), and thalamus

Neurotransmitters

Name the NT described below:

Major NT of the parasympathetic nervous system	ACh
NT which is increased in the CNS of patients with schizophrenia	Dopamine
NT believed to cause panic attacks when released suddenly by the locus coeruleus	NE
Major NT of the preganglionic sympathetic nervous system	ACh
NT highly concentrated in the substantia nigra that plays a key role in pain transmission	Substance P

Major NT of the postganglionic sympathetic neurons supplying sweat glands and certain blood vessels	ACh
NT which is depleted from the basal nucleus of Meynert in Alzheimer disease	ACh
NT which is depleted from the substantia nigra in patients with Parkinson disease	Dopamine
NT that causes renal vasodilation	Dopamine
Two NTs believed to be depleted in depression	1. NE 2. Serotonin
Powerful analgesic NT found exclusively in the hypothalamus	β-Endorphin
Opiate peptides which play a role in pain suppression	Enkephalins
NT that regulates release of GH and TSH; markedly ↓ Alzheimer disease	Somatostatin
Major inhibitory NT of the cortex	GABA
Major inhibitory NT of the spinal cord	Glycine
Major excitatory NT of the brain	Glutamate
Gaseous, vasoactive NT involved in memory	Nitrous oxide
NT important in the initiation of sleep	Melatonin
NT which inhibits the reticular activating center, thereby increasing total sleep time	ACh
Which two amino acids can serve as a precursor for the synthesis of catecholamines?	1. Phenylalanine 2. Tyrosine

Cerebral Cortex

Name the site of a lesion, within the cortex, capable of causing each of the following deficits:

Right-sided flaccid hemiparalysis	Left primary motor area
Left-sided pronator drift	Right primary motor area
Loss of abstract thought and self-restraint	Bilateral loss of frontal lobes anterior to the frontal eye fields

Slowed speech without any impairment of language comprehension	Broca speech area
Loss of right-sided tactile sensation and proprioception	Left somesthetic area
Cortical deafness	Bilateral destruction of the auditory areas; unilateral destruction of the auditory area causes a slight ↓ in hearing
Inability to understand spoken language and verbalize coherent thoughts	Wernicke speech area in the dominant hemisphere, usually left
Ipsilateral anosmia (inability to smell)	Primary olfactory area (Brodmann area 34)
Alexia and agraphia (inability to read and write)	Angular gyrus (Brodmann area 39)
Loss of ability to transfer information from short-term to long-term memory	Bilateral destruction of the hippocampal cortex
Psychic blindness, hyperphagia, docility, and hypersexuality (Klüver-Bucy syndrome)	Bilateral destruction of the anterior temporal lobes (amygdala)
Loss of ability to recognize faces	Inferomedial right occipitotemporal area
Loss of vision in the right visual field with macular sparing	Destruction of the left primary visual area (Brodmann area 17)
Name the term used to describe a deficit in the ability to draw a geometric figure:	Construction apraxia
Name the term used to describe a "magnetic gait," commonly seen in normal pressure hydrocephalus:	Gait apraxia
What part of the nervous system is involved in maintaining wakefulness?	Reticular activating system and bilateral cortex

PATHOLOGY OF THE NERVOUS SYSTEM

Cerebral Cortex

Identify the type of aphasia:	
Impaired repetition, nonfluent with comprehension intact	Broca (expressive) aphasia

Impaired repetition, fluent with impaired comprehension	Wernicke (receptive) aphasia
Impaired repetition, fluent with intact comprehension	Conduction aphasia
Impaired repetition, nonfluent with impaired comprehension	Global aphasia
Intact repetition, nonfluent with comprehension intact	Transcortical motor
Intact repetition, fluent with impaired comprehension	Transcortical sensory
Intact repetition, nonfluent with impaired comprehension	Transcortical mixed

Congenital Disorders

Name the type of neural tube defect with the following features:

Failure of posterior vertebral arch closure (not evident on clinical examination)	Spina bifida occulta
Failure of posterior vertebral arch closure accompanied by herniation of the meninges	Spina bifida cystica
Herniation of the meninges outside of the spinal canal	Meningocele
Herniation of nervous tissue and meninges outside of the spinal canal	Myelomeningocele
Complete cerebral agenesis due to lack of closure of the anterior neuropore	Anencephaly
Diverticulum of malformed CNS tissue	Encephalocele

What factor is used to screen pregnant mothers for neural tube defects?	α-Fetoprotein
What is the most common cause of mental retardation?	Fetal alcohol syndrome, often associated with cardiac and facial anomalies
What are two common chromosomal genetic causes of mental retardation?	1. Trisomy 21 2. Fragile X

Name the condition characterized by an excess of CSF in the cranial cavity:

Hydrocephalus

What type of hydrocephalus is characterized by obstruction in the flow of CSF through the ventricular system and subarachnoid space?

Noncommunicating hydrocephalus

What type of hydrocephalus is characterized by free flow of CSF but abnormal CSF absorption?

Communicating hydrocephalus

What congenital malformation of the CNS is characterized by herniation of the cerebellar tonsils and medulla through the foramen magnum (which may result in obstruction of CSF circulation)?

Arnold-Chiari malformation (type 1)

What congenital malformation of the CNS is associated with syringomyelia (central cavitation of the spinal cord)?

Arnold-Chiari malformation (type 2)

What congenital malformation of the CNS is characterized by cystic dilation of fourth ventricle, agenesis of vermis, and associated with hydrocephalus?

Dandy-Walker malformation

What complication of premature babies usually results in hypoxic/ischemic injuries of brain?

Subependymal germinal matrix bleed

Stroke

Describe the artery that has been occluded in each of the following stroke syndromes:

Paresis and sensory loss of contralateral lower extremity

ACA

Hemiparesis, contralateral hemisensory loss, homonymous hemianopia, aphasia

MCA supplying the dominant hemisphere, usually left hemisphere

Loss of consciousness, hemisensory loss, homonymous hemianopia with macular sparing

PCA

Amaurosis fugax

Ophthalmic artery (branch of internal carotid artery)

Vertigo, CN palsies, impaired level of consciousness, dysarthria	Vertebrobasilar artery
Sensory neglect and apraxia	MCA supplying the nondominant hemisphere, usually right hemisphere
Urinary incontinence, suck and grasp reflexes	Middle or ACA supplying the frontal lobe
Ipsilateral loss of pain and temperature for face, contralateral pain and temperature for body, dysphagia, hoarseness, absent gag reflex	PICA—Wallenberg syndrome (lateral medulla)
Ipsilateral facial droop, ipsilateral loss of pain and temperature for face, contralateral pain and temperature for body	AICA—Lateral pontine syndrome

What are the most frequent sites of thrombotic occlusion in the cerebral vasculature?	Carotid bifurcation, MCA, and basilar artery
What is the most frequent site of embolic occlusion in the cerebral vasculature?	MCA
Which cardiac arrhythmia is associated with embolic stroke?	Atrial fibrillation
What type of stroke, associated with hypertension, causes the formation of small, cystic, moon-shaped pits?	Lacunar infarctions
Where do lacunar strokes usually occur?	Basal ganglia, thalamus, internal capsule, white matter, pons, cerebellum
Name the term used to describe small aneurysms of the cerebral vasculature, caused by long-standing HTN, that may result in intracerebral hemorrhage:	Charcot-Bouchard aneurysms
What are the most common locations for Charcot-Bouchard aneurysms?	Thalamus and basal ganglia
Within the cerebral vasculature, what are the most common sites of berry aneurysm formation?	At the bifurcations of the circle of Willis
What is the most common complication of berry aneurysms?	Rupture causing subarachnoid hemorrhage

What are three disorders that predispose to the formation of berry aneurysms?

1. Polycystic kidney disease
2. Ehlers-Danlos syndrome
3. Marfan syndrome

Which CN palsy is associated with internal carotid or posterior communicating artery aneurysms?

CN III palsy causing papillary dilation

Name the term used to describe paroxysmal, self-limiting episodes of neurologic deficit, commonly including transient aphasia:

Transient ischemic attack

Which syndrome is characterized by loss of all motor function except that of CN III and IV?

Locked-in syndrome (usually a result of infarction or tumor at the base of the pons)

Seizures

Name the type of seizure associated with the following clinical findings:

Loss of consciousness followed by loss of postural control, a tonic phase of muscle contraction and clonic limb jerking

Tonic-clonic seizure

A child who appears to be daydreaming in class and is found to have a 3-second spike-and-wave pattern on EEG

Absence seizure

Sudden, brief muscle contractions

Myoclonic epilepsy

Motor, sensory, visual, psychic, or autonomic phenomena with preserved level of consciousness

Simple partial seizure

Seizure begins with behavioral arrest, which is followed by auditory or visual hallucination, automatisms, and finally by postictal confusion

Complex partial seizure

What biomarker can discriminate epileptic seizure from non-epileptic seizure (ie, pseudoseizure)?

Prolactin

What disorder is characterized by paroxysmal episodes of sharp, shooting facial pain in the distribution of one or more branches of CN V?

Trigeminal neuralgia

What is the drug of choice for trigeminal neuralgia?

Carbamazepine

What is the triad of cerebellar dysfunction?

1. Loss of balance (disequilibrium)
2. Hypotonia
3. Loss of coordinated muscle activity (dyssynergia)

Intracranial Hemorrhage

Name the type of intracranial hemorrhage associated with the following features:

Bloody or xanthochromic CSF on lumbar puncture

Subarachnoid hemorrhage

Hematoma following the contour of a cerebral hemisphere on computed tomography (CT) scan

Subdural hematoma

Laceration of bridging cerebral veins

Subdural hematoma

Laceration of middle meningeal artery due to fracture of the temporal bone

Epidural hematoma

Lucid interval followed by rapid decline in mental status

Epidural hematoma

Most common type of intracranial hemorrhage resulting from trauma

Subdural hematoma

Ruptured berry aneurysm or arteriovenous malformation

Subarachnoid hemorrhage

Seen in patients with long-standing, poorly controlled HTN

Intraparenchymal hemorrhage

Lens-shaped hematoma on CT scan

Epidural hematoma

Crescentic hematoma on CT scan

Subdural hematoma

Seen more commonly in alcoholics and the elderly

Subdural hematoma

What is the most common cause of subarachnoid hemorrhage?

Trauma

What is the most common acute complication of a subarachnoid hemorrhage?

Rebleed

What is the most common delayed complication of a subarachnoid hemorrhage?

Vasospasm, prophylaxis using nimodipine

Meningitis/Encephalitis

Name the type of meningitis associated
with the following CSF findings:

Greater than 1000 polymorpho-   Bacterial meningitis
nuclear mononuclear leukocytes, ↓
glucose, increased protein

Increased lymphocytes, minor   Viral or aseptic meningitis
elevation in protein, normal CSF
pressure

Increased lymphocytes, minor   Fungal meningitis
elevation in protein, elevated CSF
pressure

Perivascular cuffing, inclusion bodies,   Viral meningoencephalitis
and glial nodules may be seen in what
cerebral infection?

Name the most common causes of
bacterial meningitis in each age group:

Neonates
1. Group B *Streptococcus*
2. *Streptococcus pneumoniae*
3. *Listeria monocytogenes*
4. *Escherichia coli*

Infants and children
1. *S. pneumoniae*
2. *Neisseria meningitidis*
3. *Haemophilus influenzae* (type B)
4. Group B *Streptococcus*

Teens and young adults
1. *N. meningitidis*
2. *S. pneumoniae*

Older adults
1. *S. pneumoniae*
2. *N. meningitidis*
3. *H. influenzae* (type B)
4. Group B *Streptococcus*
5. *L.* monocytogenes

Name the parasite spread from cats   *Toxoplasma gondii*
to humans that causes periventricular
calcifications and congenital disorders
in offspring of infected mothers:

Name the fungal meningitis most   Mucormycosis
commonly associated with diabetics
in DKA:

Bullet-shaped intracytoplasmic   Rabies
inclusions, Negri bodies are characteristic of which CNS viral infection?

Hemorrhagic necrosis of temporal lobes is most commonly associated with which viral encephalitis?	HSV-1
Which infectious disease is characterized by neuronal vacuolization leading to small cysts in the gray matter of the brain *without* an associated inflammatory response?	Spongiform encephalopathy
Which disease is characterized by progressive ataxia, dementia, and spongiform gray matter changes?	Creutzfeldt-Jakob disease

Demyelinating Disorders

Name the demyelinating disorder associated with the following clinical and pathologic features:	
Most common demyelinating disorder	Multiple sclerosis
Associated with JC virus infection in AIDS patients	Progressive multifocal leukoencephalopathy
Periventricular calcification; spinal lesions typically in the white matter of the cervical cord	Multiple sclerosis
Postviral autoimmune syndrome causing demyelination of peripheral nerves, especially motor fibers	Guillain-Barré syndrome
May present with intranuclear ophthalmoplegia (MLF syndrome) or sudden visual loss due to optic neuritis	Multiple sclerosis
Ascending paralysis, facial diplegia, and autonomic dysfunction	Guillain-Barré syndrome
Oligoclonal bands in the CSF	Multiple sclerosis
Albuminocytologic dissociation (↑CSF protein with normal cell count)	Guillain-Barré syndrome
↑ CSF protein, normal glucose, ↑ lymphocytes	Multiple sclerosis

Leukodystrophies and Neurocutaneous Syndromes

Name the type of leukodystrophy
associated with the following features:

Globoid bodies in white matter	Krabbe disease
Deficiency of β-galactocerebrosidase	Krabbe disease
Deficiency of arylsulfatase A	Metachromatic leukodystrophy
Nervous tissue demonstrates loss of myelin and appears yellowish brown, buildup of cerebroside in myelin sheath	Metachromatic leukodystrophy
Peroxisomal deficiency, demyelination starts in occipital lobe and moves anteriorly	Adrenoleukodystrophy (X-linked)

Name the type of neurocutaneous
syndromes associated with the
following features:

Cutaneous and plexiform neurofibromas, Lisch nodules on iris, café au lait spots, axillary freckling	Neurofibromatosis (NF1)
Bilateral schwannomas, meningioma, ependymoma	NF2
Capillary hemangiomas, hemangioblastomas in cerebellum and retina, increased incidence of renal cell carcinoma	von Hippel-Lindau
Nasolabial subcutaneous angiofibroma, epilepsy, subependymal nodules, ungula fibroma, shagreen patch, ash leaf spots	Tuberous sclerosis

What is the inheritance pattern of neurocutaneous syndromes?	Autosomal dominant (AD) with exception of Sturge-Weber (congenital and noninherited)
What is the inheritance pattern of leukodystrophies?	Autosomal recessive (AR)

Neurodegenerative disorders

What are the two most common causes of dementia in the elderly?

Alzheimer dementia and multi-infarct dementia

Name the neurodegenerative disorder associated with the following clinical and pathologic features:

Neurofibrillary tangles, senile plaques (accumulations of β-amyloid protein)

Alzheimer dementia

Stepwise dementia in a patient with focal neurologic deficits

Multi-infarct (AKA vascular) dementia

Thiamine deficiency from alcohol abuse causing ophthalmoplegia, ataxia, nystagmus

Wernicke encephalopathy

Long-term alcohol abuse causing retrograde and anterograde amnesia, confabulation, and shrunken, petechial hemorrhage in mammillary bodies

Korsakoff psychosis

Progressive dementia with predominantly frontal and temporal gliosis and neuronal loss

Pick disease

Degeneration of the caudate nucleus

Huntington disease

Lewy bodies and depigmentation of the substantia nigra

Parkinson disease

Parkinsonian symptoms with autonomic dysfunction, including orthostatic hypotension

Shy-Drager syndrome

Resting tremor, cogwheel rigidity, akinesia, postural instability

Parkinson disease

Can be caused by MPTP use

Parkinson disease

Slowly progressive ataxia, dysarthria associated with kyphoscoliosis, diabetes, and hypertrophic cardiomyopathy due to triplet repeat GAA on chromosome 9

Friedreich ataxia

AD inheritance and anticipation (worsening of disease in future generations) due to increasing number of CAG repeats on chromosome 4

Huntington disease

UMN and LMN signs due to loss of myelinated fibers of the corticospinal tract	Amyotrophic lateral sclerosis (ALS)
Viral infection → inflammatory response in anterior horn of the spinal cord → LMN loss	Poliomyelitis
Childhood ataxia associated with telangiectasias of the skin and conjunctiva associated with *ATM* gene mutation	Ataxia-telangiectasia
Floppy baby (hypotonia) due to LMN degeneration, tongue fasciculation	Werdnig-Hoffman disease
Which protein gives rise to the amyloid fibrils of Alzheimer disease?	A-β
Which is the conformation of A-β protein in neuritic plaques?	β-Pleated sheet
The A-β protein is derived from processing of which larger molecule?	Amyloid precursor protein (APP)

Brain Tumors

Where are the majority of adults versus children CNS tumors found?	Supratentorial for adults, infratentorial for children
Name the brain tumor associated with each of the following clinical or pathologic findings:	
Most common pediatric intracranial tumor	Juvenile pilocytic astrocytoma
Most common pituitary tumor	Pituitary adenoma
Most common pituitary adenoma	Prolactinoma
Most common pediatric supratentorial tumor	Craniopharyngioma
Most common primary brain tumor	Glioblastoma multiforme
Most common intracranial tumor	Metastases
Malignant pediatric tumor which metastases through CSF pathways	Medulloblastoma
Malignant pediatric tumor found exclusively in the posterior fossa	Medulloblastoma

Vascular tumor of cerebellum and retina in patients with von Hippel-Lindau syndrome	Hemangioblastoma
Abundant capillaries and vacuolated foam cells	Hemangioblastoma
Type of tumor that is found bilaterally in patients with neurofibromatosis II	Vestibular schwannoma
Tumor of the dorsal root that may grow in a dumbbell configuration through a vertebral foramen	Schwannoma
Tumor which originates from the vestibular division of CN VIII	Schwannoma
Small round blue cell tumor	Medulloblastoma
Bipolar cells, Rosenthal fibers, and microcysts	Juvenile pilocytic astrocytoma
Verocay bodies	Schwannoma
Tumor derived from Rathke pouch	Craniopharyngioma
Two tumors often presenting with bitemporal hemianopia	Pituitary adenoma and craniopharyngioma
Tumor characterized by concentric whorls and calcified psammoma bodies	Meningioma
Tumor arising from ependymal lining of ventricular system	Ependymoma
Tumor commonly arising in the pineal region causing obstructive hydrocephalus by compromising the aqueduct of Sylvius	Germinoma
EBV positive B-cell tumor of the CNS in AIDS patients	CNS lymphoma
Tumor of the foramen of Monro causing obstructive hydrocephalus	Colloid cyst of the third ventricle
Benign tumor characterized by calcifications and cells with fried-egg appearance or perinuclear halos	Oligodendroma
Tumor characterized by highly malignant cells bordering necrotic areas	Glioblastoma multiforme
Benign tumor derived from arachnoid cap cells with well-delineated margins	Meningioma

Disorders of the Spinal Cord

Name a disease of the spinal cord associated with each of the following neurologic findings:

Loss of all spinal modalities except actile discrimination, vibratory sensation, and proprioception — Ventral spinal artery occlusion

Impaired tactile discrimination, vibratory sensation, and proprioception — Tabes dorsalis

Loss of pain and temperature sensation in a cape-like distribution and flaccid paralysis of the intrinsic muscles of the hand — Syringomyelia

Impaired tactile discrimination, vibratory sensation and proprioception, UMN signs, and ataxia — Vitamin B_{12} deficiency

Miscellaneous

What complication affecting the brainstem can be caused by rapid correction of hyponatremia? — Central pontine myelinolysis

Describe how transtentorial herniation causes contralateral hemiparesis — Compresses the crus cerebri → corticospinal and corticobulbar fibers are compromised (Kernohan notch)

Describe how transtentorial herniation causes pupillary dilation — Tension on external parasympathetic fibers of CN III causes papillary dilation

Name a life-threatening complication of transforaminal or tonsillar herniation: — Compression of the medullary respiratory center → respiratory insufficiency

What is the term used to describe brainstem hemorrhages caused by transtentorial and transforaminal herniation? — Duret hemorrhages

What is the systemic response to increased intracranial pressure (Cushing triad)?
1. HTN
2. Bradycardia
3. Irregular respirations

What is the most common reversible cause of dementia in the elderly?	Normal pressure hydrocephalus
Normal pressure hydrocephalus is a common complication of what type of intracranial pathology?	Subarachnoid hemorrhage
What is the triad of normal pressure hydrocephalus?	1. Ataxic, magnetic gait (**Wobbly**) 2. Dementia and/or short-term memory loss (**Weird**) 3. Urinary incontinence (**Wet**)
What diuretic is commonly used to manage increased intracranial pressure?	Mannitol (provides osmotic diuresis)
What is the protein change associated with prion diseases?	Conformational change in PrPc (α-helix isoform) to PrPsc (β-pleated sheet isoform)

PHARMACOLOGY OF THE NERVOUS SYSTEM

Antiepileptics

For each of the following drugs, provide:
1. The mechanism of action (MOA)
2. Indication(s) (IND)
3. Significant side effects or important toxicity (TOX) (if any)

Carbamazepine	**MOA:** Na^+ channel blocker **IND:** tonic-clonic, partial, and Jacksonian seizures, trigeminal neuralgia **TOX:** $\uparrow$ LFT, agranulocytosis, aplastic anemia
Ethosuximide	**MOA:** may block T-type Ca^{2+} channels in thalamus **IND:** absence seizures **TOX:** GI upset, Stevens-Johnson syndrome
Diazepam, lorazepam	**MOA:** facilitates GABA action by $\uparrow$ frequency of Cl channel opening **IND:** status epilepticus **TOX:** sedation

Gabapentin	**MOA:** modulates GABA activity in CNS **IND:** antiepileptic, postherpetic neuralgia, diabetic neuralgia (off-label) **TOX:** sedation
Lamotrigine	**MOA:** blocks Na^+ channels **IND:** adjuvant antiepileptic agent **TOX:** Stevens-Johnson syndrome
Levetiracetam	**MOA:** binds to synaptic vesicle protein SV2A, modulating synaptic transition **IND:** antiepileptic agent **TOX:** hypertension (primarily children), headache
Phenytoin	**MOA:** Na^+ channel blocker **IND:** tonic-clonic, partial, and status **TOX:** nystagmus, ataxia, gingival hyperplasia, hirsutism, megalobastic anemia, teratogenic (fetal hydantoin syndrome)
Phenobarbital	**MOA:** facilitates GABA action by ↑ duration of Cl channel opening **IND:** tonic-clonic seizures **TOX:** induces P-450, drowsiness
Valproic acid	**MOA:** Na^+ channel inactivation, facilitate GABA action by inhibiting GABA transaminase **IND:** myoclonic seizures **TOX:** "fat, shaky, bald, and yellow"—weight gain, tremor, alopecia, hepatotoxicity (jaundice); also GI toxicity, inhibits P-450, thrombocytopenia

Name the drug(s) of choice for each of the following types of epilepsy:

Simple and complex partial	Lamotrigine, carbamazepine, levetiracetam
Absence	Ethosuximide
Febrile	Phenobarbital
Myoclonic	Valproic acid, clonazepam
Status epilepticus	Phenytoin, diazepam
Tonic-clonic	Lamotrigine, valproate, levetiracetam

Antiparkinsonian Agents

For each of the following drugs,
provide:
1. The mechanism of action (MOA)
2. Indication(s) (IND)
3. Significant side effects or important
   toxicity (TOX) (if any)

Amantidine	**MOA:** may enhance dopamine release **IND:** helpful for rigidity and bradykinesia **TOX:** acute psychosis (rare)
Benztropine	**MOA:** antimuscarinic **IND:** adjuvant therapy **TOX:** similar to atropine
Bromocriptine	**MOA:** dopamine receptor agonist **IND:** used with levodopa **TOX:** hypotension, confusion, hallucinations, nausea
Levodopa	**MOA:** dopamine precursor converted to dopamine in CNS **IND:** combined with carbidopa, levodopa is the most efficacious regimen for Parkinson disease **TOX:** nausea, tachycardia, hypotension, hallucinations, dyskinesias
Carbidopa	**MOA:** inhibition of dopamine decarboxylase $\rightarrow \uparrow$ levodopa availability in CNS **IND:** used with levodopa **TOX:** spasms of the eyelid, irregular heartbeat, confusion, agitation, hallucinations
Tolcapone	**MOA:** peripheral and central COMT inhibitor, prevent L-dopa breakdown into 3-O-methyldopa (3-OMD) **IND:** increases levodopa availability **TOX:** see Levodopa toxicity
Entacapone	**MOA:** peripheral COMT inhibitor **IND:** increases levodopa availability **TOX:** see Levodopa toxicity

Anesthetics

For each of the following drugs,
provide:
1. The mechanism of action (MOA)
2. Indication(s) (IND)
3. Significant side effects or important
   toxicity (TOX) (if any)

Halothane

MOA: CNS depression
IND: prototype general anesthetic;
potent anesthetic but weak analgesic
TOX: arrhythmias, $\downarrow$ cardiac output,
hypotension, hepatotoxicity

Nitrous oxide

MOA: CNS depression
IND: weak general anesthetic, strong
analgesic
TOX: anoxia, vitamin B_{12} deficiency
(with chronic use)

Thiopental

MOA: prolongs inhibitory postsynaptic
potentials by $\uparrow$ GABA levels (similar to
phenobarbital)
IND: surgical anesthesia
TOX: laryngospasm

Benzodiazepines (diazepam,
midazolam)

MOA: facilitates GABA action by $\uparrow$
frequency of Cl channel opening
IND: sedative, hypnotic, anxiolytic
TOX: sedation

Ketamine

MOA: PCP analog (NMDA receptor
blocker)
IND: general anesthetic
TOX: postoperative hallucinations,
amnesia, respiratory depression

Propofol

MOA: facilitates GABA action
IND: general anesthetic—rapid onset
and clearance
TOX: cannot be given to patients with
egg or soybean allergies

Local anesthetics (procaine, cocaine,
tetracaine, lidocaine, bupivacaine)

MOA: block Na^+ channels
IND: anesthetic for minor procedures,
spinal blocks
TOX: arrhythmias, HTN; cardiotoxicity
(bupivacaine), seizures

Succinylcholine	**MOA:** depolarizing neuromuscular blocker **IND:** rapid sequence induction **TOX:** hyperkalemia; malignant hyperthermia when given with halogenated inhaled anesthetic; contraindicated in patients with glaucoma because of ↑ intraocular pressure (IOP)
Tubocurarine	**MOA:** nondepolarizing neuromuscular blocker **IND:** adjuvant to general anesthesia **TOX:** hypotension
Dexmedetomidine	**MOA:** α_2 agonist **IND:** sedation during mechanical ventilation **TOX:** bradycardia, hypotension
Why is epinephrine commonly combined with local anesthetics?	To prolong the duration of the anesthetic effect by causing local vasoconstriction
What types of fibers are affected most by local anesthetic agents?	Pain > temperature > touch > pressure; small unmyelinated fibers most affected; large, myelinated fibers least affected
Which drug is used to reverse the effects of the nondepolarizing muscle blockers?	Neostigmine (cholinesterase inhibitor)
Which drug is used to treat malignant hyperthermia?	Dantrolene (ryanodine receptor antagonist)

Analgesics

For each of the following drugs, provide:
1. **The mechanism of action (MOA)**
2. **Indication(s) (IND)**
3. **Significant side effects and unique toxicity (TOX) (if any)**

Acetaminophen	**MOA:** COX-3 inhibitor (mechanism not known with certainty) **IND:** pain, fever (but not used as anti-inflammatory) **TOX:** overdose causes hepatic necrosis

Aspirin	**MOA:** irreversible inhibition of COX-1 and COX-2 **IND:** antiplatelet drug; not commonly anymore used as analgesic or antipyretic due to better alternatives **TOX:** GI ulcers, bleeding, hypersensitivity reactions, bronchoconstriction, tinnitus, Reye syndrome in children
Celecoxib	**MOA:** COX-2 inhibitor **IND:** osteoarthritis, rheumatoid arthritis **TOX:** similar to aspirin but less GI toxicity, increased risk of thrombosis
Gabapentin	**MOA:** modulates GABA activity in CNS **IND:** antiepileptic, postherpetic neuralgia, diabetic neuralgia (off-label) **TOX:** sedation
Indomethacin	**MOA:** reversible inhibition of COX-1 and COX-2 **IND:** acute gout, neonatal patent ductus arteriosus **TOX:** GI upset, headache
Meperidine	**MOA:** μ opioid receptor agonist **IND:** analgesic **TOX:** seizures; side effects similar to morphine
Morphine	**MOA:** μ opioid receptor agonist; opioid receptor binding activates G proteins and adenylyl cyclase **IND:** analgesic, cough suppressant **TOX:** constipation, emesis, sedation, respiratory depression, miosis, urinary retention **Note:** these symptoms are typical for heroin overdose
Naloxone	**MOA:** μ opioid receptor antagonist **IND:** used to reverse the effects of opioid agonists **TOX:** CNS depression
Buprenorphine-naloxone (Suboxone)	**MOA:** long-acting partial opioid agonist (μ receptors) combined with opioid antagonist (naloxone); the naloxone portion has negligible bioavailability and only acts if the medication is abused by being injected **IND:** opioid use disorder **TOX:** sedation, headache, nausea, respiratory depression

Methadone

MOA: long-acting opioid agonist
(μ receptors)
IND: opioid use disorder
TOX: cardiac arrhythmia, respiratory
depression

What two types of opioid receptors mediate analgesia, respiratory depression, and physical dependence?

1. μ
2. δ

What type of opioid receptors mediates spinal analgesia and the sedative effects of opioids?

κ

CHAPTER 5

Cardiovascular

EMBRYOLOGY

What are the five dilatations of the primitive heart tube?	1. Truncus arteriosus 2. Bulbus cordis 3. Primitive ventricle 4. Primitive atrium 5. Sinus venosus
Name the structures in the mature heart that are derived from the following embryonic structures:	
Truncus arteriosus	Ascending aorta and pulmonary trunk
Bulbus cordis	Smooth parts of left (aortic vestibule) and right (conus arteriosus) ventricle
Primitive ventricle	Trabeculated parts of left and right ventricle
Primitive atria	Trabeculated parts of left and right atria
Left horn of sinus venosus	Coronary sinus
Right horn of sinus venosus	Smooth part of right atrium (sinus venarum)
Transient common pulmonary vein	Smooth part of left atrium
Right common cardinal vein and right anterior cardinal vein	Superior vena cava
Which embryonic layer gives rise to most of the cardiovascular system?	Mesoderm
What structure divides the truncus arteriosus and bulbus cordis?	Aorticopulmonary septum
Name the structure between the atria that develops from the walls of the septum primum and septum secundum:	Foramen ovale

Name the three physiologic shunts in the fetal circulation and the structures they shunt between:

1. Foramen ovale (right to left atrium)
2. Ductus arteriosus (pulmonary artery to aortic arch)
3. Ductus venosus (umbilical vein to IVC)

ANATOMY

What are the two anatomic divisions of the pericardium?

1. Serous pericardium (made of visceral epicardial layer and parietal layer)
2. Fibrous pericardium

Which nerve lies between the fibrous pericardium and mediastinal pleura?

Phrenic nerve (runs with pericardiophrenic vessels)

Name the major artery that commonly supplies each of the following structures:

Right atrium and right ventricle

Right coronary artery (RCA)

Sinoatrial (SA) and atrioventricular (AV) nodes

RCA

Left atrium and left ventricle

Left main coronary artery (LMCA)

Anterior 2/3 of interventricular septum

1. Left anterior descending (LAD) artery

Posterior 1/3 of interventricular septum

2. Posterior descending artery (PDA)

Which artery determines dominance of cardiac blood supply?

PDA

Trace the general pathway of venous drainage from myocardium

Great, middle, and small cardiac veins → coronary sinus → right atrium

Trace the conduction pathway of a cardiac impulse

SA node → AV node → bundle of His → right and left bundle branches → Purkinje fibers

Which nerve supplies parasympathetic input to heart?

Vagus nerve

Which syndrome is characterized by arm claudication, syncope, vertigo, nausea, and a supraclavicular bruit?

Subclavian steal syndrome (occlusion in subclavian artery proximal to take vertebral artery take-off → "stealing" of blood from vertebral artery to distal subclavian artery)

Describe the best location for auscultation of the following cardiac valves:

Tricuspid valve	Left sternal border, fifth intercostal space
Pulmonary valve	Left sternal border, second intercostal space
Mitral valve	Apex of heart, fifth intercostal space
Aortic valve	Right sternal border, second intercostal space

PHYSIOLOGY

Cardiac Electrophysiology

Name the electrical event in the heart associated with each feature of a normal electrocardiogram:

P wave	Atrial depolarization
PR interval	Atrial depolarization and conduction delay through AV node
QRS complex	Depolarization of the ventricles
T wave	Ventricular repolarization

What conduction abnormality results in a prolonged (wide) QRS complex?	Bundle branch block, metabolic disturbance resulting in slowed conduction (eg, hyperkalemia), ventricular tachycardia
Which ion primarily dictates the resting membrane potential of a myocyte?	Potassium; membrane has high K^+ permeability through K^+ channels
Which membrane protein maintains the ion gradient?	Sodium-potassium ATPase
What is the effect of potassium efflux from a myocardial cell?	Hyperpolarization
What is the effect of potassium influx into a myocardial cell?	Depolarization

Describe the electrochemical events that cause the following phases of the cardiac myocyte action potential:

Phase 0 (the upstroke)

Influx of Na^+ into cell

Phase 2 (the plateau)

Influx of Ca^{2+} into cell, efflux of K^+ out of cell

Phase 3 (repolarization)

Efflux of K^+ out of cell

Phase 4 (resting membrane potential)

Equilibrium potential, balance between K^+ leak current and Na^+/K^+ ATPase

What unique electrochemical feature of SA node allows it to act as a pacemaker for the heart?

Spontaneous Phase 4 depolarization causing **automaticity**

What ion and channel are responsible for automaticity?

Na^+ conductance via I_f channel

Describe the electrochemical events that cause the following phases of the SA nodal action potential:

Phase 0 (the upstroke)

Influx of Ca^{2+} into cell

Phase 3 (repolarization)

Efflux of K^+ out of cell

Phase 4 (slow depolarization)

Increasing Na^+ influx into cell

What phase 4 characteristic determines heart rate?

Slope of depolarization; a steeper slope reaches threshold sooner resulting in a faster heart rate

Name the component of the cardiac conduction system where phase 4 depolarization is *fastest*:

SA node

Name the components of the cardiac conduction system where phase 4 depolarization is *slowest*:

Bundle of His, Purkinje fibers, myocardium

What is the intrinsic rate of depolarization of the SA node?

100 beats per minute

Define conduction velocity

The rate at which an impulse spreads throughout cardiac tissue

What determines conduction velocity?

Rate of depolarization (phase 0 upstroke)

Where is conduction velocity *fastest*?

The Purkinje system

Where is conduction velocity *slowest*?   The AV node

What is the significance of the conduction delay at the AV node?   The delay in conduction allows for ventricular filling

Cardiac Contractility and Output

Describe the function of each myocardial cellular component:

    Sarcomere   Contractile unit

    Intercalated disks   Cell adhesion

    Gap junction   Electrochemical communication between myocardial fibers

    T tubules   Carry action potentials into the cell interior

    Sarcoplasmic reticulum   Storage and release of calcium

Which ion determines the magnitude of tension in a contracting myocardial cell?   Amount of intracellular calcium

Describe the effect of each of the following on contractility:

    Increased heart rate   Increased contractility

    Catecholamines   Increased contractility

    Digoxin   Increased contractility

    Acetylcholine (ACh)   Decreased contractility

What is the Frank-Starling relationship?   The greater the end-diastolic volume (preload), the greater is the stroke volume

How does contractility affect cardiac output?   Cardiac output increases as contractility increases

Name the four factors that determine myocardial oxygen consumption:
1. Afterload (wall tension)
2. Size of heart
3. Contractility
4. Heart rate

Provide formulas for each of the following:

    Stroke volume   End-diastolic volume – end-systolic volume

    Cardiac output   Stroke volume × heart rate

Ejection fraction	Stroke volume/end-diastolic volume
Cardiac output based on Fick principle	O_2 consumption/(arterial O_2 − venous O_2)
Coronary perfusion pressure	CPP = Diastolic blood pressure − LV end diastolic pressure (LVEDP)

Heart Sounds

Name the event associated with each heart sound:

S_1	Closure of the AV (tricuspid, mitral) valves
S_2	Closure of semilunar (aortic, pulmonary) valves
S_3	Flow of blood from atria into ventricles during diastole (often seen with large ventricular volumes, ie, CHF; often benign in youth and trained athletes)
S_4	Flow of blood from atria into ventricles during atrial systole (often present in patient with stiffened ventricle)

Maintenance of Blood Pressure

What is the site of highest resistance in the cardiovascular system?	Arterioles
Which vascular bed has the largest cross-sectional and surface areas?	Capillaries
Which vascular bed contains the largest volume of blood at any given time?	Veins

Define the following terms:

Systolic blood pressure	Highest arterial blood pressure during a cardiac cycle
Diastolic blood pressure	Lowest arterial blood pressure during a cardiac cycle
Pulse pressure	Difference between systolic and diastolic blood pressure
Mean arterial pressure	$1/3 \times$ systolic blood pressure $+ 2/3 \times$ diastolic blood pressure

What is the most important determinant of pulse pressure?	Stroke volume
What is the effect of aging on pulse pressure?	Aging widens pulse pressure due to ↓ capacitance of blood vessels
How is left atrial pressure determined clinically?	Pulmonary capillary wedge pressure
Where are the carotid baroreceptors located?	Bifurcation of common carotid arteries
What is the function of the carotid baroreceptors?	Minute to minute regulation of blood pressure
Which nerve carries information from baroreceptors to the vasomotor center in the brainstem?	Cranial nerve IX (glossopharyngeal)
Name two ways that the vasomotor center responds to decreased mean arterial pressure:	1. ↓ Parasympathetic output 2. ↑Sympathetic output
Name the hormone(s) responsible for each of the following functions:	
Long-term regulation of blood pressure	Renin-angiotensin-aldosterone system
Stimulation of aldosterone secretion and arterial vasoconstriction	Angiotensin II
Water retention and direct arteriolar vasoconstriction causing an increase in blood pressure	Vasopressin
Inhibition of renin release, stimulation of salt and water excretion, and vascular smooth muscle relaxation	Atrial natriuretic peptide
Name three stimuli for renin secretion:	1. ↓ Renal blood pressure 2. ↓ Na^+ delivery to macula densa of JGA 3. ↑ Sympathetic tone
What is the effect of cerebral ischemia on blood pressure and heart rate?	Cushing reflex: blood pressure ↑ and heart rate ↓
What is the mechanism of increased blood pressure in cerebral ischemia?	Chemoreceptors in the vasomotor center stimulate increased sympathetic outflow

What is the mechanism of decreased heart rate in cerebral ischemia?

Baroreceptor reflex to increase in BP leads to increased parasympathetic outflow to heart

Where are the carotid chemoreceptors located?

Bifurcation of common carotid arteries and the aortic arch at carotid body

What do chemoreceptors sense?

Oxygen, CO_2, pH, and temperature

What is the Starling equation?

$J_v = K_f [(P_c - P_i) - (\pi_c - \pi_i)]$

Describe the effect of each of the following on capillary filtration:

Increased capillary hydrostatic pressure

Increased fluid filtration

Increased interstitial hydrostatic pressure

Decreased fluid filtration

Increased capillary oncotic pressure

Decreased fluid filtration

Increased interstitial oncotic pressure

Increased fluid filtration

Define autoregulation

The capacity of an organ to maintain constant blood flow despite changes in mean arterial pressure

Name the primary mechanism of blood flow regulation in the following tissues:

Coronary arteries

Local metabolic control

Cerebral vasculature

Local metabolic control

Muscle

Local metabolic control

Skin

Sympathetic control

Pulmonary

Local metabolic control

Name five key metabolites which cause vasodilation:

1. Lactate
2. K^+
3. Adenosine
4. CO_2
5. H^+

Name the primary vasoactive metabolite in the following tissues:

Coronary arteries

O_2, adenosine

Cerebral vasculature

CO_2 (most important), H^+

Muscle

Lactate, K^+, adenosine

Pulmonary

O_2

CARDIOVASCULAR PATHOLOGY AND PATHOPHYSIOLOGY

Murmurs

Name the valvular defect causing each
murmur described below:

Harsh midsystolic murmur in the left second intercostal space at the left sternal border	Pulmonic stenosis
Harsh midsystolic murmur in the right second intercostal space at the right sternal border, radiating to the neck (carotid arteries) and apex	Aortic stenosis
Harsh midsystolic murmur at the left third and fourth interspaces radiating down the left sternal border; murmur louder with decreased preload (ie, on Valsalva); S_4 and biphasic apical impulse often present	Hypertrophic cardiomyopathy
Blowing holosystolic murmur at apex radiating to the left axilla with increased apical impulse	Mitral regurgitation
Blowing holosystolic murmur at the lower left sternal border radiating to the right of the sternum; may ↑ with inspiration	Tricuspid regurgitation
Soft, late systolic murmur at the left sternal border or apex, accompanied by midsystolic click	Mitral valve prolapse
Harsh holosystolic murmur at the lower left sternal border, accompanied by a thrill	Ventricular septal defect (VSD)
Blowing, high-pitched diastolic murmur at the left second to fourth interspaces radiating to the apex	Aortic regurgitation
Low-pitched diastolic murmur at the apex that gets louder prior to S_1; an opening snap is often present just after S_2	Mitral stenosis
Systolic flow murmur at left upper sternal border; fixed splitting of S_2	Atrial septal defect (ASD)

What congenital valvular defect is associated with aortic stenosis?	Bicuspid aortic valve

What are two common manifestations of aortic stenosis?

Angina and syncope

Which disorder results from myxomatous degeneration of the mitral valve?

Mitral valve prolapse

Patients with mitral valve prolapse are at increased risk of which infection?

Infective endocarditis

Heart Failure

What are the most common causes of left-sided heart failure?

Ischemic heart disease, HTN, mitral and aortic valvular disease, primary myocardial disease (cardiomyopathy, myocarditis)

Name four key mechanisms of compensation in congestive heart failure (CHF):

1. Hypertrophy
2. Ventricular dilation
4. Blood volume expansion
5. Tachycardia

Name two major clinical signs/ symptoms of left-sided heart failure:

1. Pulmonary congestion
2. Pulmonary edema causing dyspnea and orthopnea

Name three consequences of suboptimal renal perfusion:

1. RAA axis activation leading to salt and water retention
2. Ischemic acute tubular necrosis (ATN)
3. Prerenal azotemia

What is the consequence of impaired cerebral perfusion in CHF?

Hypoxic encephalopathy

What is the most common cause of right-sided heart failure?

Left-sided heart failure

Name two major pulmonary causes of right-sided heart failure:

1. Interstitial fibrosis
2. Pulmonary HTN

Name four key clinical signs of right-sided heart failure:

1. Portal, systemic, peripheral congestion, and edema
2. Hepatomegaly
3. Congestive splenomegaly
4. Renal congestion

Describe the phases of pathologic change in the liver that result from chronic right-sided heart failure.

Nutmeg appearance → centrilobular necrosis → central hemorrhagic necrosis → cardiac sclerosis (cirrhosis)

What is the most common cause of acute right-sided heart failure in a patient with a deep venous thrombosis?

Massive pulmonary embolus

What ECG findings may be seen with acute right-sided heart stress?

$S_1Q_3T_3$: S wave in lead 1, Q wave in lead 3, T-wave inversion in lead 3

What is the most common ECG finding in acute pulmonary embolism?

Sinus tachycardia

Ischemic Heart Disease

Name four important manifestations of ischemic heart disease:

1. Angina
2. Myocardial infarction (MI)
3. Arrhythmia (which can lead to sudden cardiac death)
4. Heart failure

What are the two major etiologies of myocardial ischemia?

1. ↓ Coronary perfusion
2. ↑ Myocardial O_2 demand

What conditions compound the consequences of impaired myocardial perfusion?

Anemia, advanced lung disease, cigarette smoking, congenital heart disease

Name the type of angina:

Pain precipitated by exertion, relieved by rest/vasodilators

Stable angina

Angina in the absence of coronary artery disease

Vasospastic (Prinzmetal) angina

Angina at rest or worsening of existing stable pattern of angina

Unstable angina

Describe the underlying pathology for each type of angina:

Stable angina

Stenosis of coronary artery exceeding the autoregulatory threshold resulting in flow-limitation (usually >70%)

Vasospastic (Prinzmetal) angina

Coronary vasospasm

Unstable angina

Plaque disruption with resulting occlusive thrombosis within a coronary artery

Describe the associations between myocardial ischemia, injury, and infarction

1. Ischemia—insufficient blood supply to the myocardium, occurs first
2. Injury—results when the ischemic process is prolonged
3. Infarction—describes necrosis or death of myocardial cells

Name the type of myocardial damage described below:

Full-thickness infarction caused by complete occlusion of a coronary artery

Transmural infarction

Infarction of the inner half (or less) of the ventricular wall supplied by a partially occluded coronary artery

Subendocardial infarction

ST depression on ECG

Subendocardial injury

ST elevation on ECG

Transmural injury

Q waves on ECG

Transmural infarction

What is the initial event in the development of a transmural infarction?

Acute plaque disruption

What are the most common symptoms of a myocardial infarct?

Crushing retrosternal chest pain or pressure, dyspnea, pain radiating into left arm or neck, diaphoresis, nausea

What type of necrosis is seen in myocardium within 24 hours of infarction?

Coagulative necrosis

What type of inflammatory cells is seen in the myocardium within 24 hours of infarction?

Neutrophils

What is the most common type of inflammatory cell seen in myocardium from the 2nd to 10th day after an infarction?

Macrophages

When is the risk of myocardial rupture greatest and why?

At 4 to 7 days; tissue is weakest following phagocytosis of debris by macrophages and prior to growth of granulation tissue

How many days does it take to form granulation tissue in a region of infracted myocardium?

7 to 10 days

How many weeks does it take to form contracted scar tissue in a region of infarcted myocardium?

7 weeks

What is the diagnostic test of choice in a patient with suspected MI?

ECG

What two classic ECG changes are seen during a transmural MI?	1. ST elevation 2. Q waves (later)
When does CK-MB begin to rise, peak, and return to normal?	Rise: 3 to 8 hours Peak: 10 to 24 hours Return to normal: 2 to 3 days
When does troponin begin to rise, peak, and return to normal?	Rise: 3 to 8 hours Peak: 24 to 48 hours Return to normal: 5 to 10 days
What are the advantages and disadvantages of the CK-MB serum cardiac marker?	Allows diagnosis of re-infarction as levels quickly return to normal; may be falsely elevated with skeletal muscle injury
What are the advantages of the troponin assay?	Very specific to cardiac injury; allows diagnosis of late presenting MI
What disease can lead to a false-positive elevated troponin?	Chronic kidney disease
What are the two most common complications of MI?	1. Cardiac arrhythmia 2. CHF
List five less common but severe complications of MI:	1. Cardiogenic shock 2. Ventricular aneurysm or rupture 3. Papillary muscle rupture 4. Mural thrombosis with resulting peripheral embolism 5. Dressler syndrome

Cardiomyopathy

How does the left ventricle respond to long-standing hypertension?	Concentric hypertrophy
What are the three types of cardiomyopathy?	1. Dilated (or non-ischemic) 2. Hypertrophic 3. Restrictive
What are the most common nongenetic etiologies of dilated cardiomyopathy?	"ABCDE" Alcohol abuse Beriberi (thiamine deficiency) Coxsackie B myocarditis, Cocaine, Chagas **disease** Doxorubicin toxicity prEgnancy

Name the type of cardiomyopathy associated with the following clinical and pathologic features:

30% to 40% of cases are genetic	Dilated
100% of cases are genetic	Hypertrophic
Associated with alcoholism and thiamine deficiency	Dilated
Associated with coxsackie virus B and with *Trypanosoma cruzi*	Dilated
Associated with doxorubicin	Dilated
Associated with eosinophilia	Restrictive (Loeffler endocarditis)
Associated with pregnancy	Dilated
Asymmetric hypertrophy without dilatation	Hypertrophic
Can be caused by sarcoidosis, amyloidosis, scleroderma, hereditary hemochromatosis, endocardial fibro-elastosis, radiation-induced fibrosis	Restrictive
Cardiomyopathy most commonly caused by endomyocardial fibrosis as seen in chronic eosinophilia	Restrictive
Causes sudden death in young, otherwise healthy athletes	Hypertrophic
Commonly inherited in an autosomal dominant (AD) fashion	Hypertrophic
Four-chamber hypertrophy and dilation	Dilated
Left ventricular outflow obstruction	Hypertrophic
Myocyte tangles, disorientation	Hypertrophic
Symptoms relieved by squatting	Hypertrophic

Pericarditis and Cardiac Tumors

Name the type of pericarditis based on the following exudates descriptions:

Clear, straw colored, minimal inflammation, decreased fibrin	Serous pericarditis
Fibrin rich	Fibrinous pericarditis
Bloody	Hemorrhagic or malignant pericarditis

What are the most common etiologies of serous pericarditis?	Uremia, systemic lupus erythematosus (SLE), rheumatic fever
What are the most common etiologies of fibrinous pericarditis?	Uremia, SLE, rheumatic fever, coxsackie viral infection, MI, trauma
What are the most common etiologies of hemorrhagic pericarditis?	Trauma, malignancy, tuberculosis
What ECG and hemodynamic findings are seen in pericarditis?	**ECG:** diffuse ST elevations in all leads **Hemodynamic:** pulsus paradoxus
What is the most common cardiac tumor of adults?	Metastases (eg, melanoma)
What is the most common primary cardiac tumor of adults?	Left-sided atrial myxoma
What is the most common primary cardiac tumor in children?	Rhabdomyoma, commonly associated with tuberous sclerosis

Congenital Heart Disease

Name the congenital heart defect associated with each of the following statements:

Three most common causes of R→L shunting	1. ASD 2. VSD 3. Patent ductus arteriosus (PDA)
Two most common defects	1. VSD 2. PDA
Five defects causing cyanosis at birth	"5 T's": 1. Tetralogy of Fallot 2. Transposition of the great vessels 3. Truncus arteriosus 4. Total anomalous pulmonary venous return 5. Tricuspid atresia
Continuous machinery-like murmur	PDA
Pulmonic stenosis, right ventricular hypertrophy, overriding aorta, VSD ("PROVe")	Tetralogy of Fallot
Boot-shaped cardiac silhouette	Tetralogy of Fallot
Defect causing lower body cyanosis	Preductal coarctation
Defect causing upper extremity HTN and diminished lower extremity pulses	Postductal coarctation (stenosis distal to the ductus arteriosus)

Associated with Turner syndrome	Coarctation of the aorta
Associated with Down syndrome	ASDs, VSDs, and AV valve abnormalities (due to endocardial cushion abnormalities)
Associated with Rubella	PDA
Associated with 22q11 syndrome	Truncus arteriosus, tetralogy of Fallot
Common cyanotic congenital heart defect in children born to diabetic mothers	Transposition of the great vessels
Aorta arises from *right* ventricle and pulmonary trunk arises from *left* ventricle	Transposition of the great vessels
Valvular defect associated with increased risk of infective endocarditis and calcification	Bicuspid aortic valve
What is the consequence of leaving a left-to-right shunting untreated?	Right → left shunting
What type of infection are patients with VSD at an increased risk for?	Infective endocarditis
What drug is used to induce closure of a PDA?	Indomethacin
What drug is used to prevent closure of a PDA?	Prostaglandins
What is the most common genetic cause of congenital heart disease?	Trisomy 21

Cardiac Infectious Disorders

What type of infection is responsible for causing rheumatic fever?	Group A streptococcal pharyngitis
How does streptococcal pharyngitis cause rheumatic heart disease?	Antistreptococcal antibodies cross-react with a cardiac antigen
What serologic test is elevated in rheumatic heart disease?	Antistreptolysin antibodies (ASO)
Name the five major Jones criteria for rheumatic heart disease:	1. Joints: migratory polyarthritis 2. ♥ (O) = pancarditis 3. Nodules: subcutaneous nodules 4. Erythema marginatum 5. Sydenham chorea

Name five minor Jones criteria for rheumatic heart disease:

1. Fever
2. Arthralgia
3. Elevated ESR/CRP
4. Leukocytosis
5. Heart block on ECG

What term is used to describe the foci of pink collagen surrounded by lymphocytes and Anitschkow cells (macrophages) that are pathognomonic for rheumatic heart disease?

Aschoff bodies

Which valve is most commonly affected in rheumatic heart disease?

Mitral valve

What is the most commonly observed valvular deformity in rheumatic heart disease?

Fishmouth stenosis of the mitral valve

What are the three major categories of endocarditis?

1. Infective
2. Nonbacterial thrombotic (marantic)
3. Libman-Sacks

What is the most common valve affected by bacterial endocarditis?

Mitral valve

What is the most common valve affected by bacterial endocarditis in IV drug users?

Tricuspid valve

Name the type of endocarditis described in each of the following vignettes:

25-year-old (y/o) IV drug user with rapid onset of high fever, rigors, malaise, and tricuspid regurgitation

Acute infective endocarditis

60-y/o woman with mitral valve prolapse, who has recently undergone dental extraction, presents with low-grade fever and flu-like symptoms

Subacute infective endocarditis

65-y/o man with metastatic colon cancer and new murmur consistent with mitral regurgitation

Nonbacterial thrombotic endocarditis

30-y/o woman with SLE

Libman-Sacks endocarditis

Which organism most often causes acute infective endocarditis?

Staphylococcus aureus

Which organism most often causes subacute infective endocarditis?	*Streptococcus viridians*
What are the clinical signs of bacterial endocarditis?	Fever Roth spots Osler nodes Murmur Janeway lesions Anemia Nail bed hemorrhages (ie, splinter) Emboli

Define the following eponyms used to describe signs of bacterial endocarditis:

Osler nodes	Tender, raised lesions on finger and toe pads; they are tender due to the presence of inflammatory immune complexes causing local vasculitis
Janeway lesions	Small, nontender erythematous lesions on palms and soles
Roth spots	Erythematous spots with white centers on retina
What are some sequelae to bacterial endocarditis?	Valvular injury, renal injury (glomerulonephritis), septic emboli to brain, kidneys causing infarction or abscess

Atherosclerosis

What are the major risk factors for coronary heart disease?	Age (men >45, women >55 or with premature menopause) Family history of premature heart attacks (MI or sudden cardiac death in men <55, women <65) Cigarette smoking Hypertension (HTN) Diabetes mellitus HDL <40, HDL >60 negates one risk factor
What are the two main histopathologic components of an atheroma?	Superficial fibrous cap overlying a necrotic core
What are the components of the fibrous cap?	Smooth muscle cells, macrophages, foam cells, lymphocytes, collagen, and elastin.
What is the pathologic precursor to atheroma?	Fatty streak

What is the term for ulcerated, calcified, hemorrhagic atheromas that predispose to thrombosis?	Complicated plaques
What is the underlying pathologic basis for the initiation of atherosclerosis?	Endothelial injury
What may produce this endothelial injury?	Hypercholesterolemia, mechanical injury, HTN, immune mechanisms, toxins, etc.
How are foam cells created?	Macrophages that ingest oxidized LDL that has accumulated in the vessel wall become foam cells
Which lipids are most commonly found in an atheromatous plaque?	Cholesterol and cholesterol esters (LDL)
What is the function of smooth muscle cells in an atheroma?	Smooth muscle cells when activated by growth factors proliferate and migrate into intima; they then secrete extracellular matrix glycoproteins
What are the major cell types associated with the formation of an atheroma?	Macrophages (foam cells), T lymphocytes (attracted to zone of injury), smooth muscle cells, and endothelial cells
What are the most common locations for atherosclerotic disease?	Abdominal aorta, coronary arteries, popliteal arteries, and carotid arteries
What are the four major clinical manifestations of atherosclerosis?	1. Arterial insufficiency (ie, stroke, MI, peripheral vascular disease, ischemic bowel disease) 2. Thrombus formation due to plaque rupture 3. Atheroembolism 4. Aneurysm, dissection, or rupture of a major vessel

Name the type of arteriolosclerosis associated with the following clinical and pathologic features:

Hyaline deposits causing thickening of arteriolar walls	Hyaline arteriolosclerosis
Onion skin arteriolar thickening	Hyperplastic arteriolosclerosis
Deposition of calcium in the medial coat of arteries of the lower extremities	Monckeberg arteriosclerosis

Pipestem arteries with ringlike calcifications	Monckeberg arteriosclerosis
Two types of arteriolosclerosis that occur in patients with long-term HTN	1. Hyaline arteriolosclerosis 2. Hyperplastic arteriolosclerosis

Hypertension

HTN is the most important risk factor in which two vascular diseases?	1. Cerebrovascular disease 2. Coronary artery disease
What percentage of hypertensive patients have essential HTN?	90% to 95%
What are two common renal causes of secondary HTN?	1. Renal artery stenosis 2. Renal parenchymal disorders
What sleep disorder is associated with HTN?	Obstructive sleep apnea
What are some common endocrine causes of secondary HTN?	1. Hyperaldosteronism (Conn syndrome) 2. Hypercortisolism (Cushing syndrome) 3. Hyperthyroidism 4. Oral contraceptive use (estrogen-containing) 5. Pheochromocytoma 6. Acromegaly
Name two common cardiac complications of long-standing HTN:	1. Left ventricular hypertrophy (LVH) 2. Left-sided heart failure (as a result of diastolic dysfunction related to LVH)

List the possible effects of malignant HTN on each organ system below:

Heart	Acute LV failure, MI
Aorta	Dissection
Lungs	Pulmonary edema
Kidneys	Acute renal failure
Eyes	Papilledema, fundal hemorrhages, blurred vision
Brain	Headache, encephalopathy, seizure, hemorrhagic cerebrovascular accident (CVA)

What is the most common cause of death in patients with untreated HTN	CHF

Aneurysms and Dissections

What is the most common site for syphilitic aneurysm?	Thoracic aorta (often ascending)
What is the mechanism of syphilitic aneurysms?	Obliteration of the arteries supplying the aorta (vasa vasorum), leading to necrosis of the media (endarteritis obliterans)
What is the most common site for atherosclerotic aneurysm? Why?	Abdominal aorta, below renal arteries and above iliac bifurcation; due to lack of vasa vasorum in this region

Name the type of aneurysm referred to in the following clinical vignettes:

55-y/o man, who is a smoker with HTN, diabetes, and coronary artery disease, is found to have a pulsatile midline abdominal mass	Atherosclerotic, abdominal aortic aneurysm
35-y/o with a family history of polycystic kidney disease presents with the worst headache of his life	Berry aneurysm rupture leading to subarachnoid hemorrhage
40-y/o sex worker with angina and shortness of breath (SOB) is found to have wide pulse pressure and a high-pitched blowing diastolic murmur	Syphilitic/luetic, dilation of aortic root leads to aortic regurgitation

What are the most common etiologies for the development of aortic dissection?	HTN and connective tissue disorders (such as Marfan syndrome)
Name two characteristic histopathologic findings in the aorta in a patient with Marfan syndrome:	1. Elastic tissue fragmentation 2. Cystic medial degeneration
What is the genetic defect in Marfan disease?	Defect in fibrillin-1 which forms a scaffold for elastic fibers
What is the classic clinical presentation of aortic dissection?	Sudden onset of severe tearing pain radiating to the back and descending as the dissection progresses
What is the underlying mechanism in the development of varicose veins?	Venous dilation or deformation leading to venous valvular incompetence
State two complications of varicose veins:	1. Varicose ulceration 2. Stasis dermatitis

Vasculitides

Name the type of vasculitis associated with the following clinical and pathologic features:

Presence of C-ANCA	Granulomatosis with polyangiitis (GPA) (ie, Wegener granulomatosis)
Presence of P-ANCA	Microscopic PolyANgiitis, PolyArteritis Nodosa (PAN), and eosinophilic granulomatosis with polyangiitis (EGPA) (ie, Churg-Strauss syndrome)
Most common vasculitis in the United States	Temporal or giant cell arteritis
Fibrous thickening of origins of the great vessels leading to absent pulses	Takayasu arteritis
Well-demarcated, segmental fibrinoid necrosis of the arterial wall and diffuse neutrophilic infiltrates in medium-sized arteries	PAN
Commonly affecting the coronary arteries and may result in coronary aneurysm	Kawasaki disease
Segmental inflammation/ thrombosis of arteries and adjacent veins, nerves, and connective tissue; results in painful ischemic disease and associated with smoking	Thromboangiitis obliterans (Buerger disease)
Vascular and mesangial deposition of IgA complexes with abdominal pain, palpable purpura especially on buttocks, glomerulonephritis, and arthritis	Henoch-Schonlein purpura

Which vessels are most commonly involved in temporal arteritis?	External carotid artery and its branches
What is the triad of GPA (ie, Wegener granulomatosis)?	1. Focal necrotizing vasculitis of upper airways and lungs 2. Necrotizing granulomas of upper and lower respiratory tract 3. Necrotizing glomerulitis

What are the six clinical signs of critical limb ischemia?

"Six P's":
1. Pain
2. Pallor
3. Poikilothermia
4. Parasthesia
5. Paralysis
6. Pulselessness

Name the type of vasculitis associated with each of the following clinical vignettes:

70-y/o white man with constitutional symptoms, headache, jaw claudication, acute onset of blindness; W/U: ↑ ESR

Temporal (giant cell) arteritis

30-y/o Korean woman with constitutional symptoms, arthritis; physical examination (PE): loss of carotid and radial pulses

Takayasu arteritis

35-y/o hepatitis B positive man with fever, HTN; W/U: neutrophilia, P-ANCA ⊕

PAN

12-y/o girl recovering from a viral infection presents with exertional chest pain; PE: febrile, conjunctival injection, cervical lymphadenopathy, strawberry tongue, diffuse erythematous rash, edema of hands and feet

Kawasaki disease

40-y/o man with asthma; PE: palpable purpura, diffuse wheezes; CBC: eosinophilia; transbronchial biopsy: upper airway granulomas and elevated P-ANCA and ESR

EGPA (ie, Churg-Strauss syndrome)

8-y/o boy presents with abdominal pain, hematuria, and recent history of URI; PE: palpable purpura, heme ⊕ stools; W/U: vascular biopsy shows perivascular granulocytes, IgA deposition

Henoch-Schonlein purpura

55-y/o man presents with chronic cough, rhinorrhea, ulcerations of nasal septum; W/U: RBC casts in urine and C-ANCA ⊕

GPA (ie, Wegener granulomatosis)

21-y/o woman smoker with pallor and cyanosis of fingertips after exposure to cold

Raynaud disease

Vascular Tumors

Name the vascular disorder associated with the following clinical or pathologic features:

Cutaneous vascular tumor commonly seen in patients with end-stage liver disease (hyperestrinism)	Spider telangiectasia
AD condition is characterized by a localized dilation of venules and capillaries in skin and mucous membrane leading to epistaxis and GI bleeding	Hereditary hemorrhagic telangiectasia (Rendu-Osler-Weber) syndrome
AD condition is characterized by the presence of multiple cavernous hemangiomas of skin, liver, pancreas, and spleen and hemangioblastomas of cerebellum with ↑ risk of renal cell carcinoma	von Hippel-Lindau disease
Vascular tumor associated with thorium contrast material and polyvinyl chloride	Hemangiosarcoma
Vascular tumor commonly seen in men of eastern European descent and in those infected with HIV consisting of red or purple cutaneous plaques on the lower extremities	Kaposi sarcoma
Vascular tumor caused by human herpesvirus (HHV) 8 or HIV	Kaposi sarcoma
Syndrome is characterized by cyanosis and edema of upper extremities, head, and neck in a patient with thoracic tumor	Superior vena cava syndrome

PHARMACOLOGY

Antianginal Agents

What are the four types of antianginal drugs?	1. Nitrates 2. β-blockers 3. Calcium channel blockers 4. Ranolazine (inward sodium current inhibitor)

How do nitrates cause vasodilation?

Nitrates are metabolized to nitric oxide (NO) → NO causes ↑ in cyclic guanosine monophosphate (cGMP) in endothelial cells → vasodilation

Describe how nitrates reduce angina

1. Vasodilation causes venous pooling, which reduces preload and consequently myocardial oxygen consumption
2. Coronary vasodilation improves perfusion and thus oxygen delivery to the myocardium

What is the most common side effect of nitrates?

Headache

Describe how each of the following drugs reduces angina:

β-Blockers

By ↓ contractility and heart rate

Amlodipine

Coronary arterial vasodilation

Diltiazem

Decreased heart rate and contractility, slowed conduction (especially through AV node), coronary arteriolar vasodilation

Ranolazine

Inhibits late inward sodium current, reducing intracellular calcium concentration, decreasing myocardial oxygen demand

What is the antianginal drug of choice for Prinzmetal angina?

Diltiazem

What antianginal drug is contraindicated in patients with reactive airway disease (asthma or COPD)?

β-Blockers

Inotropic Support

Name the only oral inotropic agent:

Digoxin

Describe the three-step mechanism by which digitalis potentiates myocardial contractility

1. Inhibition of Na^+/K^+ ATPase.
2. Buildup of intracellular Na^+.
3. High intracellular Na^+ impairs Na^+-Ca^{2+} antiport, causing increased intracellular Ca^{2+}

What is the most worrisome side effect of digoxin on the heart?

Arrhythmias

Which agent can be used to counteract the cardiac toxicity of digoxin? By what mechanism?

K^+ supplementation; digoxin binds near K^+ site on Na^+/K^+ ATPase; when K^+ is low, digoxin has better access and vice versa

What are the unique neurotoxicities of digoxin?

Headache, nausea, altered color perception, blurred vision, tinnitus

For which arrhythmia is digoxin commonly used?

Atrial fibrillation

What is the β-agonist of choice for inotropic support in heart failure?

Dobutamine

Which antiarrhythmic is useful for abolishing torsades de pointes?

Mg^{2+}

By which mechanism do β-agonists and phosphodiesterase inhibitors potentiate myocardial contractility?

These agents increase cAMP which promotes increased intracellular Ca^{2+}

Antiarrhythmics

For each antiarrhythmic agent, name the unique toxicity/toxicities:

Quinidine

Cinchonism—headache, tinnitus, thrombocytopenia, torsades de pointes

Procainamide

Reversible drug-induced lupus

Lidocaine

CNS depression, cardiac depression, local anesthetic

Flecainide

Proarrhythmic

Amiodarone

Interstitial pulmonary fibrosis, thyroid dysfunction, hepatotoxicity, tremor, ataxia, neuropathy, bluish discoloration of skin, corneal deposits

What is the drug of choice for abolishing acute supraventricular tachycardia (SVT)?

Adenosine

Antihypertensives

For each of the following drugs,
provide:
1. The mechanism of action (MOA)
2. Indication(s) (IND)
3. Significant side effects and unique
   toxicity (TOX) (if any)

ACE inhibitors

MOA: ↓ vasoconstriction, ↓ aldosterone
secretion, ↓ renal Na^+ reabsorption
IND: essential HTN (first-line)
TOX: acute kidney injury,
hyperkalemia, cough, angioedema

Sacubitril

MOA: ↓ neprolysin (normally
degrades ANP) → ↓ atrial natriuretic
peptide (ANP)
IND: systolic heart failure
TOX: acute kidney injury,
hyperkalemia, hypotension

Amlodipine

MOA: dihydropyridine Ca^{2+} blockers,
selective for vascular smooth muscle
IND: essential HTN (first-line)
TOX: lower-extremity edema,
bradycardia, hypotension, metabolic
acidosis

Diltiazem, verapamil

MOA: nondihydropyridine Ca^{2+}
blockers, verapamil is cardioselective,
diltiazem has intermediate affinity for
heart and vascular smooth muscle
IND: essential HTN (first-line)
TOX: constipation, mild LFT
abnormality, sexual dysfunction

Hydrochlorothiazide

MOA: ↓ renal NaCl reabsorption
IND: essential HTN (first-line)
TOX: hypokalemia, hypovolemia

β-Blockers

MOA: β-blockade ↓ cAMP
IND: intravenous agent for the short-
term management of HTN
TOX: impotence, asthma, mask signs of
hypoglycemia, CV effects (bradycardia,
CHF, AV block), sedation, seizures
(propranolol only since lipophilic,
crosses blood-brain barrier)

Prazosin, terazosin, doxazosin

MOA: α-blocker
IND: essential HTN, benign prostatic
hypertrophy
TOX: first-dose hypotension

Phentolamine	**MOA:** reversible α-blocker **IND:** diagnosis of pheochromocytoma, ischemia from accident injection of epinephrine (EPI) into soft tissue
Phenoxybenzamine	**MOA:** irreversible α-blocker **IND:** diagnosis of pheochromocytoma
Clonidine	**MOA:** centrally acting α_2-agonist that decreases sympathetic outflow **IND**: essential HTN (second-line) **TOX:** dry mouth, rebound HTN with sudden withdrawal
α-Methyldopa	**MOA:** converted to α-methyl norepinephrine (NE) to act centrally as an α-agonist and decrease sympathetic outflow **IND**: pregnant patients with HTN **TOX:** positive Coombs test, drowsiness
Hydralazine	**MOA:** causes arteriolar vasodilation by increasing cGMP in vascular smooth muscle **IND:** essential HTN (second-line) **TOX:** drug-induced lupus, angina
Nitroprusside	**MOA:** metabolism of nitroprusside releases NO which causes vasodilation via cGMP **IND**: malignant HTN **TOX:** cyanide toxicity (avoided if drug is mixed just prior to administration)

For each situation listed below, select the best antihypertensive agent(s):

Angina pectoris	β-Blockers, Ca^{2+} channel blockers
Diabetes	Angiotensin-converting enzyme inhibitors (ACEi), Ca^{2+} blockers, β-blockers
SVT	β-Blockers
Heart failure	Diuretics, ACEi, β-blockers, dihydropyridine CCB
History of MI	β-Blockers, ACEi
Chronic kidney disease	ACE inhibitors, diuretics, Ca^{2+} blockers
Anxiety	β-Blockers
Benign prostatic hyperplasia	α_1-Selective antagonist
Pheochromocytoma	Phenoxybenzamine, phentolamine

Hypertrophic obstructive cardiomyopathy	β-Blockers
Asthma, COPD	Diuretics, Ca^{2+} blockers
Hyperthyroidism	β-Blockers
Pregnancy	α-Methyldopa
African descent	Thiazide diuretics
Migraine headaches	β-Blockers

For each condition listed below, list the antihypertensive agent that should be avoided:	
CHF	Non-dihydropyridine CCB (eg, diltiazem, verapamil)
Severe reactive airway disease (COPD, asthma)	β-Blockers
What class of antihypertensives is useful in patients who cannot tolerate the side effects of ACEi?	Angiotensin receptor blockers (ARBs)
What classes of antihypertensive agents are absolutely contraindicated in pregnant patients?	ACEi and ARBs
List three agents useful in the management of malignant HTN:	1. Sodium nitroprusside 2. Hydralazine 3. Labetalol

Lipid-lowering Agents

Cholestyramine	**MOA:** bile acid–binding resin, ↓ bile acid stores, ↑catabolism of plasma LDL **IND:** adjuvant therapy for patients with familial hypercholesterolemia, ↓ LDL **TOX:** constipation, GI discomfort, may interfere with intestinal absorption of other drugs, LFT changes, myalgias
Statins	**MOA:** hydroxymethylglutaryl-CoA (HMG-CoA) reductase inhibitors, rate-limiting step of XOL synthesis **IND:** hypercholesterolemia: to ↓ LDL **TOX:** myalgias, hepatotoxicity (rare), rhabdomyolysis (rare)

Ezetimibe	**MOA**: inhibit intestinal absorption of cholesterol **IND**: refractory hyperlipidemia, familial hyperlipidemia **TOX**: diarrhea, hepatotoxicity
PCSK-9 inhibitors	**MOA**: inhibit PCSK-9 binding to LDL-C, ↑ LDL receptors on liver, ↓ LDL in blood **IND**: refractory hyperlipidemia, familial hyperlipidemia **TOX**: rash, urticaria
Gemfibrozil, clofibrate	**MOA:** stimulate lipoprotein lipase to increase catabolism of VLDL and triglycerides (↓ VLDL, ↓ TGs) **IND:** hypertriglyceridemia; dramatically ↓ TGs, ↑ HDL **TOX:** myositis, hepatoxicity

Autonomics

Direct cholinergic agonists

Ach	**MOA**: physiologic cholinergic agonist **IND:** no clinical use; ACh decreases heart rate, cardiac output, and blood pressure **TOX (for all direct cholinergic agonists):** 1. Diarrhea 2. Diaphoresis 3. Miosis (pupillary constriction) 4. Nausea 5. Urinary urgency
Bethanechol	**MOA**: binds primarily at muscarinic receptors; stimulates bowel and bladder smooth muscle contraction **IND**: postoperative ileus and urinary retention
Pilocarpine	**MOA**: direct cholinergic agonist that activates ciliary muscle of the eye and pupillary sphincter **IND**: glaucoma

Indirect cholinergic agonists (anticholinesterases)

Neostigmine, physostigmine	**MOA:** inhibitor of acetylcholinesterase → accumulation of ACh at synapses **IND:** postoperative ileus, urinary retention, myasthenia gravis, reversal of neuromuscular blockade; atropine overdose (physostigmine) **TOX:** generalized convulsions (rare)
Edrophonium, pyridostigmine	**MOA:** inhibitor of acetylcholinesterase **IND:** diagnosis (edrophonium) and treatment (pyridostigmine) of myasthenia gravis
Echothiophate	**MOA:** irreversible inhibitor of acetylcholinesterase **IND:** treatment of organophosphate overdose, glaucoma
List the toxicities of acetylcholinesterase poisoning (caused by parathion or organophosphates):	"DUMBELS" Diarrhea Urination Miosis (pupillary constriction) Bronchoconstriction Excitation of skeletal muscles Lacrimation Sweating and salivation
Atropine	**MOA:** nonselective muscarinic antagonist **IND:** pupillary dilation, reduction of gastric acid secretion, reduction of GI motility, reduction of airway and salivary secretions, organophosphate/cholinergic poisoning **TOX: "Dry as a bone, Red as a beet, Blind as a bat, Mad as a hatter, Hot as a hare"** **Dry as a bone:** ↓ perspiration, lacrimation, salivation **Red as a beet:** dry, red skin **Blind as a bat:** blurry vision (from miosis) **Hot as a hare:** hyperthermia
Describe how atropine acts on the following organs or systems:	
Eyes	Pupillary dilation (bella donna alkaloid), mydriasis, cycloplegia
Airways	Blocks bronchial secretion, bronchodilation
Salivary glands	Blocks salivary secretion

Heart	Tachycardia
Scopolamine	**MOA:** nonselective muscarinic antagonist **IND:** motion sickness, vertigo
Ipratropium	**MOA:** nonselective muscarinic antagonist **IND:** bronchodilator used for asthma or COPD
Benztropine	**MOA:** centrally acting antimuscarinic agent **IND:** adjuvant therapy for Parkinson disease
Succinylcholine	**MOA:** depolarizing neuromuscular blocker (nicotinic antagonist) **IND:** neuromuscular blockade during general anesthesia **TOX:** malignant hyperthermia when combined with halogenated anesthetic agents in susceptible patients (treat with dantrolene)
Tubocurarine, atracurium, vecuronium	**MOA:** nondepolarizing neuromuscular blocker **IND:** neuromuscular blockade during general anesthesia; atracurium and vecuronium are degraded in the plasma and therefore preferred in patients with renal failure **TOX:** may cause histamine release resulting in bronchospasm, skin wheals, and hypotension
Pralidoxime	**MOA:** cholinesterase regenerator **IND:** used for organophosphate poisoning

State the MOA for each of the following agents:

Botulinum	Inhibits release of ACh in cholinergic neurons
Amphetamine	Stimulates release of NE from adrenergic neurons (indirect-acting amines)
Cocaine, tricyclic antidepressants	Inhibit reuptake of NE from synapse

Direct adrenergic agonists

EPI	**MOA:** agonist at α_1, α_2, β_1, β_2 receptors **IND:** acute, refractory asthma (bronchodilator), open angle glaucoma, anaphylactic shock, used with local anesthetic to ↑ duration of action (local vasoconstriction) **TOX:** CNS disturbance, HTN, arrhythmia, pulmonary edema

Describe the effect of EPI on each of the following organs or tissues:

Myocardium	Positive inotropic and chronotropic effects (β_1)
Blood vessels	Overall ↑ blood pressure (vasoconstriction of cutaneous mucous membrane and visceral vasculature; vasodilation of liver and skeletal muscle vasculature) ($\alpha_1 > \beta_2$)
Lungs	Bronchodilation (β_2)
Liver	Increased glycogenolysis, increased insulin release (β_2)
Adipose tissue	Increased lipolysis (α_2, β_1, β_2, β_3)
Pupils	Mydriasis (α_1 radial dilator muscle contraction); accommodation for far vision (β_2 ciliary muscle relaxation)
Skin	Piloerection(α_1)
NE	**MOA:** selective adrenergic agonist; strong α-agonist that also stimulates β_1 receptors; NE produces only minimal stimulation of β_2 receptors **IND:** useful in maintaining blood pressure in shock

Compare the effects of NE and EPI at the different adrenergic receptors.	α_1 EPI $\geq$ NE α_2 EPI $\geq$ NE β_1 EPI = NE β_2 EPI $>>$ NE creates difference
Phenylephrine	**MOA:** direct adrenergic agonist; stimulates $\alpha_1 > \alpha_2$ **IND:** nasal decongestant **TOX:** causes HTN

Clonidine	**MOA:** direct adrenergic agonist; stimulates $\alpha_2 > \alpha_1$
	IND: HTN (especially in pregnant patients), nicotine, heroin, and cocaine withdrawal
	TOX: rebound HTN, dry mouth, drowsiness
Isoproterenol	**MOA:** direct adrenergic agonist; stimulates β_1 and β_2 receptors equally
	IND: bradycardia, bronchodilator used in asthma
Dobutamine	**MOA:** direct adrenergic agonist; stimulates $\beta_1 > \beta_2$
	IND: positive inotropic agent used to improve cardiac output in heart failure
	TOX: arrhythmias
Albuterol, terbutaline	**MOA:** direct adrenergic agonist; $\beta_2 > \beta_1$
	IND: bronchodilator used in asthma; slows preterm labor by inhibiting uterine contraction (terbutaline)
	TOX: tremor, tachycardia
Dopamine	**MOA:** direct adrenergic agonist; stimulates D_1 and D_2 receptors equally
	IND: maintenance of blood pressure in shock
	TOX: arrhythmia
What is the toxicity of most adrenergic agonists?	1. CNS disturbance—fear, anxiety, tension, headache 2. HTN 3. Arrhythmia 4. Pulmonary edema

Indirect adrenergic agonists

Amphetamine	**MOA:** stimulates release of NE from adrenergic neurons
	IND: attention deficit hyperactivity disorder, narcolepsy, appetite control
	TOX: psychosis, anxiety
Ephedrine	**MOA:** stimulates release of NE from synaptic vesicles in adrenergic neurons
	IND: nasal decongestant, enhances athletic performance
	TOX: causes HTN

Cocaine	**MOA:** inhibition of catecholamine reuptake
	IND: local anesthetic
	TOX: arrhythmias, MI, seizures

Adrenergic antagonists

Phenoxybenzamine	**MOA:** irreversible adrenergic antagonist; blocks $\alpha_1 > \alpha_2$
	IND: HTN 2° to pheochromocytoma
	TOX: nasal congestion, postural hypotension, compensatory tachycardia
Phentolamine	**MOA:** reversible adrenergic antagonist; blocks α_1 and α_2 receptors equally
	IND: diagnosis of pheochromocytoma; management of intraoperative HTN
Prazosin, terazosin	**MOA:** adrenergic antagonist; selectively blocks α_1 receptors
	IND: treatment of HTN and benign prostatic hypertrophy
	TOX: orthostatic hypotension
Propranolol	**MOA:** adrenergic antagonist, blocks both β_1 and β_2 receptors
	IND: HTN, angina prophylaxis, antiarrhythmic, anxiety, thyroid storm, migraine prophylaxis
	TOX: bronchoconstriction, arrhythmias, sexual dysfunction, CNS sedation, and fatigue

Describe the effect of propranolol on each of the following tissues:

Heart	Decreased cardiac output
Blood vessels	Reflex peripheral vasoconstriction
Kidneys	Increased Na^+ retention
Lungs	Bronchoconstriction
Metoprolol, atenolol, esmolol	**MOA:** adrenergic antagonist; selectively blocks β_1 receptors
	IND: HTN, angina prophylaxis, MI, superventricular tachycardia
	TOX: hypotension, bradycardia, hyperglycemia

List two β-blockers with intrinsic sympathomimetic activity:

1. Acebutolol
2. Pindolol

Which β-blockers also block α_1 receptors?	Labetalol and carvedilol
What are the six common side effects of β-blockers?	1. Bronchoconstriction/asthma attack 2. Arrhythmia 3. Sexual dysfunction 4. Fasting hypoglycemia, masking of hypoglycemic signs 5. CNS sedation, fatigue 6. Hypotension

Describe the effect of dopamine on each of the following organs or tissues:

Myocardium	Positive inotropic and chronotropic effects
Blood vessels	Vasoconstriction →↑ BP
Kidneys	Increases renal blood flow at low and moderate doses

CHAPTER 6

Pulmonary

EMBRYOLOGY

From what structure does the lung bud arise?	Foregut
From which embryonic layer is the lining of the respiratory tract derived?	Endoderm
From which embryonic layer is the muscle and connective tissue of the respiratory tract derived?	Mesoderm
What is the consequence of incomplete separation of the lung bud from the esophagus?	Tracheoesophageal fistula (TEF)
What is the most typical type of TEF?	Esophageal atresia (ends in blind pouch) with distal TEF
What other constellation of developmental abnormalities should you look for with TEF?	**VATER** syndrome: Vertebral, Anal, Tracheal, Esophageal, Radial/Renal
At what gestational age is a human capable of respiration?	25 weeks
In what period do the majority of alveoli develop?	Postpartum
What histology is typical of cells lining the conducting airway?	Pseudocolumnar ciliated cells
Which cells produce surfactant?	Type II pneumocytes
List the structures the diaphragm is derived from:	"Several Parts Build Diaphragm"— Septum transversum, Pleuroperitoneal folds, Body wall, Dorsal mesentery of esophagus

Which disorder results from abnormal development of the diaphragm?

Diaphragmatic or hiatal hernia

Where can pain from the diaphragm refer?

To the shoulder

ANATOMY

Which nerve provides motor innervations to the diaphragm?

Phrenic nerve ("C3, C4, C5 keep the diaphragm alive")

Which muscles are involved in respiration?

Diaphragm (most important), external intercostals, sternocleidomastoids, anterior and medial scalene

What area of the left lung is most similar to the right middle lobe?

Lingula (technically part of the left upper lobe)

Which lobe does foreign body aspiration most commonly affect when supine?

Superior segment of right lower lobe (because right main stem bronchus is wider, more vertical, and the superior segment ostium is posteriorly located)

The bifurcation of the trachea occurs at the level of which vertebral body?

Intervertebral disk T4 to T5

What four structures make up a bronchopulmonary segment?

1. Segmental bronchus
2. Branch of the pulmonary artery
3. Branch of the bronchial artery
4. Tributaries of the pulmonary vein

Which syndrome can result from a malignant tumor in the region of the superior pulmonary sulcus?

Pancoast syndrome (lower trunk brachial plexopathy and Horner syndrome)

Most common site of epistaxis

Kiesselbach plexus (anterior nostril)

Name the three structures that pass through the diaphragm:

Vena cava (T8), esophagus (T10), aorta (T12)

Cellular precursor to Type I and Type II pneumocytes

Type II pneumocytes

Lung malformation associated with Potter sequence

Pulmonary hypoplasia

PHYSIOLOGY

Lung Volumes and Capacities

Name the lung volume defined below:

Expired volume with each normal breath	Tidal volume (TV)
Volume that can be inspired beyond the TV	Inspiratory reserve volume (IRV)
Volume that can be expired beyond the TV	Expiratory reserve volume (ERV)
Volume that remains in the lungs after maximal expiration	Residual volume (RV)

Name the lung capacity defined below:

TV + IRV	Inspiratory capacity (IC)
ERV + RV	Functional residual capacity (FRC)
TV + IRV + ERV	Vital capacity (VC)
Volume which can be forcibly expired in 1 second after maximal inspiration	Forced expiratory volume (FEV1)
Total volume which can be forcibly expired	Forced VC (FVC)
TV + IRV + ERV + RV	Total lung capacity (TLC)

What is the formula for minute ventilation?	TV × respiratory rate (breaths per minute)

Lung Compliance and Resistance

What is the relationship between compliance and elasticity?	Compliance and elasticity are inversely related
Name five common causes of decreased lung compliance:	1. Pulmonary fibrosis 2. Atelectasis 3. Acute respiratory distress syndrome (ARDS) 4. Neonatal respiratory distress syndrome 5. Pulmonary edema
What is a common smoking-related cause of increased lung compliance?	Emphysema, normal aging lungs

What is the effect of surfactant on alveolar surface tension and lung compliance?

Surfactant decreases surface tension to allow small alveoli to stay open and increases compliance

What is the law of Laplace?

Pressure = 2 × surface tension/radius; the larger the radius of the vessel/airway, the more stable and less likely it is to collapse

What is the relationship between airflow and resistance?

Airflow is inversely proportional to airway resistance

What is the relationship between airway radius and resistance?

Resistance is inversely proportional to the fourth power of the radius (Poiseuille law)

Hemoglobin

For each factor below, state whether airway resistance will be increased or decreased:

Bronchoconstriction

Increased (↑)

Parasympathetic stimulation

Increased (↑)

Sympathetic stimulation

Decreased (↓)

High lung volumes

Decreased (↓)

Low lung volumes

Increased (↑)

For each of the factors below, determine whether the hemoglobin dissociation curve will be shifted to the left or to the right?

Increased P_{CO_2}

Right (decreased affinity)

Increased pH

Left (increased affinity)

Decreased temperature

Left (increased affinity)

Increased 2,3-bisphosphoglycerate (2,3-BPG) concentration

Right (decreased affinity)

Fetal hemoglobin

Left (increased affinity)

Carbon monoxide poisoning

Left (increased affinity)
Note: ↑ in any factor (except pH) results in right shift

What is the mnemonic for right shift?

CADET face RIGHT (CO_2, Acid/ Altitude, DPG (2,3-DPG), Exercise, Temperature

Which quaternary conformation of Hb has the highest affinity for oxygen?

The R (relaxed form)

How does hemoglobin's affinity for O_2 compare to that of CO?

The affinity of CO is 200 times as great as that of O_2

What are the signs and symptoms of carbon monoxide toxicity?

Headache, nausea/vomiting, loss of consciousness, confusion; blood samples are bright red due to high affinity for oxygen

What are the three ways in which CO_2 is transported from the tissues to the lungs (listed in order of importance)?

1. As HCO_3^- in erythrocytes
2. Bound to hemoglobin (carbaminohemoglobin)
3. Dissolved in blood (P_{CO_2})

Which enzyme catalyzes the conversion of CO_2 into HCO_3^-?

Carbonic anhydrase

Which protein is the main buffer within erythrocytes?

Deoxyhemoglobin

Acclimatization to High Altitude

For each of the values below, determine how they are affected by high altitude *acutely*:

Ventilation

Increased ($\uparrow$)

PaO2

Decreased ($\downarrow$) (due to decreased partial pressure of atmospheric O_2)

$PaCO_2$

Decreased ($\downarrow$) (due to hyperventilation)

Systemic arterial pH

Increased ($\uparrow$)

Hemoglobin saturation

Decreased ($\downarrow$)

Hemoglobin concentration

No change

For each of the values below, determine how they are affected by high altitude *chronically*:

Ventilation

Increased ($\uparrow$)

PaO_2

Decreased ($\downarrow$) (due to decreased partial pressure of atmospheric O_2)

$PaCO_2$

Decreased ($\downarrow$) (due to hyperventilation)

Systemic arterial pH

Increased ($\uparrow$) (but closer to normal due to renal excretion of bicarbonate)

Hemoglobin saturation	Decreased ($\downarrow$)
Hemoglobin concentration	Increased ($\uparrow$) (polycythemia due to increased erythropoietin production)

Lung Zones

Choose the zone or region of the lungs that fits each description below:

Alveolar pressure > arterial pressure > venous pressure	Zone 1
Arterial pressure > alveolar pressure > venous pressure	Zone 2
Arterial pressure > venous pressure > alveolar pressure	Zone 3
V/Q ≈ 3 → wasted ventilation	Apex
V/Q ≈ 0.6 → wasted perfusion	Base

What is the effect of hypoxia on pulmonary blood vessels?	Vasoconstriction **Note:** hypoxia causes vasodilation in all other vascular beds
What is the quotient of V/Q in a lung where the pulmonary artery is completely occluded (shunt-unventilated blood)?	∞
What is the quotient of V/Q in complete airway obstruction (physiologic dead space)?	0

Neurologic Regulation of Respiration

Describe the function of each of the following neural structures in the control of respiration:

Medullary respiratory center	Determines the rhythm of breathing by controlling inspiration and expiration
Pontine apneustic center	Stimulates inspiration
Cerebral cortex	Voluntary control of respiration
Lung stretch receptors in bronchial smooth muscle	Reflexive slowing of respiratory frequency (Hering-Breuer reflex)
Irritant receptors in airway epithelial cells	Initiate coughing

Juxtacapillary (J) receptors in alveolar walls	Cause dyspnea when stretched due to pulmonary edema
Joint and muscle receptors	Stimulate respiration at the initiation of exercise
Medullary chemoreceptors	Increase breathing rate in response to low pH
Peripheral chemoreceptors in the carotid and aortic bodies	Increase breathing rate in response to low arterial P_{O_2}, low pH, and high P_{CO_2}

PATHOLOGY

Pulmonary Edema, ARDS, and Neonatal RDS

Which syndrome is characterized by diffuse alveolar damage, pulmonary edema, and respiratory failure?	Acute respiratory distress syndrome
What type of material is seen in the alveoli of a patient in the acute phase of ARDS?	Hyaline membranes formed by a fibrinous exudate and necrotic cellular debris
What are some of the causes of ARDS?	Shock of any etiology, fat embolism, gram-negative sepsis, severe bacteria/viral infections, near-drowning, aspiration of GI contents, acute pancreatitis, heroin overdose, oxygen toxicity, cytotoxic drugs, snake bite
What is the most common cause of respiratory failure in the newborn and also of death in premature infants <28 weeks gestational age?	Neonatal respiratory distress syndrome (hyaline membrane disease)
What is the typical clinical presentation of neonatal respiratory distress syndrome?	Preterm infants with initially normal respirations followed by cyanosis, tachypnea, and signs of respiratory distress
What is the pathogenesis of neonatal respiratory distress syndrome?	Deficiency of pulmonary surfactant leading to increased surface tension
What type of cells produces pulmonary surfactant?	Type II pneumocytes
What is the predominant chemical in pulmonary surfactant?	Dipalmitoyl phosphatidylcholine (lecithin)

What is the diagnostic test of choice to judge fetal lung maturity?	Amniotic fluid lecithin: sphingomyelin ratio (a ratio of 2:1 implies adequate surfactant is present)
What are the three strongest risk factors for neonatal respiratory distress syndrome?	1. Prematurity 2. Maternal diabetes 3. Delivery by C-section
What is the classic pathologic finding in the alveoli of an infant with neonatal respiratory distress syndrome?	Intra-alveolar hyaline membranes
Infants surviving an initial bout of neonatal respiratory distress syndrome are at risk for which five complications?	1. Bronchopulmonary dysplasia (resulting in part from oxygen therapy) 2. Retinopathy of prematurity (resulting from oxygen therapy) 3. Patent ductus arteriosus 4. Intraventricular cerebral hemorrhage 5. Necrotizing enterocolitis
What medications can you give to prevent neonatal respiratory distress syndrome?	Glucocorticoids given to the mother can accelerate fetal lung maturation and reduce the risk of neonatal respiratory distress syndrome

Pulmonary Embolism

What are the most common clinical presentations of PE?	Tachycardia, tachypnea, dyspnea, pleuritic chest pain
What is the etiology of 95% of pulmonary emboli?	Dislodged deep venous thromboses (DVT) from the deep veins of the thigh or pelvis
What factors favor the development of a DVT?	Virchow triad: (1) stasis, (2) hypercoagulability, (3) endothelial dysfunction
How do you diagnose a PE radiographically?	CT angiogram (1st line), V/Q scan, or pulmonary angiography (gold standard)
What type of tumors commonly causes a DVT by inducing a hypercoagulable state?	Adenocarcinomas
What is the most common genetic disease that predisposes to the development of DVT?	Factor V Leiden
What type of embolism can develop uniquely in a peripartum woman?	Amniotic fluid embolism

For what type of embolism is a patient with a long bone fracture at risk?	Fat emboli from bone marrow, pulmonary thromboembolism due to trauma and stasis
What type of infarction results from a PE?	Hemorrhagic infarction (appears as wedge-shaped opacity on chest x-ray [CXR])
What therapy is indicated for high-risk patients during the workup of PE and for patients diagnosed with PE?	Full treatment doses of heparin (unfractionated or low molecular weight)
What is used for long-term prophylaxis for patients at risk of developing DVT?	Anticoagulants (ie, Vitamin K antagonists, Factor Xa antagonists, direct thrombin inhibitors)

Obstructive Lung Disease

What are the most common disease categories causing pulmonary hypertension?	1. Chronic obstructive pulmonary disease (COPD) 2. Left-sided heart disease 2. Recurrent PE 3. Collagen vascular disease
How is the heart affected by long-standing pulmonary hypertension?	Pulmonary hypertension causes right ventricular hypertrophy and dilatation
What is the reversal of a left-to-right shunt to a right-to-left shunt due to long-standing pulmonary hypertension?	Eisenmenger syndrome
What is the effect of COPD on hematocrit (Hct)?	Chronic hypoxia leads $\rightarrow\uparrow$ Hct (ie, secondary polycythemia)
What is the effect of COPD on FEV_1/FVC?	$\downarrow FEV_1/FVC$ <0.8
Name the obstructive pulmonary disorder described by the following pathologic features:	
Smooth muscle and goblet cell hyperplasia; mucus-plugged airways containing Curschmann spirals, eosinophils, and Charcot-Leyden crystals	Bronchial asthma
Hyperplasia of bronchial submucosal glands, hypersecretion of mucus, squamous metaplasia, or dysplasia of bronchial epithelium	Chronic bronchitis

Permanent airway dilation and scarring; inflammation and necrosis of bronchial walls and alveolar fibrosis	Bronchiectasis
Alveolar enlargement due to alveolar wall destruction; ↓ lung elasticity	Pulmonary emphysema
Diagnosed clinically by productive cough for >3 consecutive months for 2+ years	Chronic bronchitis
Name the chronic disorder characterized by increased airway reactivity, resulting in paroxysmal bronchial contraction:	Bronchial asthma
What type of hypersensitivity response is seen in atopic asthma?	Type I hypersensitivity response mediated by IgE and mast cells, eosinophils, and basophils
What other conditions are typically seen in association with atopic asthma?	Allergic rhinitis, eczema
Name several common triggers of atopic asthma:	Dust, pollen, food, and animal dander
Name several triggers of nonatopic asthma:	Respiratory tract infection, cold, chemical irritants, exercise
What are the two common presenting features of bronchial asthma?	1. Dyspnea 2. Wheezing
What are the three common presenting features of bronchiectasis?	1. Abundant, copious, often foul-smelling sputum 2. Chronic cough 3. Hemoptysis
What are the components of an acinus of the lungs?	Alveoli, air ducts, respiratory bronchioles, terminal bronchioles
Name the type of emphysema described below:	
Enlargement of bronchioles, typically in the upper lobes and apices (most often associated with smoking)	Centriacinar emphysema
Destruction and dilation of entire acinus, typically in the lower lobes; associated with α_1-antitrypsin deficiency	Panacinar emphysema

Destruction of the distal acinus occurring typically near the pleura and areas of fibrosis that may cause pneumothorax	Paraseptal emphysema
How does smoking cause emphysema?	Smoke particles recruit inflammatory cells, promote the release and enhance the activity of elastase, and inhibit the activity of α_1-antitrypsin
What is the role of α_1-antitrypsin deficiency in the development of emphysema?	The lack of this protease inhibitor results in the digestion of the elastin in alveolar walls by elastase
What is the effect of emphysema on the anteroposterior diameter of the chest and the TLC?	Both are increased

Restrictive Lung Disease

What general category of pulmonary disease is characterized by dyspnea, decreased lung volumes, and decreased compliance?	Restrictive lung disease
What is the effect of restrictive lung disease on FEV_1/FVC?	$\downarrow FEV_1/FVC \geq 0.8$
What are the two categories of restrictive lung disease?	1. *Pulmonary*: interstitial lung disease or pneumonitis, resulting in poor lung expansion 2. *Extrapulmonary*: extrapulmonary disease associated with disorders of the chest wall, obesity, pleura, or respiratory muscles
Name the specific type of restrictive lung disease described below:	
65-year-old (y/o) hay farmer with recent exposure to moldy hay presents with chronic dry cough, chest tightness; physical examination (PE): bilateral diffuse rales; bronchoscopy: interstitial inflammation; bronchioalveolar lavage: lymphocyte and mast cell predominance	Hypersensitivity pneumonitis
35-y/o man presents with intermittent hemoptysis and hematuria; W/U demonstrates alveolar hemorrhage and acute glomerulonephritis	Anti-glomerular basement membrane (Anti-GBM) disease (Goodpasture syndrome)

40-y/o with progressive hypoxemia and cor pulmonale; lung biopsy demonstrates chronic inflammation of the alveolar wall in a pattern consistent with honeycomb lung; bronchioalveolar lavage: mild eosinophilia	Idiopathic pulmonary fibrosis
58-y/o former shipbuilder presents with the insidious onset of dyspnea; transbronchial biopsy demonstrates interstitial pulmonary fibrosis, ferruginous bodies; chest CT scan demonstrates pleural effusion and dense pleural fibrocalcific plaques	Asbestosis
55-y/o miner (nonsmoker) presents with dyspnea and dry cough; pulmonary function tests (PFTs) show both obstructive and restrictive pattern; chest x-ray (CXR): hilar lymphadenopathy with eggshell calcifications	Silicosis
60-y/o male with 100 pack-year history of (h/o) smoking presents with pleuritic chest pain, hemoptysis, and dyspnea; PE: dullness to percussion and absent breath sounds in the right lower lung field	Pleural effusion (secondary to malignancy)
50-y/o former heavy smoker presents with multiple lung and rib lesions; biopsy: cells (similar to the Langerhans cells of the skin) containing tennis racket–shaped Birbeck granules	Eosinophilic granuloma
30-y/o black female presents with DOE, fever, arthralgia; PE: iritis, erythema nodosum; W/U: eosinophilia, ↑ serum ACE levels; PFT: restrictive pattern; CXR: bilateral hilar lymphadenopathy interstitial infiltrates; lymph node biopsy: non-caseating granulomas	Sarcoidosis
Which typically asymptomatic disorder causes visible black deposits in the lungs of coal workers?	Anthracosis
Which three medications are known to commonly cause interstitial lung disease?	Bleomycin, methotrexate, and amiodarone

Pulmonary Infections

What infection is characterized by fever >39°C, chills, cough productive of blood-tinged, purulent sputum, pleuritic pain, hypoxia, and lobar infiltrate on CXR?

Acute pneumonia

What infection is characterized by fever <39°C, nonproductive cough, GI upset, and diffuse patchy infiltrates on CXR?

Atypical pneumonia

Name the most common organism(s) associated with the pulmonary infection described below:

Community-acquired acute pneumonia

Streptococcus pneumoniae and viruses

Commonly follow a viral respiratory infection

Staphylococcus aureus and *Haemophilus influenzae*

Interstitial pneumonia

Mycoplasma pneumoniae (most common), *Chlamydia pneumoniae*

Fungal pneumonia in an AIDS patient

Pneumocystis jirovecii (previously *Pneumocystis carinii*)

Typical pneumonia in neonate

Streptococcus agalactiae (group B streptococcus)

Typical pneumonia in an alcoholic after aspiration

Klebsiella pneumoniae

Atypical pneumonia in patient with positive cold agglutinin test

M. pneumoniae

Atypical pneumonia in a neonate with trachoma

Chlamydia trachomatis

Atypical pneumonia in a dairy worker

Coxiella burnetii

Atypical pneumonia in a rabbit hunter

Francisella tularensis

Pneumonia in a bird owner with splenomegaly and bradycardia

Chlamydia psittaci

Hospitalized patient with lobar pneumonia

S. pneumoniae > *S. aureus*

Pneumonia in an IV drug user

S. pneumoniae, *K. pneumoniae*, and *S. aureus*

Atypical pneumonia in a spelunker from the Ohio river valley

Histoplasma capsulatum

Atypical pneumonia in a patient from the southwestern United States	*Coccidioides immitis*
Associated with spread by inhalation of contaminated water droplets from air conditioners	*Legionella pneumophila*

Name the most common causative pathogen(s) of pneumonia for each age group below:

Neonates	Group B *streptococci, Escherichia coli, Listeria*
Children (6 weeks–18 years)	RSV and other viruses, *M. pneumoniae, C. pneumoniae, S. pneumoniae*
Adults (18–40 years old)	*M. pneumoniae, C. pneumoniae, S. pneumoniae*
Adults (45–65 years old)	*S. pneumoniae, H. influenzae,* anaerobes, viruses, *M. pneumoniae*
Adults (>65 years old)	*S. pneumoniae,* viruses, anaerobes, *H. influenzae,* gram-negative rods

Name three common complications of lobar pneumonia:	1. Abscess formation (especially *S. aureus* and anaerobes) 2. Empyema or spread of infection to the pleural cavity 3. Sepsis
What type of pulmonary infection is characterized by localized suppurative necrosis of lung tissue?	Lung abscess
Name several bacterial pathogens capable of causing lung abscess:	*S. aureus,* aerobic and anaerobic streptococci, gram-negative bacilli, and anaerobic oral flora

Cystic Fibrosis

What is the most common lethal genetic disease in Caucasians?	Cystic fibrosis (CF)
What is the mode of inheritance of CF?	Autosomal recessive (chromosome 7)
Which membrane protein is defective in CF?	The cystic fibrosis transmembrane conductance regulator (CFTR), a chloride channel protein

What is the function of CFTR?

Regulation of sodium, chloride, and bicarbonate transport across the plasma membrane

What is the most common genetic lesion causing CF?

Deletion of three nucleotides encoding phenylalanine 508 in the CFTR; ΔF508 prevents the normal expression of CFTR

Describe how the ΔF508 mutation prevents normal expression of CFTR:

Altered membrane folding precludes glycosylation and transport to the plasma membrane

What is the end result of the ΔF508 mutation of the *CFTR* gene?

Complete loss of CFTR in the plasma membrane

How does a defect in the CFTR affect exocrine glands?

Altered CFTR activity causes the accumulation of hyperviscid mucus that blocks the secretions of exocrine glands

What tests are used to diagnose CF in infants?

Sweat chloride test (positive if elevated [Cl⁻] in sweat), measurement of nasal potential difference, genotyping (definitive)

How does CF typically present in an infant?

Failure to thrive, meconium ileus, mother complains child "tastes salty"

Describe the effect of CF on each of the following organs:

Lungs

Recurrent pulmonary infections, bronchiectasis; ↑ RV and TLC in chronic disease; ↓ FEV_1/FVC in acute exacerbation; pulmonary hemorrhage may occur

Pancreas

Variable defects in pancreatic exocrine function; may cause pancreatic insufficiency and diabetes mellitus

Intestines

Mucus plugs → small bowel obstruction; meconium ileus in some infants

Liver

Plugging of bile canaliculi → cirrhosis

Epididymis and ductus deferens

Bilateral absence of the vas deferens

Salivary glands

Ductal dilation; squamous metaplasia of ductal epithelium and glandular atrophy

Which organisms are commonly responsible for pulmonary infections in CF?

Pseudomonas aeruginosa, *S. aureus*, and *Pseudomonas cepacia*

What is a common nutritional deficiency in CF?	Deficiency of the fat-soluble vitamins (vitamins A, D, E, and K) due to malabsorption from pancreatic insufficiency
What type of heart disease is common in patients with CF?	Cor pulmonale

Lung Cancer

What is the most common cause of cancer deaths in the United States for both men and women?	Lung cancer
What is the most common type of malignant tumor in the lungs?	Metastasis from non-lung primary malignancies
What are the most common primary lung tumors?	Adenocarcinoma is slightly more common than squamous cell carcinoma

Name the type(s) of primary lung cancer associated with the following features:

Central location	Squamous cell and small (oat) cell carcinomas
Peripheral location	Adenocarcinoma, large cell carcinoma, bronchioalveolar carcinoma
Dysplasia and carcinoma in situ precede development of this tumor	Squamous cell carcinoma
Strongest link to smoking	Squamous cell and small (oat) cell carcinomas
Least linked to smoking, frequently seen in nonsmoking women	Bronchioalveolar carcinoma
Most aggressive tumor	Small (oat) cell carcinoma
Associated with production of PTH-related peptide, hypercalcemia	Squamous cell carcinoma
Associated with production of ADH (SIADH) and ACTH (Cushing syndrome)	Small (oat) cell carcinoma
Carcinoembryonic antigen (CEA) positive	Adenocarcinoma
Secretion of 5-hydroxytryptamine (5-HT, serotonin)	Carcinoid
Oat-like, dark blue cells	Small (oat) cell carcinoma
Tumor cells lining alveolar walls	Bronchioalveolar adenocarcinoma

Giant pleomorphic cells, poor prognosis, and high likelihood of cerebral metastasis	Large cell carcinoma
Tumor at apex of lung causes Horner syndrome or lower brachial plexopathy	Pancoast tumor
Rare pleural tumor is found in patients with a h/o exposure to asbestos	Malignant mesothelioma
Most common cancer in patients with h/o exposure to asbestos	Lung cancer (not mesothelioma)

OTHER PATHOLOGY

Immotile cilia secondary to a dynein arm defect, associated with situs inversus, infertility, bronchiectasis	Kartagener syndrome
Causes stridor, toxic presentation, may be life threatening, thumbprint sign on x-ray, caused by *H. influenzae*	Acute epiglottitis
Causes stridor, nontoxic presentation, steeple sign on x-ray, caused by parainfluenza virus	Laryngotracheobronchitis, croup
Name the diagnosis: patient with hypoxia and dyspnea, no breath sounds on right, right-sided hyperresonance to percussion	Tension pneumothorax, requires emergent needle decompression
What lung pathology shows psammoma bodies on histologic examination?	Mesothelioma

PHARMACOLOGY

For each of the following drugs, provide:
1. The mechanism of action (MOA)
2. Indication(s) (IND)
3. Significant side effects and unique toxicity (TOX) (if any)

Albuterol	**MOA:** β_2-agonist $\rightarrow$ bronchodilator, short acting **IND:** asthma **TOX:** tachycardia, arrhythmias, tremor, hyperglycemia

Inhaled corticosteroids (beclomethasone, fluticasone, triamcinolone)	**MOA:** anti-inflammatory; inhibits smooth muscle hyperreactivity **IND:** moderate-to-severe asthma **TOX:** oropharyngeal thrush, dysphonia
Cromolyn	**MOA:** anti-inflammatory; inhibits histamine release from mast cells **IND:** prophylaxis for asthmatic attack **TOX:** laryngeal edema (very rare)
Ipratropium	**MOA:** bronchodilator; cholinergic antagonist **IND:** COPD **TOX:** Rare—minor systemic manifestations of anticholinergic effect
Leukotriene inhibitors (zileuton, zafirlukast, montelukast)	**MOA:** inhibits leukotriene synthesis (zileuton) or blocks leukotriene receptors (zafirlukast, montelukast) **IND:** prophylaxis for asthmatic attack **TOX:** elevation of liver enzymes
Theophylline	**MOA:** bronchodilator; exact mechanism unknown **IND:** asthma **TOX:** seizures and arrhythmias
What is the drug of choice for mild asthma?	Inhaled albuterol as needed
What is the drug of choice in an asthmatic requiring daily albuterol use?	Inhaled glucocorticoids
Describe how glucocorticoids act on airways to control asthma:	Glucocorticoids reduce inflammation and decrease the reactivity of airways to irritants such as cold, cigarette smoke, allergens, and exercise
Name three agents used in the treatment of allergic rhinitis:	1. Antihistamines (eg, diphenhydramine, loratadine, terfenadine) 2. α-Agonist aerosols (eg, phenylephrine) 3. Corticosteroid nasal sprays (eg, beclomethasone, fluticasone, triamcinolone)
Which class of bronchodilators is useful in patients who cannot tolerate β-agonists?	Anticholinergic agents (eg, ipratropium)
Treatment for methemoglobinemia (oxidized form of hemoglobin, Fe 3+)	Methylene blue
Antibiotic for lung abscess	Clindamycin (or other anaerobic coverage)

CHAPTER 7

Gastroenterology

EMBRYOLOGY

What portion of the GI tract is derived from the embryonic foregut?	From the intra-abdominal esophagus → pancreas (distal to sphincter of Oddi)
What portion of the GI tract is derived from the embryonic midgut?	From the second part of the duodenum → proximal two-thirds of the colon (at the splenic flexure)
What portion of the GI tract is derived from the embryonic hindgut?	From the distal one-third of the colon → rectum (proximal to the pectinate line)
What GI structures are derived from the embryonic ectoderm?	Oropharynx (anterior two-thirds of tongue, lips, parotids, tooth enamel), anus, and rectum (distal to the pectinate line)
Name the embryonic layer supplied by the following arteries:	
Celiac trunk	Foregut
Inferior mesenteric artery	Hindgut
Superior mesenteric artery	Midgut
What embryonic structure gives rise to the anterior two-thirds of the tongue?	First branchial arch
What embryonic structure gives rise to the posterior one-third of the tongue?	Third and fourth branchial arches
What disorder results from failure of fusion of the maxillary and medial nasal processes?	Cleft lip
What disorder results from failure of fusion of the nasal septum, lateral palatine processes, and/or median palatine process?	Cleft palate

What is Meckel diverticulum?	Persistence of the vitelline duct or yolk stalk that may contain ectopic tissue **Remember: "the rule of 2's": 2** in long, **2%** of population, **2** ft from ileocecal valve, presents within **2** years of life, can contain **2** types of epithelia (gastric, pancreatic)
What primordial embryonic structures give rise to the pancreas?	Ventral bud → pancreatic head, uncinate process, main duct Dorsal bud → everything else (body, tail, isthmus, accessory duct)
What congenital defect is caused by abnormal fusion of the ventral and dorsal buds of the pancreas?	Annular pancreas (leads to ring around duodenum and obstruction)
What congenital defect results from failure of migration of neural crest cells, causing an absence of parasym-pathetic ganglion cells in the distal colon?	Hirschsprung (congenital aganglionic) megacolon
What congenital defect results from incomplete canalization of the bile ducts during development and presents shortly after birth with clay-colored stools and jaundice?	Biliary atresia

ANATOMY

What are the four main layers of the wall of the digestive tract?	1. Mucosa 2. Submucosa 3. Muscularis 4. Serosa
Name the enteric plexus associated with the following descriptions:	
Located between mucosa and inner layer of smooth muscle in GI tract wall	Submucosal (Meissner) plexus
Located between inner (circular) and outer (longitudinal) layer of smooth muscle in GI tract wall	Myenteric (Auerbach) plexus
Coordinates motility along the entire gut wall	**M**yenteric plexus = **M**otility

Controls local secretions, absorption, and blood flow	Submucosal plexus = Secretions
Name the lymphoid tissue found in lamina propria and submucosa of small intestine:	Peyer patches
What is the major function of the Peyer patch?	Detect antigens → secrete IgA into lumen
In the liver, which zone of the portal acinus contains the highest O_2 concentration and nutrients?	Zone 1
Which zone of the portal acinus contains the lowest O_2 concentration and nutrients?	Zone 3
Name the three major branches of the abdominal aorta and their approximate vertebral level:	1. Celiac trunk (T12) 2. Superior mesenteric artery (L1) 3. Inferior mesenteric artery (L3)
What structure provides collateral venous drainage to the superior vena cava (SVC) when there is obstruction of the inferior vena cava (IVC)?	Azygous vein
Name the four key sites for portal-systemic shunt and the veins involved:	1. Esophagus (left gastric → esophageal) 2. Umbilicus (paraumbilical → superficial/inferior epigastric) 3. Rectum (superior rectal → middle/inferior rectal) 4. Posterior abdominal wall (colic → lumbar)
Which two vessels merge to form the portal vein?	Splenic (inferior mesenteric vein has already joined the splenic vein) and superior mesenteric veins
What important neural structure traverses the parotid gland?	Facial nerve (CN VII)
What are the muscles of mastication?	Three open: masseter, temporalis, and medial pterygoid; one close: lateral pterygoid
What types of muscle are found in the esophagus?	Proximal 1/3 = skeletal; distal 1/3 = smooth; middle 1/3 = both

What is the function of the pylorus? — Acts as muscular sphincter to regulate movement of food out of the stomach and prevents reflux of duodenal contents

Which blood vessel lies posterior to the first part of the duodenum? — Gastroduodenal artery (a concern in cases of posterior perforation due to ulcers)

The common bile duct and main pancreatic duct empty into what portion of the duodenum? — Second (descending) part

The common bile duct and pancreatic duct drain into the duodenum through what structure? — Hepatopancreatic ampulla (of Vater)

What structure controls the release of bile into the duodenum? — Sphincter of Oddi

Which two ducts combine to form the common bile duct?
1. Common hepatic
2. Cystic duct

What structures make up the porta hepatis? — Hepatic artery, portal vein, common bile duct (in gastroduodenal ligament)

What is the "bare area" of the liver? — A portion of the diaphragmatic surface of the liver that is devoid of peritoneum

What divides the left and right lobes of the liver? — Interlobar fissure (an invisible line running from the gallbladder to the IVC)

What structure supports the duodenum at the duodenojejunal flexure? — Suspensory ligament (of Treitz)

Name the intestinal structures (duodenum, ileum, jejunum, or colon) associated with each of the following characteristics:

Brunner's glands — Duodenum

Greatest number of goblet cells in the small intestine — Ileum

Long, finger-shaped villi — Jejunum

Intestinal glands (crypts) and <3 cm luminal diameter — Ileum

No villi, large crypts, and 6 to 9 cm luminal diameter — Colon

Large, numerous, plicae circularis	Jejunum
Accounts for the terminal three-fifths of the small intestine	Ileum
Contains fatty tags (appendices epiploicae)	Colon
Contains prominent Peyer patches	Ileum
Contains long vasa recta	Jejunum
What term is used to describe the three longitudinal bands of smooth muscle in the colon?	Teniae coli
What is the name for the wall sacculations in the colon that are separated by the plicae semilunares?	Haustra
What anatomic feature divides the upper and lower anal canal?	Pectinate line
Describe the arterial supply, venous drainage, and innervation of internal hemorrhoids:	Vasculature = superior rectal artery/vein (drains to portal circulation); visceral innervation → not painful
Describe the arterial supply, venous drainage, and innervation of external hemorrhoids:	Vasculature = inferior rectal artery/vein (drains to systemic circulation via IVC); somatic innervation → painful
Describe the lymphatic drainage of internal hemorrhoids	Internal iliac nodes
Describe the lymphatic drainage of external hemorrhoids	Superficial inguinal nodes
What type of muscle is found in the internal anal sphincter?	Smooth muscle (under involuntary control via autonomic innervation)
What type of muscle is found in the external anal sphincter?	Striated muscle (under voluntary control via the pudendal nerve)
What are the boundaries of Hesselbach triangle?	Inferior epigastric artery, inguinal ligament, lateral border of rectus abdominus muscle
Name the types of hernia:	
Peritoneum protrudes through Hesselbach triangle, medial to the inferior epigastric artery	Direct hernia

Retroperitoneal structures to enter the thorax because of defective development of pleuroperitoneal membrane	Diaphragmatic hernia
Peritoneum protrudes through both the internal (deep) and external (superficial) inguinal rings	Indirect hernia
Stomach herniates upward through the esophageal hiatus of the diaphragm	Hiatal hernia
Occurs in infants as a result of failure of processus vaginalis to close	Indirect hernia
Protrudes below the inguinal ligaments and lateral to the pubic tubercle; more common in females	Femoral hernia

PHYSIOLOGY

Saliva

Which three glands produce saliva?	1. Parotid 2. Submandibular 3. Sublingual
Name three important functions of saliva:	1. Protection of dental health by buffering oral bacterial acids 2. Digestion (starches by α-amylase); triglycerides (TGs) by lingual lipase 3. Lubrication of food with mucins
What determines the relative composition of salivary contents?	Flow rate
How is the regulation of saliva production unique?	It is stimulated by *both* parasympathetic and sympathetic activity

GI Hormones and Secretions

Name the source of the following GI secretory products:

Intrinsic factor (IF)	Parietal cells (stomach)
Pepsinogen	Chief cells (stomach)
Histamine	Mast cells (stomach)

Gastric acid (H$^+$)	Parietal cells (stomach)
Gastrin	Antral G cells and duodenum
Bicarbonate	Surface mucosal cells (of stomach and duodenum)
Secretin	S cells (duodenum)
Somatostatin	D cells (duodenum)
Cholecystokinin (CCK)	I cells (duodenum) and jejunum
Gastric inhibitory peptide (GIP)	Duodenum and jejunum

For each of the following substances, state the factors that regulate its secretion:

Gastric acid (H$^+$)	↑ By histamine, acetylcholine (ACh), gastrin; ↓ by prostaglandin, somatostatin, GIP
Pepsinogen	↑ By vagal stimulation (ACh) and low pH
Gastrin	↑ By small peptides and amino acids (AAs) (Phe and Trp = most potent), gastric distention, and vagus (via gastrin-releasing peptide[GRP]); ↓ by pH <3.0 and secretin
Bicarbonate in pancreatic secretions	↑ By secretin (potentiated by CCK and vagal input)
Secretin	Acid (H$^+$ and fatty acids [FAs]) in the duodenum
Somatostatin	↑ By acid; ↓ by vagus
CCK	↑ By FAs, AAs, and small peptides
GIP	↑ By FAs, AAs, and oral glucose

List the most important functions of the following GI secretions:

Intrinsic factor (IF)	Binds vitamin B$_{12}$ for uptake in terminal ileum
Gastric acid (H$^+$)	Converts pepsinogen to pepsin and sterilizes chyme **Note:** inadequate acid production →↑ risk of *Salmonella* infections
Pepsinogen	Digests protein
Gastrin	↑ Secretion of IF, HCl, and pepsinogen; stimulates gastric motility and growth of gastric mucosa

Bicarbonate	Neutralizes acid → prevents autodigestion
Secretin	↑ Pancreatic HCO_3^- secretion; ↓ gastric acid secretion
Vasoactive intestinal peptide (VIP)	↑ Secretion of water into pancreatic juice, ↓ absorption
Somatostatin	↓ H^+ and pepsinogen secretion, ↓ pancreatic and SI secretions, ↓ gallbladder contraction, ↓ release of both insulin and glucagon
CCK	↑ Gallbladder contraction, ↑ pancreatic enzyme secretion, ↓ gastric emptying
GIP	↑ Insulin (especially in response to oral glucose); ↓ H^+ secretion

What mechanisms regulate the release of gastric acid by parietal cells?	1. Paracrine (histamine) 2. Neural (vagus innervation) 3. Hormonal (gastrin)
Which enzyme in the parietal cell catalyzes the production of H^+ and HCO_3^- from CO_2 and H_2O?	Carbonic anhydrase
How is H^+ secreted into the lumen of the stomach?	H^+/K^+ ATPase pumps H^+ out of cells and Cl^- diffuses concurrently to maintain electrical neutrality forming HCl
Which chemical potentiates the actions of ACh and gastrin in stimulating H^+ secretion?	Histamine; (this is why H^+ receptor blockers are so effective in treating ulcers)
Which prototypical drug blocks the effects of histamine at the level of the parietal cell?	Cimetidine (an H_2 receptor blocker)
Why does not atropine block vagally mediated gastrin secretion?	Vagal stimulation of acid production is independent of Ach; (it is mediated by GRP)
Which GI hormone is released by the small intestine in response to fats, proteins, and carbohydrates?	GIP

GI Motility

What are the two main divisions of the enteric nervous system?	1. Extrinsic (parasympathetic and sympathetic nervous systems) 2. Intrinsic (enteric nervous systems)

Parasympathetic innervation of the GI tract occurs via which nerves and has what general effect?	Vagus and pelvic → usually stimulatory
Sympathetic innervation of the GI tract occurs via which nerves and has what general effect?	Fibers originate in spinal cord and synapse in the celiac and superior mesenteric ganglia → usually inhibitory
What disorder is characterized by delayed gastric emptying, commonly seen in diabetic patients?	Gastroparesis
What two centers of the brain are integral to vomiting?	1. Chemoreceptor trigger zone (floor of the fourth ventricle) 2. The vomiting center of the medulla (area postrema)
What pacemaker cells in the GI tract regulate the basal rate of gut contraction?	Interstitial cells of Cajal (ICC)
What are the frequencies of ICC's pacemaker activities?	Stomach—3/min, duodenum—12/min, ileum—10/min, colon—3/min

Miscellaneous GI Physiology

What part of the pancreas is responsible for synthesizing and releasing zymogens?	Secretory acinar cells
Which two chemicals stimulate the release of zymogens?	1. Ach 2. CCK
Which hormone acts on the pancreatic ductal cells to increase mucus and HCO_3^- secretion?	Secretin
Name the pancreatic enzymes responsible for the following actions:	
Starch digestion	α-Amylase (secreted in active form)
Protein digestion	Proteases (eg, trypsin, chymotrypsin, elastase, carboxypeptidases—secreted as proenzymes)
Fat digestion	Lipase, phospholipase A, colipase
Which enzyme catalyzes the conversion of trypsinogen into trypsin?	Enterokinase (a brush-border enzyme)

Why is the conversion of trypsin an important part of protein digestion?	Trypsin converts proenzymes to their active forms (including trypsinogen to form a positive-feedback loop)
What is the rate-limiting step in carbohydrate digestion?	Production of monosaccharides by oligosaccharide hydrolases (at brush border)
What are the five major components of bile?	1. Water (97%) 2. Bile salts 3. Phospholipids 4. Cholesterol 5. Bilirubin (BR)
What property of bile salts allows them to solubilize lipids into micelles for absorption?	They are amphipathic (contain *both* hydrophilic and hydrophobic regions)
Where is bile produced and stored?	It is produced continuously by hepatocytes and stored in gallbladder
What is the role of intestinal bacteria in the synthesis of bile acids?	They convert primary (1°) bile acids to secondary (2°) bile acids
Which membrane protein is essential for bile acids recirculation?	Na^+-bile cotransporter in terminal ileum
Why does ileal resection result in steatorrhea?	Lack of bile acid recirculation → depletion of the bile acid pool → impaired fat absorption
What types of carbohydrates can be absorbed?	Monosaccharides only (eg, glucose, galactose, fructose)
By what mechanism are carbohydrates absorbed?	Glucose/galactose: Na^+-dependent cotransport; fructose: facilitated diffusion
How are fats absorbed?	Lipase breaks triglycerides into glycerol and FAs; short- and medium-chain FAs undergo passive diffusion; long-chain FAs form micelles with bile salts for passive diffusion
What metabolites of protein can be absorbed by the GI tract and what type of transport molecules are involved in their absorption?	AAs, dipeptides, and tripeptides; Na^+-dependent cotransporters

PATHOLOGY

Nonneoplastic Disorders of the Upper GI Tract

Name the nonneoplastic disorder of the upper GI tract with the following pathologic and clinical features:

Common vesicular circumoral lesion with eosinophilic intranuclear inclusions

Herpes labialis (usually herpes simplex virus [HSV]-1)

Connective tissue disorder characterized by xerostomia, keratoconjunctivitis sicca, and autoantibodies to SS-A (Ro) and SS-B (La)

Sjögren syndrome

Esophageal dysmotility caused by inability of the lower esophageal sphincter to relax (due to loss of ganglion cells in the myenteric plexus)

Achalasia

Eosinophilic infiltrate with dysphagia, esophageal rings seen on endoscopy

Eosinophilic esophagitis

Linear esophageal erosions in HIV patient with CD4 <100

CMV esophagitis

Disease characterized by dysphagia, iron-deficiency anemia, glossitis, cheliosis, and esophageal webs

Plummer-Vinson syndrome

Type of hiatal hernia in which the stomach and the cardioesophageal junction slide in and out of the thorax

Sliding (axial) hernia

Pharyngeal outpouching involving >1 layer of the esophageal wall; results in food accumulation and chronic halitosis

Zenker (pharyngoesophageal) diverticulum

Retching-induced laceration of gastroesophageal (GE) junction resulting in hematemesis and mediastinitis; ↑ incidence in alcoholics

Mallory-Weiss tear

Complete rupture of the esophagus (all layers), often due to severe retching

Boerhaave syndrome

May result from Chagas disease causing the loss of myenteric plexus in the esophagus	2° achalasia
Hyperplasia of gastric surface mucosal cells	Ménétrier disease
Postvagotomy, unimpeded passage of hypertonic food to SI → distention and diarrhea	Dumping syndrome

Neoplastic Disorders of the Upper GI Tract

Name the neoplastic disorder of the upper GI tract described by each of the following statements:

Most common salivary gland tumor; contains a mix of epithelial and mesenchymal elements	Pleomorphic adenoma (mixed tumor)
Irregular, unscrapable white mucosal patches in the mouth of an AIDS patient as a result of Epstein-Barr virus (EBV)	Oral hairy leukoplakia
Accounts for 95% of oral cancers	Squamous cell carcinoma
Benign salivary tumor containing cystic spaces lined by double-layered eosinophilic epithelium (oncocytes) embedded in dense lymphoid tissue	Warthin tumor (papillary cystadenoma lymphomatosum)
Most common esophageal carcinoma; usually in proximal two-thirds; associated with alcohol and tobacco use	Squamous cell carcinoma
Intestinal metaplasia of squamous epithelium in distal esophagus in response to prolonged injury (often due to GERD)	Barrett esophagus
Mucin-producing glandular tumor of the distal 1/3 of the esophagus	Adenocarcinoma
Infiltrating carcinoma, causing extensive thickening of stomach wall; "leather-bottle stomach"	Linitis plastica (signet ring carcinoma)
Gastric carcinoma that has metastasized to the bilateral ovaries	Krukenberg tumor

Name six important risk factors for gastric carcinoma:

These ↑ your **"CHANSE"** for gastric cancer:
1. **C**hronic gastritis
2. *Helicobacter pylori* infection
3. **A** blood type
4. **N**itrosamines
5. **S**ex (men >50 years old)
6. **E**ating habits (low-fiber diet)

Name six important risk factors for esophageal carcinoma:

"ABCDEF"
1. **A**chalasia
2. **B**arrett esophagus
3. **C**orrosive esophagitis
4. **D**iverticuli
5. **E**sophageal webs
6. **F**amilial

What is the name for metastatic spread of gastric cancer to the supraclavicular node?

Virchow node

What is the name of the subcutaneous periumbilical metastasis in the context of gastric cancer?

Sister Mary Joseph node

Sudden appearance of multiple seborrheic keratoses, sign of underlying malignancy

Leser-Trelat sign

Pediatric GI Disorders

Name the GI disorder commonly diagnosed in the pediatric population with the following findings:

Difficulty with feeding starting from birth, excessive oral secretions, inability to pass NG tube, no gas in abdomen, early pneumonia

Tracheoesophageal fistula

Nonbilious projectile vomiting, abdominal "olive" in epigastric region

Pyloric stenosis

Bilious vomiting, "double bubble," associated with Trisomy 21

Duodenal atresia

Commonly occurs at ileocecal junction, most common cause of small bowel obstruction in toddlers

Intussusception

Failure to pass meconium in the first 48 hours of birth, abdominal distention, associated with CF

Meconium ileus

Gastritis

Name the type of gastritis associated
with the following findings:

Autoimmune disorder with auto-
antibodies to parietal cells and IF,
achlorhydria, pernicious anemia,
and aging

Type A (fundal) chronic gastritis
(**Remember:** the 5 A's for type A)

"Coffee-ground emesis" from
mucosal inflammation

Acute (erosive) gastritis

Helicobacter pylori **infection**

Type B (antral) chronic gastritis
(**B = bug**)

Left shoulder pain

Perforation of ulcer → irritation of
left diaphragm → referred pain from
phrenic nerve

Peptic Ulcer Disease

Name the type of peptic ulcer (gastric
or duodenal) disease associated with
each of the following findings:

Pain is greater with meals

Gastric ulcer (pain is Greater with
meals) → weight loss

Pain decreases with meals

Duodenal ulcer (pain Decreases with
meals) → weight gain

Almost 100% associated with
H. pylori **infection**

Duodenal ulcer

Due to ↓ mucosal protection against
gastric acid

Gastric ulcer

Associated with nonsteroidal anti-
inflammatory drug (NSAID) and
steroid use

Gastric ulcer

Hypertrophy of Brunner glands

Duodenal ulcer

Elevated gastrin levels

Duodenal ulcer

Name four common complications of
peptic ulcer disease:

1. Bleeding
2. Penetration
3. Perforation
4. Obstruction

Name a classic complication of posterior duodenal ulcers:

Massive hemorrhage from erosion of the
gastroduodenal artery

Malabsorption

Name the malabsorption syndrome associated with each of the following pathologic and clinical findings:

Gluten sensitivity	Celiac disease (nontropical sprue)
Brush-border enzyme deficiency resulting in bacterial digestion of unabsorbed disaccharide, causing osmotic diarrhea	Disaccharidase deficiency (#1 = lactase deficiency)
Steatorrhea, weight loss, hyperpigmentation, polyarthritis, fever, and lymphadenopathy in an older, white male; infectious etiology	Whipple disease (caused by *Tropheryma whipplei*)
Increased risk of T-cell lymphoma, GI, and breast malignancy	Celiac disease
Autosomal recessive (AR) defect in chylomicron assembly resulting in an absence of chylomicrons, very low-density lipoproteins (VLDLs), or low-density lipoprotein (LDL) in blood	Abetalipoproteinemia
Crypt hyperplasia, interepithelial lymphocytosis and marked villous blunting	Celiac disease
Distinctive periodic acid–Schiff (PAS)-positive macrophages in intestinal mucosa	Whipple disease
Associated with HLA-DQ2 and HLA-DQ8	Celiac disease
Gram-positive actinomycetes	Whipple disease
Acanthocytes (*burr* cells) in blood	Abetalipoproteinemia

Diverticular Disease

What is the most common cause of painless bleeding from the lower GI tract?	Diverticulosis
What part of the colon is most frequently affected by diverticulosis?	Sigmoid colon

Name the disorder characterized by diverticular inflammation causing left lower quadrant (LLQ) pain, anorexia, nausea, and vomiting:	Diverticulitis
Name four complications of diverticulitis:	1. Perforation 2. Peritonitis 3. Abscess 4. Obstruction
What part of the GI tract is most commonly affected by ischemic bowel disease?	"Watershed" areas (splenic flexure, rectosigmoid junction)
Define intussusception	Telescoping of the intestines resulting in intestinal obstruction
Define volvulus	Complete twisting of the bowel around its mesenteric base
Where does volvulus most commonly occur?	Sigmoid colon (more common in elderly)
Name the inflammatory bowel disease which is often characterized by overgrowth of exotoxin-producing bacteria:	Pseudomembranous colitis
Which organism is responsible for pseudomembranous colitis?	*Clostridium difficile*
What disorder is characterized by nausea, vomiting, anorexia, leukocytosis, and pain at McBurney point?	Appendicitis

Inflammatory Bowel Disease

Ulcerative colitis or Crohn's disease?	
Pancolitis with crypt abscesses	Ulcerative colitis (UC)
Fistulas and fissures	Crohn's disease
Associated with ankylosing spondylitis	Both
Associated with sclerosing cholangitis	UC
Amyloidosis	Crohn's disease
Can lead to toxic megacolon	UC
Longitudinal ulcers	Crohn's disease

Punched-out aphthous ulcers	Crohn's disease
Increased risk of colorectal carcinoma	UC >>> Crohn's disease
Skip lesions	Crohn's disease
Can involve any portion of the GI tract (usually terminal ileum and colon)	Crohn's disease
"String sign" on x-ray (due to bowel wall thickening)	Crohn's disease
Associated with pyoderma gangreosum	Both
Transmural inflammation	Crohn's disease
Noncaseating granulomas	Crohn's disease
Cobblestone mucosa	Crohn's disease
Surgery is curative	UC

Neoplastic Disorders of the Lower GI Tract

What is the most common histologic type of GI lymphomas?	95% are B cell (MALTomas)
What is the most common tumor of the appendix?	Carcinoid tumor
What type of cells gives rise to carcinoid tumors?	Neuroendocrine cells
What substances are secreted from carcinoid tumors?	Serotonin, histamine, and prostaglandins
Metastases to which organ result in carcinoid syndrome?	Liver; carcinoid tumors elsewhere in the GI tract secrete hormones that are metabolized by the liver before they can exert effects
Name five clinical findings of carcinoid syndrome:	1. Vasomotor dysfunction 2. GI hypermotility 3. Bronchoconstriction 4. Hepatomegaly 5. Right-sided heart valve stenosis
What laboratory test is used in the diagnosis of carcinoid syndrome?	5-Hydroxyindoleacetic acid (5-HIAA) in urine

Name the types of neoplastic polyp:

Usually benign and pedunculated; most common	Tubular adenoma (75%)
Highly malignant; sessile tumor >4 cm with fingerlike projections	Villous adenoma
Shares features of both other types of polyps	Tubulovillous adenoma

Name five major risk factors for colon cancer:

1. Presence of colonic villous adenomas
2. Inflammatory bowel disease
3. Low fiber, high animal fat diet
4. Age (>60)
5. Positive family/personal history

How does colorectal carcinoma classically present?

Left side lesions → change in stool caliber, hematochezia; right side lesions → anemia (from occult blood loss)

Where is the most common site for colorectal cancer?

Sigmoid colon

Name the autosomal dominant (AD) polyposis syndrome associated with each of the following findings:

Colonic polyps, osteomas, and soft tissue tumors; associated with abnormal dentition	Gardner syndrome
Hundreds of colonic polyps; malignant potential ~100%	Familial adenomatous polyposis (FAP)
Colonic polyps and CNS tumors; malignant potential ~100%	Turcot syndrome
Defect in DNA mismatch repair → many colonic lesions (especially proximal); malignant potential ~50%	Hereditary nonpolyposis colorectal carcinoma (HNPCC)
Benign, hamartomas of GI tract; melanotic pigmentation of hand, mouth, and genitalia; no malignant potential (but ↑ risk of other tumors)	Peutz-Jeghers syndrome

What are the three tumor syndromes in which the *APC* gene is mutated?

1. FAP
2. Gardner syndrome
3. Turcot syndrome

Pancreatitis and Pancreatic Cancer

Name nine causes of acute pancreatitis:	**"GET SMASHeD"** 1. **G**allstones (major cause) 2. **E**thanol (major cause) 3. **T**rauma 4. **S**teroids 5. **M**umps 6. **A**utoimmune disorder 7. **S**corpion sting 8. **H**yperlipidemia 9. **D**rugs (especially ddI) Other causes: ischemia, infections, pancreatic cancer, and peptic ulcer disease
Name seven possible sequelae of acute pancreatitis:	1. Progression to chronic pancreatitis 2. Necrotizing pancreatitis 3. Pseudocyst 4. Hypocalcemia 5. Focal fibrosis and diffuse fat necrosis 6. Acute respiratory distress syndrome (ARDS) 7. Disseminated intravascular coagulation (DIC)
Name four common laboratory abnormalities in acute pancreatitis:	1. ↑ Serum amylase (within 24 hours) 2. ↑ Serum lipase (72–96 hours) 3. Hypocalcemia 4. Glycosuria
Name five causes of chronic pancreatitis:	**"ABCCD"** 1. **A**lcoholism (#1 in adults) 2. **B**iliary tract disease 3. **C**ystic fibrosis (#1 in kids) 4. **C**a^{2+} (hypercalcemia) 5. **D**ivisum (pancreas divisum)
Most pancreatic tumors are found in what region of the pancreas?	Two-thirds of pancreatic tumors are found in the pancreatic head
What is a common clinical presentation of a mass in the pancreatic head?	Painless jaundice causing malabsorption and Courvoisier (enlarged, palpable) gallbladder
What is Trousseau syndrome?	Migratory thrombophlebitis associated with visceral cancer, commonly pancreatic adenocarcinoma
What are the two most commonly mutated genes causing pancreatic adenocarcinoma?	1. *K-ras* (>90% mutated) 2. *p53* (60%–80% mutated)

What is the prognosis for pancreatic adenocarcinoma?	Averages 6 months or less (very aggressive)

Disorders of Bilirubin Metabolism

What type of hyperbilirubinemia results from cholestasis?	Conjugated

Name the hereditary hyperbilirubine-mia described in each of the following statements:

Mildly ↓ UDP-glucuronyl transfer-ase; asymptomatic; associated with stress in 6% of people	Gilbert syndrome
AR defect causing ↓ canalicular excretion of BR conjugates → grossly black liver; asymptomatic	Dubin-Johnson syndrome
AR absence UDP-glucuronyl transferase → ↑ unconjugated BR → jaundice, kernicterus, early death	Crigler-Najjar syndrome, type I
AR defect causing asymptomatic, conjugated bilirubinemia	Rotor syndrome

Liver Disorders

What three pathologic characteristics define cirrhosis?	1. Fibrosis 2. Nodular regeneration of hepatocytes 3. Disruption of parenchymal architecture
Name four common causes of micronodular cirrhosis:	1. Chronic alcoholism (think of a **micro**brewery) 2. Hereditary hemochromatosis 3. Primary biliary cirrhosis 4. Wilson disease (hepatolenticular degeneration)
Name four common causes of macronodular cirrhosis:	1. Hepatitis B virus (HBV) 2. Hepatitis C virus (HCV) 3. α_1-Antitrypsin deficiency 4. Wilson disease (hepatolenticular degeneration)

List the effects of cirrhosis on the following body systems:

Eye	Conjunctival icterus

Neurologic	Coma, hepatic encephalopathy (asterixis, hyperreflexia, behavioral changes)
Systemic	Peripheral edema, malnutrition
Skin	Jaundice, palmar erythema, spider angiomata, caput medusae
Reproductive	Testicular atrophy, gynecomastia, loss of pubic hair
Hematopoietic	Anemia, bleeding tendency ($\downarrow$ coagulation factors), splenomegaly
Renal	Hepatorenal syndrome (2° to hypoperfusion)
GI	Fetor hepaticus, ascites, esophageal varices, hemorrhoids

Name the liver disorder associated with each of the following findings:

Mallory bodies	Alcoholic hepatitis
Occlusion of IVC or hepatic veins with centrilobular congestion $\rightarrow$ congestive liver disease; associated with polycythemia, pregnancy, and hepatocellular carcinoma	Budd-Chiari syndrome
Obliteration of hepatic vein radicals following bone marrow transplant	Veno-occlusive disease
Copper deposition in liver, kidneys, brain, and cornea $\rightarrow$ asterixis, basal ganglia degeneration, dementia	Wilson disease (hepatolenticular degeneration)
AST:ALT ratio >1.5	Alcoholic hepatitis
Lymphoid aggregates and interface hepatitis	Chronic hepatitis
May be incidental finding in young woman taking oral contraceptives	Hepatic adenoma
Hemolysis, elevated LFTs, and low platelets in a pregnant woman	**HELLP** syndrome (hepatic disease of pregnancy)
Elevated α-fetoprotein (AFP)	Hepatocellular carcinoma

Name the etiology of cirrhosis associated with each of the following findings:

Panacinar emphysema	α_1-Antitrypsin deficiency
Decreased ceruloplasmin	Wilson disease (hepatolenticular degeneration)

Triad of bronze diabetes, skin pigmentation, and Prussian blue stain-positive deposits in the liver	Hemochromatosis
Antimitochondrial antibodies	Primary biliary cirrhosis
Nutmeg liver	Congestive heart failure (also called congestive hepatopathy)
Kayser-Fleischer rings	Wilson disease (hepatolenticular degeneration)
Micronodular fatty liver; portal hypertension, asterixis, jaundice, and gynecomastia	Chronic alcohol abuse
↑ Ferritin, transferrin, and total iron; ↓ total iron-binding capacity (TIBC)	Hereditary hemochromatosis **Note:** total body iron is sometimes high enough to trigger metal detectors
Name the major risk factors for hepatocellular carcinoma:	**"WATCH for ABC"** **W**ilson's disease α_1-**A**ntitrypsin deficiency **C**arcinogens (eg, aflatoxin B, polyvinyl chloride) **H**emochromatosis **A**lcoholic cirrhosis **B**Hepatitis B **C**Hepatitis C
Hepatocellular carcinoma tends to spread through which route?	Hematogenous
What is the most common type of malignancy in the liver?	Metastasis
Which primary tumors tend to metastasize to the liver?	Colon > Stomach > Pancreas > Breast > Lung (**Remember:** "**C**ancer **S**ometimes **P**enetrates **B**enign **L**iver!")
Name the hepatobiliary disorder associated with the following:	
Associated with *Clonorchis sinensis* (liver fluke) infection in Asia	Cholangiocarcinoma
Inflammation of the bile duct; commonly due to *Escherichia coli* infection	Ascending cholangitis

Disorders of the Gallbladder

What is Courvoisier law?	An enlarged, palpable gallbladder with jaundice is likely the result of an underlying malignancy (often in head of the pancreas) and not from a stone in the common duct (because gallbladder is typically too scarred from infection)
What is Charcot triad?	Spiking fevers with chills, jaundice, and right upper quadrant (RUQ) pain (biliary colic); strongly suggests cholangitis
What is Reynold's pentad?	Charcot triad + shock and altered mental status; strongly suggests cholangitis
What are the risk factors for cholelithiasis?	4 F's: Fertile, Fat, Forty-year-old Female
What is the most common type of gallstone?	Mixed stone (components of pigment and cholesterol stones)
Name six complications of cholelithiasis:	1. Biliary colic and common bile duct obstruction 2. Cholecystitis (acute or chronic) 3. Ascending cholangitis 4. Acute pancreatitis 5. Gallstone ileus 6. Malignancy (adenocarcinoma)

Viral Hepatitis

Name the hepatitis virus (viruses) associated with the following features:

Fecal-oral transmission	Hepatitis A virus (HAV)
Water-borne transmission	Hepatitis E virus (HEV)
Infection may lead to a carrier state	HBV, HCV, and hepatitis D virus (HDV, delta agent)
Defective virus requiring HBsAg as its envelope	HDV (delta agent)
Sexual, parenteral, and transplacental transmission	HBV, HCV, HDV
DNA hepadnavirus	HBV
High mortality rate in pregnant women	HEV

Associated with IV drug use	HCV
Long incubation (~3 months)	HBV
Increased risk of hepatocellular carcinoma	HBV, HCV
Immune globulin vaccine available	HAV, HBV (and HDV)
Short incubation (~2 weeks)	HAV

Name the hepatitis serologic marker described below:

Antigen found on surface of HBV; continued presence suggests carrier state	HBsAg
Antigen associated with core of HBV	HBcAg
Antigen in the HBV core that indicates transmissibility	HBeAg
Antibody suggesting low HBV transmissibility	HBeAb
Acts as a marker for HBV infection during the "window" period (acute phase)	IgM-HBcAb
Provides immunity to HBV	HBsAb

What is the "window" period of a hepatitis infection?	Period during acute infection when HBsAg has become undetectable, but HBsAb has not yet appeared

Infectious Diarrhea

Name six infectious causes of bloody diarrhea:	1. *Salmonella* 2. *Shigella* 3. *Campylobacter jejuni* 4. Enteroinvasive and enterohemorrhagic *E. coli* 5. *Yersinia enterocolitica* 6. *Entamoeba histolytica*

Name the diarrhea-causing organism associated with the following statements:

Most common cause of diarrhea in infants globally	Rotavirus
Ten to twelve loose, bloody, and mucous diarrhea stools per day due to ingestion of cysts	*E. histolytica*

Comma-shaped organisms causing rice-water stools	*Vibrio cholerae*
Second to rotavirus as a cause of gastroenteritis in kids	Caliciviruses (Norwalk-like and Sapporo-like)
Bloody diarrhea; very low ID_{50} (small numbers of organisms can cause disease); nonmotile	*Shigella*
Usually transmitted from pet feces	*Y. enterocolitica*
Motile; lactose nonfermenter; causes bloody diarrhea	*Salmonella*
Comma- or s-shaped organisms causing bloody diarrhea; grows at 42°C; can cause Guillain-Barre syndrome	*C. jejuni*
Watery diarrhea with extensive fluid loss in AIDS patient	*Cryptosporidium*
Foul-smelling diarrhea after returning from a camping trip	*Giardia lamblia*
Watery diarrhea caused by antibiotic-induced suppression of colonic flora	*C. difficile*

Name the organism responsible for food poisoning from the following items:

Reheated rice	*Bacillus cereus*
Reheated meat dishes	*Clostridium perfringens*
Improperly canned food	*Clostridium botulinum*
Contaminated seafood or raw oysters	*Vibrio parahaemolyticus* and *Vibrio vulnificus*
Meats, mayonnaise, custards	*Staphylococcus aureus* **Note:** starts and ends quickly *due to pre-formed toxin*
Undercooked beef products	*E. coli* O157:H7
Raw poultry, milk, eggs, and meat	*Salmonella*
Proposed non-antibiotic treatment to prevent recurrent *C. difficile* infection	Fecal microbiota transplant

PHARMACOLOGY

For each of the following drugs, provide:
1. The mechanism of action (MOA)
2. Indication(s) (IND)
3. Significant side effects and unique toxicity (TOX) (if any)

Omeprazole, pantoprazole, lansoprazole

MOA: irreversibly inhibits H+/K+-ATPase in parietal cells (proton pump inhibitor)
IND: peptic ulcer disease, Zollinger-Ellison syndrome, erosive esophagitis
TOX: liver toxicity, pancreatitis, agranulocytosis (rare), ↑ risk of pneumonia and *C. difficile* infection

Cimetidine, ranitidine, famotidine, nizatidine

MOA: H_2 receptor antagonist in parietal cell
IND: GE reflux disease
TOX: endocrine effects (gynecomastia—primarily caused by cimetidine, galactorrhea, ↓ sperm count), potent inhibitor of P-450, ↓ renal creatinine clearance

Misoprostol

MOA: PGE_1 analog →↑ secretion of gastric mucus and bicarbonate
IND: prophylaxis for NSAID-induced peptic ulcer disease (PUD); maintenance of a patent ductus arteriosus (PDA)
TOX: abortifacient

Octreotide

MOA: somatostatin analog
IND: VIPoma, carcinoid syndrome, bleeding esophageal varices
TOX: hyperglycemia, constipation, headache

Aluminum sucrose sulfate (sucralfate)

MOA: polymerizes in stomach → binds to injured tissue, forming a protective coating over ulcers
 (**Note**: requires an acidic environment)
IND: peptic ulcer disease
TOX: osteodystrophy, osteomalacia (mainly in pts with renal failure)

Dicyclomine

MOA: muscarinic agonist
IND: irritable bowel syndrome
TOX: atropine-like (dry mouth, blurry vision, tachycardia, constipation)

Ondansetron

MOA: $5\text{-}HT_3$ receptor antagonist
IND: postoperative nausea/vomiting, chemotherapy-induced emesis
TOX: headache, diarrhea

Meclizine

MOA: H_1 receptor antagonist
IND: motion sickness
TOX: teratogenic

Loperamide, diphenoxylate

MOA: antimotility agents (opioid analogs) with limited transit into CNS
IND: diarrhea
TOX: toxic megacolon in kids (loperamide)

Budesonide	**MOA:** glucocorticoid steroid anti-inflammatory; limited systemic absorption and thus limited side effects **IND:** inflammatory bowel disease, lymphocytic colitis, microscopic colitis **TOX:** adrenal suppression, osteoporosis (but less than with glucocorticoids with more systemic absorption, ie, prednisone)
Metoclopramide	**MOA:** stimulates ACh release →↑ upper GI motility **IND:** nausea, ileus **TOX:** sedation, diarrhea, and extrapyramidal symptoms (EPS) (especially in kids)
Lactulose	**MOA:** osmotic laxative **IND:** hepatic encephalopathy, colonic lavage precolonoscopy **TOX:** dehydration with overuse
What is "triple therapy" for *H. pylori*?	Proton pump inhibitor (PPi), bismuth salicylate, and two of the following antibiotics: metronidazole, amoxicillin, clarithromycin, or tetracycline
What is the most important approach to healing peptic ulcers?	Eradicating *H. pylori*
Antacids	Hypokalemia, alter absorption of other drugs
Sodium bicarbonate	Systemic alkalinization
Aluminum hydroxide	Constipation
Magnesium hydroxide	Diarrhea
Name the therapy of choice for each of the following disorders:	
Hereditary hemochromatosis	Repeated phlebotomy and deferoxamine
Wilson disease	Chelation therapy (with penicillamine)
Acute cholecystitis from gallstones	Cholecystectomy

CHAPTER 8

Reproductive and Endocrine

EMBRYOLOGY

During embryogenesis, when is male/female phenotypic differentiation complete?	By week 20
Which gene determines phenotypic differentiation?	*Sry* gene (encodes for a protein called testis-determining factor [TDF])
Which cells secrete Müllerian-inhibiting factor (MIF) during fetal development?	Sertoli cells
What factors are required to direct the indifferent embryo into a male phenotype?	TDF, MIF, testosterone, and dihydrotestosterone (DHT)
In what structure, within the testes, does spermatogenesis occur?	Seminiferous tubules
What molecule is the primary (1°) source of energy for sperm?	Fructose
Give the number of chromosomes and amount of DNA found in each of the following cell types:	
Spermatogonia	46,2N
1° spermatocyte/oocyte	46,4N
Secondary (2°) spermatocyte/oocyte	23,2N
Spermatid/ovum	23,1N

What stage is each cell type halted in and when is the stage finally completed?

1° oocyte — Prophase I, just prior to ovulation

2° oocyte — Metaphase II, at fertilization

Name the structure of the mature sperm associated with each of the following statements:

Contains mitochondria — Middle piece (neck)

Derived from one of the centrioles — Flagellum (tail)

Name the congenital disorder that results from each of the following aberrations:

Complete lack of fusion of paramesonephric ducts — Double uterus with double vagina

Partial fusion of the paramesonephric ducts — Bicornate uterus

Testes fail to descend into the scrotum — Cryptorchidism (bilateral → sterility)

Patency of processus vaginalis — If small → hydrocele; if large → congenital inguinal hernia

Failure of urethral folds to close — Hypospadias (penile urethra opens on inferior/ventral side)

Faulty positioning of genital tubercle — Epispadias (penile urethra opens on superior/dorsal side)

Name the embryonic structure that gives rise to each of the following tissues:

Thyroid gland — Thyroid diverticulum

Thymus, inferior parathyroids — Third branchial pouch

Superior parathyroids and the parafollicular "C" cells — Fourth branchial pouch (fourth is *superior* to third)

Chromaffin cells of adrenal medulla — Neural crest cells

Adrenal cortex — Mesoderm

What is the most common site for ectopic thyroid tissue and why? — The tongue; during development, the thyroid migrates caudally from the level of the developing tongue

| Which syndrome is caused by a failure of the development of the third and fourth pharyngeal pouches? | DiGeorge syndrome |

| Describe the clinical features of DiGeorge syndrome | "CATCH 22" |

ANATOMY

| Name the five types of endocrine cells found in the pars distalis of the anterior pituitary: | 1. Somatotrophs (~50%)
2. Mammotrophs
3. Thyrotrophs
4. Corticotrophs
5. Gonadotrophs |

| Where is antidiuretic hormone (ADH) primarily produced? | Supraoptic nucleus of hypothalamus |

| Where is oxytocin primarily produced? | Paraventricular nucleus of hypothalamus |

| What part of the pituitary stores and releases ADH and oxytocin? | Neurohypophysis (posterior pituitary) |

| Where is the hypophyseal portal system located? | Adenohypophysis (in the pars tuberalis) |

| What is the 1° arterial supply to the gonads? | Testicular/ovarian arteries (directly from abdominal aorta branches) |

| What is the 1° venous drainage of the gonads? | Left testicular/ovarian vein → left renal vein; right testicular/ovarian vein → inferior vena cava (IVC) |

| Which lymph nodes filter lymph from the gonads? | Deep lumbar/para-aortic nodes |

| Which lymph nodes filter lymph from the scrotum? | Superficial inguinal nodes |

| What are the two pathways for venous drainage from the prostate gland? | 1. Prostatic venous plexus → internal iliac veins → IVC
2. Prostatic venous plexus → vertebral venous plexus → cranial dural sinuses |

Describe the type of innervations for each phase of the male sexual response cycle:

Erection	Parasympathetic nerves (**P**oint)
Emission	Sympathetic nerves (**S**hoot)
Ejaculation	Visceral autonomic and somatic nerves

Name the structure(s) contained in the following uterine ligaments:

Transverse cervical (cardinal) ligament	Uterine vessels
Suspensory ligament of ovaries	Ovarian vessels, lymphatics, autonomic nerves
Broad ligament	Round ligaments of the uterus, ovarian ligament, ureters, uterine tubes, and uterine vessels

What is the anatomic relationship of the ureter and the uterine artery?

Ureter lies posterior and inferior to uterine artery; **"Water (ureter) under the bridge (uterine artery)"**

What is the normal position of the uterus?

Anteverted (uterus to cervix) and anteflexed (cervix to vagina)

What is the landmark for a pudendal nerve block?

Ischial spine

Name the part of the fallopian tube described below:

Opens into the peritoneal cavity	Infundibulum
Site of fertilization	Ampulla
Opens into the uterine cavity	Intramural
Majority of the length of the tube	Isthmus

Describe the venous drainage of the adrenal glands

Right adrenal vein → IVC; left adrenal vein → left renal vein

What type of nerves synapse in the adrenal medulla?

Preganglionic sympathetic (through splanchnic nerves)

In the adrenal medulla, onto what cells do the preganglionic sympathetic nerves synapse?

Chromaffin cells → secrete catecholamines

Describe the clinical features of Turner syndrome (45 XO)

Short stature, shield-shaped chest, widely spaced nipples, ovarian dysgenesis, webbed neck, bicuspid aortic valve, horseshoe kidney

PHYSIOLOGY

Second Messengers

Name the second messenger
mechanism used by each of the
following hormones:

Hypothalamic hormones— gonadotropin-releasing hormone (GnRH), thyrotropin-releasing hormone (TRH), growth hormone– releasing hormone (GHRH), oxytocin, ADH (V_1 receptor)	Inositol triphosphate (IP_3)
Hypothalamic hormones— corticotropin-releasing hormone and ADH (V_2 receptor)	cAMP
Anterior pituitary hormones— luteinizing hormone (LH), follicle-stimulating hormone (FSH), adrenocorticotropic hormone (ACTH), thyroid-stimulating hormone (TSH)	Cyclic adenosine monophosphate (cAMP)
Growth hormone (GH)	Tyrosine kinase activation
Insulin	Tyrosine kinase activation
Melanocyte-stimulating hormone (MSH)	cAMP
Angiotensin II	IP_3
Calcitonin	cAMP
Glucagon	cAMP
Parathyroid hormone (PTH)	cAMP
Insulin-like growth factor (IGF)-1	Tyrosine kinase activation
Atrial natriuretic peptide (ANP)	Cyclic guanosine monophosphate (cGMP)
Nitric oxide	cGMP

Steroid Hormones

How do steroid hormones circulate in the body?	They are bound to specific globulin carrier proteins (which ↑ solubility and delivery to target organs)
How are the cellular effects of steroids mediated?	Steroids pass through the cell membrane, bind cytoplasmic receptors, and translocate to the nucleus where they influence gene expression

Adrenal Glands

Name the three layers of the adrenal cortex and their major secretory products:	**GFR** (from outside to inside), "the deeper you go, the sweeter it gets: salt, sugar, sex" 1. Zona **G**lomerulosa—mineralocorticoids 2. Zona **F**asciculata—glucocorticoids 3. Zona **R**eticularis—androgens
How does the secretion of glucocorticoids vary throughout the day?	Highest before waking and lowest at midnight
What is the effect of glucocorticoids on ACTH and cortisol secretion?	Potent glucocorticoids inhibit ACTH and cortisol secretion (a negative feedback mechanism)
What test is used to evaluate the response of the hypothalamic-pituitary axis (HPA) to glucocorticoids?	Dexamethasone suppression test
Name four general actions of cortisol:	1. Stimulates gluconeogenesis (↑ protein catabolism and lipolysis) 2. Anti-inflammatory effects (block arachidonic acid pathway) 3. Acute exposure enhances immune response; chronic exposure suppresses immune response (inhibits interleukin [IL]-2 production) 4. Maintains vascular responsiveness to catecholamines
Name three specific actions of aldosterone:	1. ↑ Renal Na^+ reabsorption 2. ↑ Renal K^+ secretion 3. ↑ Renal H^+ secretion

Sex Hormones

What is the function of LH in male reproduction?	LH acts on Leydig cells → stimulates cholesterol desmolase → testosterone
What is the function of FSH in male reproduction?	FSH acts on Sertoli cells → spermatogenesis and secretion of inhibin (inhibits FSH)
How does testosterone regulate LH secretion?	Acts to ↓ release of GnRH from hypothalamus and to release of LH from adenohypophysis
Which enzyme is required to convert testosterone to its active form, DHT?	5-α-Reductase
Which enzyme catalyzes conversion of testosterone to estrogen?	Aromatase
Name three androgens (in order of decreasing potency) and where they are produced:	1. DHT (prostate, peripheral tissues) 2. Testosterone (testes, adrenals) 3. Androstenedione (adrenals)
Name five important functions of testosterone:	1. Sexual differentiation during development 2. 2° Sexual development, growth spurt, and fusion of epiphyseal plates 3. ↑Libido 4. Anabolic effects 5. Spermatogenesis maintenance
What is the average age of menarche?	Between 11 and 14 years (in the United States)
How does GnRH release change during puberty?	Pulsatile release of GnRH begins and it upregulates its own receptors in the adenohypophysis
What is the function of LH in female reproduction?	LH acts on theca cells → stimulates cholesterol desmolase → testosterone
What is the function of FSH in female reproduction?	FSH acts on granulosa cells → stimulates aromatase → estrogen
What happens to LH:FSH ratio during puberty?	LH >> FSH
Where is estrogen made?	Blood (via aromatase), ovaries (estradiol), placenta (estriol), and testes

What is the relative potency of the major estrogens?	Estradiol > estrone > estriol
Which estrogen is an indicator of fetal well-being?	Estriol ($\uparrow$1000 $\times$ in pregnancy)
Where is progesterone produced?	Corpus luteum, adrenal cortex, placenta, and testes

Decide whether each of the following are characteristics of estrogen, progesterone, or both:

Development of genitalia	Estrogen
Growth of follicle	Estrogen
Proliferation of endometrium	Estrogen
Maintains endometrium	Progesterone
Maintains pregnancy	Both
Produces thick cervical mucus	Progesterone
Hepatic synthesis of transport proteins	Estrogen
$\downarrow$ Myometrial excitability	Progesterone
Development of breasts	Both
$\uparrow$ Body temperature	Progesterone
Spiral artery development	Progesterone
LH surge	Estrogen
Typical female fat distribution	Estrogen
Uterine smooth muscle relaxation (prevents contractions)	Progesterone
Decreases endometrial sloughing	Progesterone
Pubertal development	Estrogen

What are the two main phases of the menstrual cycle and when do they occur?	1. Follicular phase (days 1–14) 2. Luteal phase (days 14–28)

Classify the following as characteristics of the follicular or luteal phase:

Graafian follicle matures	Follicular phase
Corpus luteum develops causing the release of estrogen and progesterone	Luteal phase (early)
Basal body temperature increases	Luteal phase

Oocyte progresses from meiosis I to meiosis II	Follicular phase
Endometrial glands grow → spiral arteries	Luteal phase
Endometrial proliferation	Follicular phase
Progesterone peaks	Luteal phase
Menses	Follicular phase (early)
When does ovulation occur?	14 days before menses (regardless of cycle length)
What changes in cervical mucus occur during ovulation?	Cervical mucus is thinnest and most penetrable during ovulation
What endocrine change induces ovulation?	Estradiol burst at end of follicular phase causes a positive feedback effect, resulting in a surge of LH
Which hormone prevents lactation during pregnancy?	High estrogen and progesterone block the effects of prolactin on the breast
Where is hCG made and what is its function?	Syncytiotrophoblast of placenta produces hCG to maintain corpus luteum so it can produce progesterone during the first trimester until placenta can produce progesterone during the second and third trimesters
Name three scenarios in which hCG is elevated:	1. Pregnancy (in urine 10 days after fertilization) 2. Hydatidiform moles 3. Choriocarcinoma
hCG peaks at what gestational age?	Gestational week 9
What happens to estrogen and progesterone just prior to delivery?	Both increase throughout; near term estrogen:progesterone ratio increases
What is the average age of menopause?	51 (tends to occur earlier in smokers)
Name four hormonal changes characteristic of menopause:	1. ↓ Estrogen 2. ↑↑ FSH 3. ↑ LH 4. ↑ GnRH

Name four clinical findings characteristic of menopause:	Menopause wreaks "HAVOC" on your body 1. Hot flashes 2. Atrophy of vagina 3. Osteoporosis 4. Coronary artery disease risk increases

Anterior Pituitary

Name the hormones produced by the anterior pituitary:	"FLAT PiG" plus melanotropin (MSH) FSH LH ACTH TSH Prolactin GH
Name four compounds derived from proopiomelanocortin (POMC):	1. ACTH 2. MSH 3. β-Lipotropin 4. β-Endorphin
Which hormones share a common α-subunit?	T.S.H. and TSH = The Sex Hormones (LH, FSH, hCG) and TSH
Which glycoprotein subunit determines hormone specificity?	β-Subunit
How is GH regulated?	↑ By GHRH, sleep, stress, exercise, hypoglycemia, and puberty; ↓ by somatomedins, somatostatin, obesity, pregnancy, and hyperglycemia
Name four direct actions of GH (somatotropin):	1. ↓ Glucose uptake into cells (diabetogenic) 2. ↑ Lipolysis 3. ↑ Protein synthesis in muscle 4. ↑ Production of somatomedins (IGF)
Name three effects of IGF on growth:	1. ↑ Linear growth (pubertal growth spurt) 2. ↑ Lean body mass 3. ↑ Organ size
Which clinical syndrome results from GH hypersecretion before puberty?	Increased linear growth (gigantism)

Which clinical syndrome results from GH hypersecretion after puberty?	Acromegaly (may include glucose intolerance)
Name four functions of prolactin:	1. Stimulates milk production 2. Inhibits ovulation 3. Stimulates breast development (with estrogen) 4. Inhibits spermatogenesis
How is prolactin regulated?	Upregulated by estrogen (pregnancy), breast-feeding, sleep, stress, TRH, dopamine (DA) antagonists Downregulated by DA and DA agonists, somatostatin, and prolactin
What are the effects of excess prolactin?	Galactorrhea, ↓ libido, and failure to ovulate
How does prolactin inhibit ovulation?	Inhibits GnRH synthesis and release

Posterior Pituitary

Which hormones are released from the posterior pituitary and what are their functions?	Oxytocin—milk ejection and uterine contraction; vasopressin (ADH)—↑ H_2O reabsorption in kidneys
How is the release of oxytocin regulated?	↑ By suckling, dilation of the cervix, and orgasm
How is the release of ADH regulated?	↑ By high serum osmolarity, volume contraction, pain, nausea, nicotine, opiates; ↓ by low serum osmolarity, ethyl alcohol, ANP, and α-agonists

Thyroid

Which cells are responsible for thyroid hormone synthesis?	Follicular cells
Thyroid hormones are synthesized from which two molecules?	1. Iodide (I^-) 2. Tyrosine
Which enzyme catalyzes the oxidation of I^- to I_2?	Thyroid peroxidase
What is the relative proportion of T_4:T_3 released into the bloodstream?	$T_4 = 90\%$, $T_3 = 10\%$

Which thyroid hormone has the greatest biological activity?	$T_3 >> T_4$ (T_4 converted into T_3 by liver and kidneys)
Which protein produced by and used entirely within the thyroid is used to produce and store T_4 and T_3?	Thyroglobulin
Which carrier protein is necessary for delivery of thyroid hormone to the tissues?	Thyroxine-binding globulin (TBG)
How is thyroid hormone production regulated?	↑ By TRH and TSH; T_3 downregulates TRH receptors in AP →↓ TSH
List four key functions of thyroid hormone:	Remember the **4 B's of T_3** 1. **B**rain maturation 2. **B**one and cartilage growth (synergistic with GH) 3. β-Agonist effects (↑ cardiac output [CO], heart rate [HR], stroke volume [SV]) 4. ↑ BMR (by ↑ Na^+/K^+ ATPase →↑ O_2 consumption)

Calcium Regulation

Which is the most important hormone in the regulation of Ca^{2+} levels and where is it made?	PTH is synthesized and secreted by the chief cells of the parathyroid gland
What is the major stimulus for PTH secretion?	↓ Serum Ca^{2+} (also mildly ↓ Mg^{2+})
Which hormone is stimulated in response to ↑ PTH levels and ↓ serum Ca^{2+}?	Vitamin D (1,25-$(OH)_2^-$ cholecalciferol is active form)
Which enzyme in the kidney catalyzes the activation of vitamin D?	1α-Hydroxylase
What factors increase 1α-hydroxylase activity?	↓ Serum Ca^{2+}, ↑ PTH, ↓ serum phosphate
What clinical syndrome results from vitamin D deficiency?	Kids → rickets; adults → osteomalacia
Which hormone is released in response to increased serum Ca^{2+} and where is it made?	Calcitonin is synthesized and secreted by the parafollicular "C" cells of the thyroid gland

What is the effect of calcitonin on bones?	Blocks PTH-mediated resorption of bones

List the effects of PTH on each of the following organs:

Kidneys	↓ Phosphate reabsorption (by ↑ urinary cAMP), ↑ Ca^{2+} reabsorption in distal convoluted tubule of kidneys
Intestines	↑ Ca^{2+} absorption (by stimulating 1α-hydroxylase to activate vitamin D)
Bone	↑ Resorption (brings Ca^{2+} and phosphate into extracellular fluid [ECF])

List the effects of vitamin D on each of the following organs:

Kidneys	↑ Ca^{2+} and phosphate reabsorption
Intestines	↑ Ca^{2+} and phosphate absorption
Bone	↑ Resorption

Pancreas

Name the three major cell types in the pancreatic islets of Langerhans, their location, and function:	1. **Alpha** (outer rim) → glucagons 2. **Beta** (central rim of islet) → insulin 3. **Delta** (intermixed) → somatostatin and gastrin
List three major actions of glucagon on the liver and adipose tissue:	1. ↑ Glycogenolysis and gluconeogenesis 2. ↑ Lipolysis and ketoacid production 3. ↑ Urea production
List five major functions of insulin:	1. ↓ Blood glucose 2. ↑ Fat deposition (↓ lipolysis) 3. ↓ Blood amino acids 4. ↓ Blood K^+ 5. ↑ Protein synthesis
What is the 2° structure of insulin?	An α-chain and a β-chain, joined by two disulfide bridges
What is C-peptide and why is it important?	A connecting peptide removed from proinsulin, packaged and secreted with insulin; serves as a useful monitor of β-cell function and exogenous insulin administration

What are some factors that ↑ insulin secretion?	↑ Blood glucose (major), ↑ AAs, ↑ FAs, GH, cortisol, glucagon, ACh
How does glucose trigger insulin release?	Binds to GLUT-2 receptor on β-cells → closes K^+ channels → cell depolarization → opens Ca^{2+} channels → insulin secretion
Which drugs mimic the action of glucose on β-islet cells?	Sulfonylurea drugs
What is the effect of starvation and obesity on insulin receptor expression?	↑ In starvation; ↓ in obesity

PATHOLOGY

Male Reproductive System

Name the male genitourinary disease characterized by each of the following statements:

Intractable, painful erection; associated with venous thrombosis, trazodone, and sickle cell disease	Priapism
Inflammation of the glans associated with poor hygiene	Balanitis
Bent penis due to acquired fibrous tissue formation	Peyronie disease
Twisting of the testicular vasculature; may be spontaneous or the result of trauma	Torsion
Collection of serous fluid in the tunica vaginalis (hint: has positive transillumination test)	Hydrocele
Palpable, "bag of worms" dilation of multiple veins of the pampiniform venous plexus of the spermatic cord	Varicocele
Acute purulent urethritis caused by gram-negative diplococci	Gonorrhea
Fever, chills, and dysuria; tender, boggy prostate; >10 WBCs per high-power field on examination of prostatic secretions	Acute bacterial prostatitis

What are the possible sequelae of cryptorchidism?	5 to 10 × ↑ risk of germ cell tumors (GCTs), atrophy, sterility, and inguinal hernias
What is the treatment for cryptorchidism?	Orchiopexy **Note:** ↓ risk of sterility, but no ↓ risk of malignancy
What are the most common etiologies of orchitis?	Mumps virus (1 week postparotiditis), gonorrhea, chlamydia, syphilis

Name the most likely organism(s) responsible for epididymitis in the following groups:

Pediatric patients	*Escherichia coli*
Sexually active, <35-year-old (y/o)	*Neisseria gonorrhoeae, Chlamydia trachomatis*
Older men	*E. coli, Pseudomonas* sp.

Name the penile neoplasm associated with each of the following:

Human papillomavirus (HPV) types 6 and 11	Condyloma acuminate
Single, grayish plaque on shaft/scrotum; associated with ↑ risk of visceral malignancy	Bowen disease
HPV types 16, 18, 31, and 33	Squamous cell carcinoma of the penis
Single erythematous plaque representing carcinoma in situ of the penis, often on glans	Erythroplasia of Queyrat

What category of testicular tumors accounts for ~95% of all cases and has a peak incidence in 15- to 34-y/o?	GCTs

Name the testicular tumor associated with each of the following:

Malignant, painless enlargement of testis; most common GCT, radiosensitive	Seminoma
Malignant, chemosensitive GCT	Nonseminoma GCT
Malignant, painful GCT that has peak incidence in childhood; ↑ α-fetoprotein (AFP)	Yolk sac tumor (endodermal sinus tumor)

Malignant GCT made of 2+ embryonic layers and multiple tissue types; more common in kids	Teratoma
Benign, androgen-producing stromal tumor with intracytoplasmic Reinke crystals	Leydig cell tumor (interstitial)
Malignant, hemorrhagic tumor arising from trophoblastic cells; ↑ β-hCG	Choriocarcinoma
Most common testicular cancer in older men	Testicular lymphoma

Benign prostatic nodular hyperplasia or prostatic carcinoma?

Commonly affects peripheral zone	Prostatic carcinoma
Caused by age-related increase in DHT, testosterone, and estrogen	Nodular hyperplasia
Associated with bladder distention and urinary tract infections (UTIs)	Nodular hyperplasia
Enlarged, firm, nodular prostate on digital rectal examination (DRE)	Prostatic carcinoma
Commonly presents with nocturia and hesitancy	Nodular hyperplasia
Primarily affects central zone	Nodular hyperplasia
Primarily affects corpora amylacea	Nodular hyperplasia
↑ Total prostate-specific antigen (PSA), with ↓ fraction of free PSA	Prostatic carcinoma
↑ Total PSA, with proportionate ↑ in fraction of free PSA	Nodular hyperplasia

Hypermethylation of which gene is commonly associated with prostatic carcinoma?	*GSTP1*
What does increased alkaline phosphatase in a prostate cancer patient suggest?	Osteoblastic lesions from bony metastasis

Female Reproductive System

Name the gynecologic infectious disorder characterized by each of the following features:

Clue cells in pap smear; ⊕ "whiff test"

Bacterial vaginosis (eg, *Gardnerella vaginitis*)

Thick, white discharge with vulvovaginal pruritis; most common form of vaginitis

Candidiasis

Fever, vomiting, diarrhea with desquamating rash; caused by exotoxins from *Staphylococcus aureus* associated with tampon use

Toxic shock syndrome

Soft, painful ulcerative lesion caused by *Haemophilus ducreyi*

Chancroid

Firm, painless chancre caused by a spirochete *Treponema pallidum*

1° syphilis

Small papule/ulcer associated with lymphadenopathy and caused by *C. trachomatis* serotypes L1, L2, or L3

Lymphogranuloma venereum

Donovan bodies on biopsy

Granuloma inguinale

Most common STD; frequent cause of pelvic inflammatory disease (PID) (though often asymptomatic); associated with Reiter syndrome

Chlamydial cervicitis (types D–K)

Sexually transmitted infection often associated with extragenital manifestations (eg, proctitis, arthritis, and neonatal conjunctivitis)

Gonorrhea

Painful vesicles/ulcers; cytologic evidence of multinuclear giant cells with viral inclusions

Herpes genitalis (most often HSV type 2)

STD caused by flagellated protozoan; #2 cause of vaginitis

Trichomoniasis

Commonly caused by *C. trachomatis* or *N. gonorrhoeae*; findings may include cervical motion tenderness, salpingitis, endometritis, or tubo-ovarian abscess

PID—at ↑ risk for ectopic pregnancy and infertility

Name the female reproductive disorder associated with each of the following features:

Triad of 2° amenorrhea, obesity, and hirsutism, ↑ testosterone, ↑ LH, ↓ FSH

Polycystic ovary (Stein-Leventhal) syndrome

Menstrual disorder associated with excessive bleeding during or between menstrual periods

Dysfunctional uterine bleeding

Cyclic pain and bleeding from proliferation of ectopic endometrial tissue

Endometriosis

Islands of endometrium found in the myometrium that may cause the uterus to grow to two to four times its normal size

Adenomyosis

Chocolate cysts

Endometriosis (in ovaries), endometrioma

Name the tumor of the vulva or vagina associated with each of the following statements:

Rare, malignant tumor of vagina associated with maternal use of diethylstilbestrol (DES) during pregnancy

Clear cell adenocarcinoma

Associated with HPV types 16, 18, 31, 33, and 45; #1 malignancy of vulva; ↑ in older women

Squamous cell carcinoma of vulva

"Bunch of grapes" protruding from vagina; usually in girls <5-y/o, desmin positive

Sarcoma botryoides

Accounts for 95% of neoplasms of vagina; usually from extension of cervical cancer

Squamous cell carcinoma of vagina

Name the uterine tumor associated with each of the following statements:

Neoplastic changes in the endometrium occurring at squamocolumnar junction; associated with HPV infection

Cervical intraepithelial neoplasia (CIN)

Invasive carcinoma evolving from CIN

Squamous cell carcinoma of the cervix

Very common, benign, estrogen-sensitive smooth muscle tumor of the uterus; usually in 20- to 40-y/o	Leiomyoma (fibroid)
Most common gynecologic malignancy; associated with prolonged estrogen exposure; usually 55- to 65-y/o	Endometrial carcinoma
Highly aggressive, bulky tumor with areas of necrosis; arises de novo; ↑ incidence in blacks	Leiomyosarcoma
What are the HPV viral proteins associated with squamous cell carcinoma?	E6 and E7
What role do HPV viral proteins play in the development of invasive cervical carcinoma?	Proteins E6 and E7 bind to and inactivate gene products of *p53* and *Rb*, respectively
What are the distinguishing histopathologic features of carcinoma in situ (CIN 3)?	Atypical changes extending through entire thickness of the epithelium
Name four factors associated with increased risk for invasive cervical carcinoma:	1. Early sexual activity 2. Multiple sex partners 3. ↓ Socioeconomic status 4. Cigarette smoking
What is the most effective screening tool for cervical cancer?	Routine pap smears
Name five factors that predispose to endometrial carcinoma:	1. Nulliparity 2. Obesity 3. Diabetes 4. Unopposed estrogen exposure (eg, estrogen-producing tumors, hormone replacement therapy [HRT]) 5. Tamoxifen
How does endometrial carcinoma typically present?	Postmenopausal vaginal bleeding
Name the ovarian cyst associated with each of the following statements:	
Distention of unruptured Graafian follicle; may be associated with ↑ estrogen endometrial hyperplasia	Follicular cyst
Hemorrhage into persistent corpus luteum; menstrual irregularity	Corpus luteum cyst

Due to gonadotropin stimulation; often bilateral/multiple; associated with choriocarcinoma and moles	Theca-lutein cyst

Name the ovarian tumor associated with each of the following statements:

Malignant tumor of epithelial origin; two-thirds are bilateral; psammoma bodies	Serous cystadenocarcinoma
Benign adenoma; frequently bilaterally; lined with fallopian tubelike epithelium	Serous cystadenoma
Malignant GCT that is homologous to seminoma and may occur in childhood	Dysgerminoma
Malignant tumor of epithelial origin; can rupture and cause pseudomyxoma peritonei	Mucinous cystadenocarcinoma
Benign multilocular cyst lined by mucus-secreting epithelium	Mucinous cystadenoma
Benign GCT with elements from multiple embryonic layers; most common GCT	Mature teratoma (dermoid cyst)
Benign tumor; cells resembling bladder transitional epithelium	Brenner tumor
GCT with Schiller-Duval bodies; ↑ AFP	Yolk sac (endodermal sinus) tumor
GCT associated with struma ovarii (mature thyroid tissue)	Teratoma (monodermal)
Malignant, aggressive tumor arising from syncytiotrophoblastic cells; ↑ serum β-hCG	Choriocarcinoma
Stromal tumor associated with Meigs syndrome (ascites, hydrothorax)	Thecoma-fibroma
Benign, estrogen-secreting tumor; Call-Exner bodies	Granulosa-theca tumor

Stromal tumor secreting androgens and causing virilization	Sertoli-Leydig cell tumor
Metastatic tumor from gastric adenocarcinoma; signet ring cells	Krukenberg tumor
Most ovarian carcinomas are associated with an increase in what serologic marker?	CA-125
What two genes are associated with a predisposition to ovarian cancer?	1. *BRCA1* 2. *HNPCC*
What is the most common type of ovarian neoplasm in women older than 20 years?	Epithelial cell neoplasms (~75% of all ovarian cancers)
What is the most common type of ovarian neoplasm in women younger than 20 years?	Germ cell neoplasms
List four physiologic adaptations to pregnancy	1. Increased cardiac output 2. Decreased hemoglobin concentration (plasma volume increases more than RBC count) 3. Hypercoagulability 4. Hyperventilation

Breast Disorders

Name the breast disease associated with each of the following statements:

Benign, firm, painless, rubbery mass; most common tumor in <25-y/o	Fibroadenoma
Inflammatory lesion caused by *S. aureus*; often occurs during nursing	Acute mastitis
"Blue-domed" cysts; usually bilateral; breast tenderness during menstruation	Fibrocystic change
Benign tumor of lactiferous ducts; most common cause of serous or bloody discharge in females <35-y/o	Intraductal papilloma
Large, malignant form of fibroadenoma	Cystosarcoma phyllodes

Invasive, malignant tumor; cells arranged in linear fashion; bloody discharge; often bilateral	Invasive lobular carcinoma
Malignant, firm mass with cells in glands; most common carcinoma of breast	Invasive ductal carcinoma
Eczematous lesion of nipple or areola containing large cells with marginal clearings	Paget disease of the breast

Name six risk factors for breast cancer:

1. Age >45-y/o
2. Early menarche and late menopause (↑ span of reproductive period)
3. Family history of (1° relative with history of [h/o]) premenopausal breast cancer
4. Personal h/o breast cancer
5. Inherited mutation (eg, HER-2/neu oncogene)
6. Obesity and high animal fat diet

Note: risk is not increased by fibroadenoma or nonhyperplastic cysts

Which disease is almost always associated with Paget disease of the breast?	Ductal carcinoma in situ
In which quadrant of the breast are most cancers located?	~50% found in upper, outer quadrant
What is the significance of estrogen/progesterone receptors on breast cancer?	Presence of estrogen and progesterone receptors reflects good prognosis (because tumor will likely respond to hormonal therapy)
What is the single most important prognostic factor in breast cancer?	Lymph node involvement (metastatic spread)
What two tumor suppressor genes are associated with a genetic predisposition for breast cancer?	1. *BRCA1* 2. *BRCA2*
What is the general function of the *BRCA1* and *BRCA2* genes?	DNA repair
Trastuzumab (Herceptin) treatment of breast cancers is directed at the protein product of which overexpressed gene?	*HER2/neu*

Pregnancy

Name the disorder of pregnancy associated with each of the following statements:

An ovum without DNA → "honeycombed uterus" and "cluster of grapes" appearance; formed from intrauterine proliferation of trophoblasts and cystic swelling of chorionic villi; serum β-hCG	Hydatidiform mole
Tear in placental membranes → sudden peripartal respiratory distress → shock → death	Amniotic fluid embolism
Placental attachment directly to myometrium → impaired separation and massive bleeding at delivery	Placenta accreta
Placental attachment to the lower uterine segment, extending to or obstructing the inner cervical os; painless bleeding in any trimester	Placenta previa
Premature detachment of a normally situated placenta; painful bleeding often in third trimester	Abruptio placentae
Hydatidiform mole with 46,XX genotype and markedly elevated β-hCG; no embryo; paternal chromosomes	Complete mole
Hydatidiform mole with triploid genotype and ↑ β-hCG; fetal parts may be present; (2 sperm + 1 egg)	Incomplete mole
Malignant, aggressive tumor that may arise from mole, ectopic, or normal pregnancy	Gestational choriocarcinoma
Toxemia of pregnancy with triad of HTN, edema, and proteinuria	Preeclampsia
Association with preeclampsia; schistocytes seen on blood smear	Hemolysis, Elevated LFTs, Low Platelets (HELLP syndrome)
Preeclampsia plus convulsions; DIC may be present	Eclampsia

What are some causes of polyhydramnios (>1.5–2 L of amniotic fluid)?	Maternal diabetes, esophageal/ duodenal atresia, anencephaly, Down syndrome

What are some causes of oligohydramnios (<0.5 L of amniotic fluid) and what sequence can result?	Genitourinary obstruction (especially posterior urethral valves in boys), bilateral renal agenesis; can result in Potter syndrome/sequence
Name the six clinically important and dangerous infections of pregnancy:	"ToRCHeS" 1. Toxoplasma 2. Rubella 3. CMV 4 and 5. HSV and HIV 6. Syphilis

Pituitary Disorders

Name the pituitary disorder associated with each of the following statements:

Most common pituitary adenoma	Prolactinoma (prolactin-secreting adenoma)
Deficiency of GnRH → lack of 2° sexual characteristics; associated with anosmia	Kallmann syndrome
Polyuria, polydipsia, hypernatremia from ↓ ADH; associated with a pituitary or hypothalamic injury	Central/neurogenic diabetes insipidus
Hypopituitarism caused by postpartum pituitary necrosis	Sheehan syndrome
Somatotrophic adenoma causing excess GH and IGF-1	Acromegaly (adults)/gigantism (kids)
Pituitary hypersecretion of ADH → hyponatremia, ↓ urine output, mental status changes	Syndrome of inappropriate antidiuretic hormone (SIADH)
What are the most important hormones to replace in Sheehan syndrome or pituitary apoplexy?	Cortisol and thyroid hormones

Name the endocrine/renal disorder associated with the following statements:

↓ sNa, ↑ Uosm with Uosm > Sosm	SIADH
High-normal sNa, ↑ Sosm, ↓ Uosm but no change in Uosm with H_2O deprivation test	Diabetes insipidus (DI)

Low-normal sNa, ↓ Uosm but
↑ Uosm toward normal w/H$_2$O
deprivation test

Primary polydipsia

**What are the two common
presentations of a pituitary tumor?**

1. Mass effect (bitemporal hemianopia, cranial nerve [CN] palsies)
2. Endocrine effects (amenorrhea, galactorrhea, hyperthyroidism, ↓ libido)

Thyroid

**What are the symptoms and physical
findings of hypothyroidism?**

Cold intolerance, ↓ HR, hypertension, hypercholesterolemia, pericardial effusion, periorbital myxedema, hypoactive deep tendon reflexes, coarse, dry skin; hair loss, weight gain, constipation, amenorrhea, ↓ pitch of voice, depression

What are symptoms and physical findings of hyperthyroidism?

Heat intolerance, hypertension, ↑ CO, ↑ HR, palpitations, cardiomegaly (long-term), staring gaze, lid lag, ↑ sympathetic activity, fine tremor, warm, moist, and flushed skin; fine hair; Graves' disease → pretibial myxedema, weight loss despite hyperphagia, ↑ motility, menstrual abnormalities, osteoporosis, anxiety

**Name four laboratory findings
common in hyperthyroidism:**

1. ↓ TSH (in 1°)
2. ↑ Free T$_4$
3. ↑ Total T$_4$
4. ↑ T$_3$ uptake

**Name four laboratory findings
common in hypothyroidism:**

1. ↑ TSH (very sensitive for 1°)
2. ↓ Free T$_4$
3. ↓ Total T$_4$
4. ↓ T$_3$ uptake

**Name the thyroid disorder associated
with each of the following statements:**

**Child with coarse facial features,
short stature, mental retardation,
and umbilical hernia**

Congenital hypothyroidism (cretinism)

**Goiter occurring with high
frequency in iodine-deficient areas**

Endemic goiter

**Painless enlargement of thyroid of
autoimmune etiology; Hürthle cells
and germinal centers; hypothyroid**

Hashimoto thyroiditis

Triad of diffuse thyroid hyperplasia, ophthalmopathy, dermopathy; hyperthyroid	Graves' disease
Normal thyroid replaced by fibrous tissue; hypothyroid	Riedel thyroiditis
Postviral, painful inflammation of thyroid; associated with HLA-B35	Subacute (granulomatous, de Quervain) thyroiditis
Thyroid-stimulating immunoglobulin (TSI) and TSH-receptor antibody (AB)	Graves' disease
Thyroid peroxidase antibody	Hashimoto disease
Extreme thyroid enlargement (>2 kg) causing mass effects; most patients euthyroid	Multinodular goiter
Most common thyroid carcinoma	Papillary carcinoma
Calcitonin-secreting tumor with amyloid deposits	Medullary carcinoma
Biopsy shows "Orphan Annie" nuclei, "fingerlike" projections, and psammoma bodies	Papillary carcinoma
Carcinoma presenting as a single nodule with uniform follicles	Follicular carcinoma
Aggressive carcinoma of older patients with pleomorphic cells; dismal prognosis	Anaplastic (undifferentiated) carcinoma
Carcinoma associated with Hashimoto thyroiditis	Lymphoma
What type of nodules is more likely to be benign: hot or cold?	Hot
Which gene is associated with medullary carcinoma of the thyroid?	*RET* (MEN 2A and 2B syndromes)
What is the function of the two genes associated with papillary carcinoma of the thyroid?	Tyrosine kinase receptors 1. RET 2. NTRK1
Name the multiple endocrine neoplasia (MEN) syndrome characterized by the following features:	
Pheochromocytoma, thyroid medullary carcinoma, and parathyroid adenomas	MEN 2A (Sipple syndrome)
Tumors of the pituitary, pancreatic islet cells, and parathyroid gland	MEN 1 (Wermer syndrome)

Mutation of RET oncogene on chromosome 10q	MEN 2A + B
Tumors in MEN 2 plus tall, thin habitus, prominent lips, and ganglioneuromas of the tongue and eyelids	MEN 3 (MEN 2b)
Mutation of *MEN 1* gene on chromosome 11q	MEN 1
Autosomal-dominant (AD) inheritance	All MEN syndromes

Parathyroid

Name the parathyroid disorder associated with each of the following statements:	
Caused by chronic renal failure or ↓ vitamin D	2° hyperparathyroidism
Most commonly due to parathyroid adenomas	1° hyperparathyroidism
Etiologies include congenital gland absence, surgically induced, and autoimmune destruction	Hypoparathyroidism
Due to autonomous hormone-secreting adenoma, often occurs after correction of chronic renal failure	3° hyperparathyroidism
Autosomal-recessive (AR) end-organ resistance to PTH → short stature and short third/fourth metacarpals	Pseudohypoparathyroidism

| What four systems are primarily targeted by hyperparathyroidism and hypercalcemia? | 1. Painful bones: osteitis fibrosa cystica, osteoporosis
2. Renal stones: nephrolithiasis, nephrocalcinosis
3. Abdominal groans: constipation, peptic ulcer disease (PUD), pancreatitis
4. Psychic moans: depression, lethargy, seizures |
| Up to 20% of parathyroid adenomas are commonly associated with altered activity of which gene? | *PRAD1* |

Adrenal Disorders

Name the four etiologies for
hypercorticism (Cushing syndrome):

1. Exogenous glucocorticoids (most
   common overall)
2. Pituitary ACTH hypersecretion
   (eg, adenoma)
3. Hypersecretion of cortisol
   (eg, adrenal hyperplasia)
4. Paraneoplastic (ectopic) ACTH
   secretion from a tumor

What is the most common cause of
endogenous hypercortisolism?

Cushing syndrome (pituitary adenoma)

What finding specific to an
ACTH-producing pituitary adenoma
differentiates it from adrenal
cortisol-producing and ectopic
ACTH-producing tumors?

↓ Cortisol level after high-dose
dexamethasone suppression test

In most cases of congenital adrenal
hyperplasia, deficiency in which
enzyme is associated with defective
conversion of progesterone to
11-deoxycorticosterone?

21-Hydroxylase

Name nine clinical findings of
Cushing syndrome:

1. Hyperglycemia (insulin resistance)
2. Virilization and menstrual
   irregularities in women
3. Moon facies
4. Truncal obesity
5. Buffalo hump
6. Skin changes (thinning, striae)
7. Osteoporosis
8. Immune suppression
9. Proximal muscle weakness

Name the adrenal disorder associated
with each of the following statements:

Aldosterone-secreting adenoma
causing HTN and hypokalemic,
metabolic alkalosis

Conn syndrome
(1° hyperaldosteronism)

Endotoxin-mediated massive
adrenal hemorrhage

Waterhouse-Friderichsen syndrome
(*Neisseria meningitidis*)

Deficiency of aldosterone and
cortisol due to adrenal atrophy or
destruction

1° chronic adrenocortical insufficiency
(Addison disease)

HPA disturbance causing failure of ACTH secretion	2° adrenocortical insufficiency
Bilateral hyperplasia of zona glomerulosa caused by stimulation of renin-angiotensin-aldosterone (RAA) system	2° hyperaldosteronism
Results from rapid steroid withdrawal or sudden ↑ in glucocorticoid requirements	1° acute adrenocortical insufficiency (adrenal crisis)
Chromaffin cell tumor usually in adults; results in episodic hyperadrenergic symptoms	Pheochromocytoma
Malignant, "small blue cell" tumor of medulla in kids associated with N-*myc* oncogene amplification	Neuroblastoma
How are 1° and 2° adrenocortical insufficiencies differentiated?	Hyperpigmentation is absent in 2° adrenocortical insufficiency (POMC is not increased)
Measurement of what substance can differentiate between 1° and 2° hyperaldosteronism?	Renin (↑ in 2° hyperaldosteronism)
What is the drug of choice for hyperaldosteronism?	Spironolactone (aldosterone antagonist)
What is the "rule of 10's" for pheochromocytomas?	10% malignant 10% bilateral 10% extra-adrenal 10% pediatric 10% familial 10% calcified
Besides MEN, name three familial syndromes associated with pheochromocytomas:	1. Sturge-Weber syndrome 2. von Recklinghausen syndrome 3. von Hippel-Lindau syndrome
What substances are secreted from pheochromocytomas and how are they detected?	Epinephrine and norepinephrine; detected by ↑ urinary secretion of catecholamines and their metabolites (metanephrine, VMA, and so forth)
Condition that causes ambiguous genitalia in males until puberty	Five Alpha reductase deficiency

Adrenogenital Syndromes

Name the enzyme deficiency responsible for each of the following androgenital syndromes:

↓ Sex hormones, ↓ cortisol, ↑ mineralocorticoids; HTN, hypokalemia, phenotypic female without maturation	17α-Hydroxylase deficiency
↓ Cortisol, aldosterone, and corticosterone; sex hormones; virilization, HTN	11β-Hydroxylase deficiency
↓ Cortisol, aldosterone, and corticosterone; sex hormones; virilization, hypotension, hyperkalemia, "salt wasting"	21-Hydroxylase deficiency

What is the phenotypic result of androgen insensitivity syndrome (testicular feminization)?

"Hairless woman"; XY with undescended testes but female genitalia (rudimentary vagina, absent uterus)

List the three syndromes associated with 21-hydroxylase deficiency:

1. Salt-wasting adrenogenitalism
2. Simple virilization adrenogenitalism (ambiguity and adrenal hyperplasia)
3. Asymptomatic

Diabetes

Describe the acute presentation of type 1 diabetes mellitus (DM)

Polydipsia, polyuria, polyphagia, weight loss, and diabetic ketoacidosis (DKA) if extreme

What causes hyperglycemia in type 1 DM?

Lack of insulin from decreased β-cell mass

What is the proposed mechanism of islet cell destruction in type 1 DM?

Environmental triggering of autoimmunity to islet β-cells

What is the theorized cause of type 2 DM?

Obesity increases insulin resistance and causes derangement of β-cell insulin secretion

What are four ways to diagnose DM?

1. Hemoglobin A1c >6.5%
2. Fasting serum glucose >126 (100–126 = impaired fasting glucose)
3. Oral glucose tolerance test >200 (148–200 = impaired glucose tolerance)
4. Symptoms + random glucose >200

What is HbA1c and what is it used for?	Percent of glycosylated hemoglobin in blood; correlates with glycemic control over the last 90 to 120 days

Type 1 or type 2 DM?

Younger average age of onset	Type 1
Associated with obesity	Type 2
Insulin treatment required from the time of diagnosis	Type 1
Associated with HLA-DR3 and -DR4	Type 1
May present with hyperosmolar coma	Type 2
May present initially as DKA	Type 1
Amyloid deposition in the islets	Type 2

What two cleavage products of proinsulin are stored in the granules of β-islet cells?	1. Insulin 2. C-peptide
Which membrane protein mediates glucose uptake by β-islet cells?	GLUT-2
Increased cytoplasmic concentration of which ion stimulates the secretion of insulin?	Calcium
By what mechanism is the cytoplasmic concentration of calcium increased in β-cells following uptake of glucose?	Decreased activation of adenosine triphosphate (ATP)-sensitive potassium channels leads to membrane depolarization, resulting in an influx of extracellular calcium via a voltage-dependent calcium channel
Glucose uptake in which organ is independent of insulin?	The brain
Activation of the PI-3K signal transduction pathway by insulin results in the translocation of what molecule to the surface of myocytes in order to transport glucose into myocytes?	GLUT-4
List four potential effects of advanced glycation end products (AGEs) in type 1 diabetes:	1. Cross-linking of collagen 2. Accumulation of extracellular matrix proteins resistant to proteolytic 3. Generation of reactive oxygen species 4. NF-κB activation

What is the most common cause of death in diabetics?	Myocardial infarction (MI) due to accelerated atherosclerosis
What is the most common morphologic change in the microvasculature of a diabetic?	Diffuse thickening of the basement membrane

Describe the long-term effect(s) of DM on each of the following organ systems

Cardiovascular (large vessels)	Atherosclerosis → cerebrovascular accident (CVA), MI, peripheral vascular disease (PVD)
Renal/urinary	**Glomerular:** glomerulosclerosis, proteinuria **Vascular:** arteriosclerosis → HTN, chronic renal failure **Infectious:** UTIs, pyelonephritis, necrotizing papillitis
Nervous	Motor and sensory peripheral neuropathy, autonomic degeneration
Eye	Retinopathy, cataract formation
Skin	Xanthomas, cutaneous infections, poor wound healing, fungal infections

Name four causes of secondary DM:	1. Pancreatic disease (eg, hemochromatosis, pancreatitis, pancreatic carcinoma) 2. Pregnancy (gestational diabetes) 3. Cushing syndrome 4. Other endocrine disorders (eg, acromegaly, glucagonoma, hyperthyroidism)

Pancreatic Endocrine Tumors

Name the islet cell tumor associated with each of the following statements:

Most common islet cell tumor	Insulinoma (β-cell tumor)
2° DM, necrolytic migratory erythema	Glucagonoma (α-cell tumor)
Associated with Zollinger-Ellison syndrome	Gastrinoma
Associated with watery diarrhea, hypokalemia, and achlorhydria (WDHA) syndrome	VIPoma

2° DM, cholelithiasis, steatorrhea	Somatostatinoma (δ-cell tumor)
Clinically characterized by Whipple triad	Insulinoma (β-cell tumor)
Name the clinical findings of Whipple triad:	Hypoglycemia, concurrent central nervous system (CNS) dysfunction, and reversal of symptoms with glucose
What is Zollinger-Ellison syndrome?	Hypersecretion of gastric HCl, recurrent PUD, and hypergastrinemia

PHARMACOLOGY

Pituitary

For each of the following drugs, provide:
1. The mechanism of action (MOA)
2. Indication(s) (IND)
3. Significant side effects and unique toxicity (TOX) (if any)

Octreotide	**MOA:** somatostatin analog **IND:** acromegaly, secretory diarrhea from VIPoma, carcinoid symptoms, high-output fistulas **TOX**: nausea, vomiting, stomach cramping, steatorrhea
Leuprolide	**MOA:** GnRH analog **Note:** given pulsatile = agonist; given continuous = antagonist **IND:** continuous → prostate cancer, endometriosis, uterine fibroids; pulsatile → infertility **TOX**: antiandrogenic effects, nausea, vomiting
Oxytocin	**MOA:** ↑ uterine contraction **IND:** induce/reinforce labor; control uterine hemorrhage **TOX:** uterine rupture, hypertensive crisis
Desmopressin	**MOA:** vasopressin analog **IND:** central diabetes insipidus, nocturnal enuresis **TOX**: HTN, overhydration, coronary constriction
Combined contraception MOA	Estrogen and progestins inhibit LH and FSH which prevents estrogen surge, resulting in LH surge, and ovulation

Thyroid and Parathyroid

For each of the following drugs,
provide:

1. The mechanism of action (MOA)
2. Indication(s) (IND)
3. Significant side effects and unique
   toxicity (TOX) (if any)

    Levothyroxine (T_4)

MOA: synthetic $T_4 \rightarrow$ converted to T_3

IND: hypothyroidism (maintenance replacement)

TOX: nervousness, palpitations, $\uparrow$ HR, heat intolerance

    Propylthiouracil/methimazole

MOA: blocks thyroid peroxidase, propylthiouracil also $\downarrow$ peripheral conversion of $T_4 \rightarrow T_3$

IND: hyperthyroidism (propylthiouracil okay in pregnancy)

TOX: rash, agranulocytosis (rare), +ANCA vasculitis, hepatotoxicity, lupuslike syndrome

    Risedronate

MOA: bisphosphonate (inhibits osteoclastic function)

IND: osteoporosis, Paget disease, metastatic bone cancer, hyperparathyroidism

TOX: GI upset, esophagitis

    Calcitonin

MOA: $\downarrow$ bone resorption, $\downarrow$ serum Ca^{2+} and phosphate

IND: acute hypercalcemia, Paget disease, osteoporosis

Which other drug is used to treat the symptoms of hyperthyroidism?

Propanolol (β-blocker)

Diabetes

Sulfonylureas (eg, glyburide)

MOA: pancreas, closes K^+ channels in β-cell membrane $\rightarrow$ depolarization $\rightarrow \uparrow$ Ca^{2+} influx $\rightarrow$ insulin release

IND: type 2 diabetes (not used in type 1 because it requires some residual β-cell activity)

TOX: hypoglycemia, weight gain

Metformin	**MOA:** liver, ↓ gluconeogenesis; ↑ glycolysis; ↓ postprandial glucose **IND:** newly diagnosed diabetic (no islet cell function required) **TOX:** potentially life-threatening lactic acidosis, ↓ vitamin B_{12} absorption, contraindicated in renal insufficiency
Glitazones (eg, rosiglitazone, pioglitazone)	**MOA:** ↑ target cell response to insulin **IND:** type 2 diabetes (monotherapy or combination) **TOX:** hepatotoxicity (troglitazone), upper respiratory infection (URI), weight gain, edema, congestive heart failure, and anemia (rosiglitazone)
α-Glucosidase inhibitor (eg, acarbose)	**MOA:** inhibits α-glucosidase at brush border → ↓ glucose absorption **IND:** type 2 diabetes **TOX:** GI upset (flatulence, diarrhea)
Glucagon-like peptide-1 (GLP-1) agonist (eg, liraglutide, semaglutide)	**MOA:** ↑ glucose-dependent insulin secretion, ↓ glucagon secretion from α cells, ↓ gastric emptying (↓ postprandial glucose, promotes satiety) **IND:** type 2 diabetes **TOX:** pancreatitis, thyroid C-cell tumor
Dipeptidyl peptidase-4 enzyme (DPP-4) antagonist (eg, sitagliptin)	**MOA:** inhibits DPP-4 which normally breaks down GLP-1 **IND:** type 2 diabetes **TOX:** pancreatitis, URI, liver injury
Sodium-glucose co-transporter 2 (SGLT2) inhibitor (eg, empagloflozin, canaglifozin)	**MOA:** ↓ reabsorption of glucose in proximal tubule of kidney → ↑ glucose excretion in urine **IND:** type 2 diabetes **TOX:** UTI, bladder cancer, hypovolemia
Amylin agonist (eg, pramlintide)	**MOA:** ↓ gastric emptying (↓ postprandial glucose, promotes satiety) **IND:** type 1 and 2 diabetes **TOX:** nausea, hypoglycemia (when used with insulin)

Insulin	**MOA:** tyrosine kinase activity $\rightarrow\uparrow$ glycogen and protein synthesis, triglyceride (TG) storage, and K^+ uptake **IND:** type 1 and refractory type 2 diabetes; life-threatening hyperkalemia **TOX:** hypoglycemia and rare hypersensitivity reaction

For each of the following types of insulin, state the peak and duration of action:

Insulin glulisine, aspart, lispro	Peak = 30 to 60 minutes; duration = 3 to 4 hours
NPH insulin	Peak = 8 to 12 hours; duration = 18 to 24 hours
Lente insulin	Peak = 8 to 12 hours; duration = 18 to 24 hours
Insulin glargine	Peak = none (peakless); duration = 20 to 24+ hours
Function of GLUT-1 transporter	Insulin-independent glucose transporter in RBCs, brain, cornea, and placenta

Adrenal Glands

Describe the mechanism of action of corticosteroids	Corticosteroids bind to cytoplasmic receptors, pass into the nucleus complexed with their receptors, and act as transcription factors for specific target genes
How do glucocorticoids affect arachidonic acid metabolism?	Glucocorticoids inhibit phospholipase A2, blocking the release of arachidonic acid and $\downarrow$ production of prostaglandins and leukotrienes

Select the most appropriate corticosteroid for each of the following clinical situations:

Diagnosis of Cushing syndrome	Dexamethasone
Autoimmune disorder	Prednisone
Addison disease	Hydrocortisone (±fludrocortisone)
Relief of inflammation	Prednisone, cortisone
Asthma/allergies	Beclomethasone or triamcinolone aerosol

Used to ↑ fetal lung maturity	Betamethasone
Cancer chemotherapy	Prednisone

List the effect of glucocorticoids on each of the following systems:

Metabolic	↑ Gluconeogenesis; net ↑ in fat deposition in prototypical areas
Muscle	↑ Muscle protein catabolism; myopathy → weakness
Bone	↑ Bone catabolism
Immune	Inhibits cell-mediated immunity; ↑ PMNs; ↓ lymphocytes, basophils, eosinophils, and monocytes; ↓ leukocyte migration
Psych	Behavioral changes, psychoses
GI	↓ Resistance to ulcers
Vascular	↓ Capillary permeability →↓ edema at sites of inflammation

What is the consequence of abrupt discontinuation of corticosteroid use?	Acute adrenal insufficiency syndrome (potentially lethal)

Name eight commonly observed effects of long-term corticosteroid use:	1. Osteoporosis 2. HTN 3. Insulin resistance 4. Edema 5. Psychoses 6. Peptic ulcers 7. ↑ Susceptibility to infections 8. Cataracts

What classic toxicity is associated with excess corticosteroid use?	Iatrogenic Cushing syndrome

For each of the following drugs, provide:
1. The mechanism of action (MOA)
2. Indication(s) (IND)
3. Significant side effects and unique toxicity (TOX) (if any)

Spironolactone	**MOA:** spironolactone binds estrogen receptors; also inhibits steroid binding **IND:** hirsutism (eg, in PCOS), prostate/breast cancer **TOX**: gynecomastia, thrombocytopenia, hepatotoxicity

Clomiphene	**MOA:** blocks negative feedback $\rightarrow \uparrow$ GnRH $\rightarrow \uparrow$ LH and FSH $\rightarrow$ ovulation **IND:** infertility **TOX:** ovarian enlargement, multiple births, hot flashes
Tamoxifen	**MOA:** competes for estrogen receptors $\rightarrow$ blocks binding to ER $\approx$ cells **IND:** breast cancer **TOX:** $\uparrow$ risk of endometrial carcinoma, hot flashes
Finasteride	**MOA:** 5α-reductase inhibitor $\rightarrow \downarrow$ DHT **IND:** benign prostatic hyperplasia (BPH), hair loss **TOX:** erectile dysfunction, gynecomastia
Mifepristone (RU486)	**MOA:** competitive progesterone receptor blocker **IND:** abortion **TOX:** GI upset, metrorrhagia
Dinoprostone	**MOA:** PGE$_2$ analog causes cervical dilation and uterine contraction **IND:** induction of labor; abortion
Ritodrine, terbutaline	**MOA:** β_2-agonists relax the uterus **IND:** preterm labor **TOX:** maternal and fetal tachycardia, fluid retention, and hyperglycemia
Sildenafil, vardenafil	**MOA:** inhibits phosphodiesterase type 5 $\rightarrow \uparrow$ cGMP $\rightarrow$ smooth muscle relaxation of corpus cavernosum **IND:** erectile dysfunction **TOX:** hypotension if also taking a nitrate, priapism, headache, color vision changes
Name five benefits of oral contraceptives (OCPs):	1. $\downarrow$ Risk of ovarian and endometrial cancer 2. $\downarrow$ Genitourinary infections 3. Regulates menstrual cycle 4. Low failure rate (if taken appropriately) 5. $\downarrow$ Risk of ectopic pregnancy
Name five disadvantages of OCPs:	1. Requires daily pill ingestion 2. Not protective against STDs 3. $\uparrow$ Triglycerides 4. $\uparrow$ Risk of hepatic adenoma 5. Induces hypercoagulable state

Name four contraindications to OCPs:

1. Pregnancy
2. H/o thromboembolism or stroke
3. H/o breast cancer or endometrial cancer
4. Smoking (in women >35-y/o)

Pheochromocytoma treatment

Phenoxybenzamine (irreversible alpha antagonist)

CHAPTER 9

Renal and Genitourinary

EMBRYOLOGY

Name the structure(s) derived from each of the following:

Nephrogenic cord (three structures)

1. Pronephros
2. Mesonephros
3. Metanephros

Ureteric bud

C CUP (*"see you pee"*): **C**ollecting tubules, **C**alyces, **U**reter, **P**elvis

Genital ridge

Gonads

Reproductive structures from the mesonephric (Wolffian) duct

"SEED" (in males *only*): **S**eminal vesicles, **E**pididymis, **E**jaculatory duct, **D**uctus deferens

Reproductive structures from the paramesonephric (Müllerian) duct

In women *only*: fallopian tubes, uterus, superior portion of vagina

Metanephros

Definitive adult kidney

Name the embryologic tissue layer that following components of the genitourinary system develop from:

Kidneys (ie, nephrons)

Mesoderm (intermediate mesoderm)

Collecting tubules, calyces, pelvis, ureters

Mesoderm (intermediate mesoderm)

Bladder, urethra

Endoderm (cloaca)

Name the parts of the external genitalia in males and females derived from the following embryologic structures:

Genital tubercle

Males: glans penis; females: glans clitoris

Urogenital sinus	Males: corpus spongiosum, bulbourethral (Cowper) glands, prostate gland; females: vestibular bulbs, Bartholin and Skene glands
Urogenital folds	Males: ventral shaft of penis; females: labia minora
Labioscrotal swelling	Males: scrotum; females: labia majora

Describe the following congenital disorders:

Exstrophy of the bladder	Congenital defect in the anterior wall of the bladder and adjacent abdominal wall causing the bladder to be exposed at birth; associated with epispadias
Horseshoe kidney	Fusion of the lower (or upper) poles of kidneys → kidney fails to ascend → often malrotated and remains in pelvis; associated with Turner syndrome
Hypospadias	Penile abnormality resulting in urethra opening on the ventral (inferior) side of penis; most common congenital penile abnormality
Epispadias	Penile abnormality resulting in urethral opening on the dorsal (superior) side of penis; associated with bladder exstrophy
Renal agenesis	Results from failure of the ureteric bud to form; associated with Potter syndrome
Potter syndrome	Renal agenesis → oligohydramnios → limb deformities and pulmonary hypoplasia

What structure limits the ascent of a fused horseshoe kidney?	Inferior mesenteric artery
What substance secreted by the testes suppresses development of paramesonephric ducts in males?	Müllerian-inhibiting substance
Promotes development of the mesonephric ducts?	Fetal androgens

Describe the gonads and external genitalia of the following:

Female (XX) infant with congenital adrenal hyperplasia (CAH)	Female gonads with masculinized genitalia

Male (XY) infant with androgen-insensitivity syndrome	Male gonads with female external genitalia, but no uterus or fallopian tubes

ANATOMY

Name the structures contained in the retroperitoneal space:	Ureters, kidneys, adrenals, pancreas, duodenum (second, third, and fourth parts), ascending/descending colon, rectum, aorta, IVC
What is the approximate vertebral level of the kidneys?	T12 to L3 (the right kidney is slightly lower because of liver)
Name the renal blood vessel that runs posterior to the superior mesenteric artery (SMA) and anterior to the aorta:	Left renal vein
What vessel does the left gonadal vein drain into?	Left renal vein
What important structures do the ureters pass *under* on their way to the bladder?	Females: uterine artery; males: ductus deferens; *water* (ureters) *under the bridge* (uterine artery, ductus deferens)
Which terminal vessels carry blood toward the glomerulus?	Afferent arterioles
What specialized cells are found between the afferent and efferent glomerular arterioles and have receptors for angiotensin II (AT II) and atrial natriuretic peptide (ANP)?	Extraglomerular mesangial cells (Lacis cells)
What makes up the juxtaglomerular apparatus (JGA)?	JG cells, extraglomerular mesangial cells (Lacis cells), and the macula densa
What hormone do the JG cells secrete?	Renin
What anatomic feature makes stress incontinence more common in women?	External urethral sphincter does not completely surround female urethra
Name the sensory and motor components of the micturition reflex:	Pelvic splanchnic nerves (parasympathetic S2–S4)

PHYSIOLOGY

What percentage of body weight is total body water (TBW)?	~60%

What proportion of TBW is accounted for by intracellular fluid (ICF) and extracellular fluid (ECF)?

Two-thirds ICF, 1/3 ECF (60 = 40 + 20; rule: 40% body weight is ICF, 20% is ECF)

Name the major cations and anions found in ICF:

Cations = K^+, Mg^{2+}; anions = proteins, organophosphates (eg, ADP, ATP)

Name the major cations and anions found in ECF:

Cations = Na^+; anions = Cl^-, HCO_3^-

What are the relative proportions of plasma and interstitial fluid in ECF?

One-fourth plasma volume, three-fourths interstitial volume

What is considered normal ECF osmolality?

~290 mOsm

Clearance of what chemical can be used to measure glomerular filtration rate (GFR)?

Inulin (inulin is freely filtered, but neither secreted nor reabsorbed)

What is a useful clinical measure to estimate GFR?

Creatinine clearance

What is considered normal GFR?

~120 mL/min

Effective renal plasma flow (ERPF) can be measured by calculating the clearance of what substance?

Para-aminohippuric acid (PAH); PAH is filtered and secreted

Complete the following calculations:

$U_x V/P_x$ **(urine concentration × urine volume/plasma concentration) =**

Renal clearance (C_x)

ERPF/(1 − hematocrit) =

Renal blood flow (RBF)

GFR/RPF (renal plasma flow) =

Filtration fraction (FF)

GFR × (plasma$_x$) =

Filtered load

$V_{urine\ flow} - (U_{osm} V/P_{osm}) =$

Free water clearance

Define GFR using the Starling formula

$K_f[(P_{GC} - P_{BS}) - (\pi_{GC} - \pi_{BS})]$, where K_f = filtration coefficient, GC = glomerular capillary, BS = Bowman space

List the three components of the glomerular filtration barrier:

1. Fused basement membrane (negative charge barrier)
2. Fenestrated capillary endothelium (size barrier)
3. Epithelial or podocyte foot process layer

If C_x > GFR then there is net ...

tubular secretion of substance X

If C_x < GFR then there is net ...

tubular absorption of substance X

If C_x = GFR then there is ...

no net tubular absorption or secretion of substance X

What proportion of total cardiac output does RBF account for?

~25%

How is RBF maintained at a constant level?

Autoregulation (via myogenic response to stretch and the activity of the JGA)

How do the following substances affect the renal arterioles, RPF, GFR, and FF?

Prostaglandins

Prostaglandins dilate afferent arterioles: ↑ RPF, ↑ GFR, thus FF stays constant

AT II

AT II constricts efferent arterioles: ↓ RPF, ↑ GFR, thus FF increases

What effect do the following have on RPF, GFR, and FF?

Afferent arteriole constriction

Decreased RPF and GFR, no change in FF

Efferent arteriole constriction

Decreased RPF, increased GFR, increased FF

Increased plasma protein concentration

No change in RPF, decreased GFR and FF

Decreased plasma protein concentration

No change in RPF, increased GFR and FF

What is the maximum plasma glucose concentration at which glucose will no longer be reabsorbed?

~200 to 250 mg/dL (concentrations of >250 mg/dL glucose will be lost in the urine)

What is the transport maximum (T_m) for glucose?

At 350 mg/min, carriers are saturated (T_m = renal threshold/GFR)

What factors cause K^+ to shift out of cells?

↓ Insulin, β-blockers, acidosis, digitalis, extreme exercise, cell lysis, hyperosmolarity

What factors cause K^+ to shift into cells?

Insulin, β-agonists, alkalosis

List four causes of decreased distal K^+ secretion:

1. Low-K^+ diet
2. Hypoaldosteronism
3. Acidosis
4. K^+-sparing diuretics

List six causes of increased distal K^+ secretion:	1. High-K^+ diet 2. Hyperaldosteronism 3. Alkalosis 4. Thiazide diuretics 5. Loop diuretics 6. Luminal anions

Describe a clinical scenario which might lead to each of the following physiologic changes:

Isosmotic volume contraction	Diarrhea
Isosmotic volume expansion	Isotonic fluid infusion (eg, normal saline IV)
Hyperosmotic volume contraction (two scenarios)	1. Profuse sweating 2. Diabetes insipidus
Hyperosmotic volume expansion	High NaCl intake, infusion of hypertonic saline
Hypo-osmotic volume contraction	Adrenal insufficiency (hypoaldosteronism)
Hypo-osmotic volume expansion	Syndrome of inappropriate antidiuretic hormone (SIADH)

Functional Regions of the Nephron

Name the part of the nephron where each of the following processes occur:

Site of reabsorption of all glucose and amino acids, and the majority of bicarbonate, sodium, and water	Proximal convoluted tubule (PCT)
Site of active reabsorption K^+, Na^+, Cl^-	Thick ascending loop of Henle
Site of 50% of urea reabsorption	PCT (passively)
Site of active reabsorption of Na^+, Cl^-	Early distal convoluted tubule (DCT)
Site of action of thiazide diuretics	DCT
Site of action of K^+-sparing diuretics	Collecting tubules
Sections that are impermeable to water	Thick ascending loop of Henle, collecting ducts (in absence of ADH)
Site where ammonia is excreted to act as a buffer for secreted H^+ ions	PCT
Portion of the nephron which is impermeable to Na^+ and passively reabsorbs water	Thin descending loop of Henle

Aldosterone-sensitive site where Na^+ is exchanged for K^+ or H^+	Collecting tubules
Site of active Ca^{2+} reabsorption that is controlled by PTH	Early DCT
Site of action of loop diuretics	Thick ascending loop of Henle
Section where reabsorption of water is regulated by vasopressin (ADH)	Collecting tubules
Site of action of carbonic anhydrase inhibitors	PCT
Section which contains principal cells and intercalated cells	Collecting tubules
Site of 85% of all phosphate reabsorption (via cotransport)	PCT

Endocrine Functions of the Kidneys

List the four main endocrine functions of the kidneys:	1. PTH-mediated conversion of 25-OH vitamin D to 1, 25-OH vitamin D by 1α-hydroxylase 2. Secretion of renin by JG cells in response to arterial pressure changes and in response to Na^+ and Cl^- delivery to the macula densa 3. Secretion of prostaglandins (to increase GFR by dilating afferent arteriole) 4. Secretion of erythropoietin in response to hypoxia by peritubular endothelial cells
Name the effect of each of the following on the kidneys:	
ANP	$\downarrow Na^+$ reabsorption, $\uparrow$ GFR
Aldosterone	$\uparrow Na^+$ reabsorption, $\uparrow K^+$ secretion, $\uparrow H^+$ secretion in distal tubules and collecting duct
Vasopressin (ADH)	$\uparrow Na^+/K^+/2Cl^-$ transporters in thick ascending limb, $\uparrow$ water permeability in principal cells (via aquaporins), $\uparrow$ urea absorption in collecting duct
Where is angiotensin-converting enzyme (ACE) primarily found?	Lung capillaries

Briefly describe the renin-angiotensin-aldosterone cascade:	↑ BP (↓ stretch of cells in afferent arterioles) → secretion of renin → conversion of angiotensinogen to angiotensin I (AT I) → AT I converted to AT II by ACE
What is the function of AT II?	Increases intravascular volume and ↑ vascular tone → ↑ BP
Name six specific actions of AT II:	1. Causes potent vasoconstriction 2. Releases vasopressin and adrenocorticotropic hormone (ACTH) from the pituitary 3. Promotes release of aldosterone from adrenal cortex 4. Stimulates hypothalamus to increase thirst 5. Stimulates catecholamine release from the adrenal medulla 6. Increases Na^+ and HCO_3^- reabsorption in proximal tubule
What cells in the kidneys produce and secrete erythropoietin?	Peritubular capillary cells
What stimulates erythropoietin production and release?	Hypoxia

PATHOLOGY

Polycystic Kidney Disease

Name the disease characterized by multiple 3 to 4 cm renal cysts, bilateral enlargement of the kidneys, and chronic renal failure in adults:	Autosomal dominant (adult) polycystic kidney disease (ADPKD)
What are the signs and symptoms of ADPKD?	Flank pain, hypertension, hematuria, and UTI
Which gene is most commonly associated with ADPKD?	*PKD1* (85% of cases)
Name three extra renal manifestations of ADPKD:	1. Liver cysts (40%) 2. Berry aneurysms (10%–30%) 3. Mitral valve prolapse (25%)
What is the prognosis of patients with autosomal recessive polycystic kidney disease (ARPKD)?	Poor; majority die in infancy or early childhood

What type of renal lesions is characteristic of ARPKD?

Multiple cylindrical cysts found perpendicular to cortex in an enlarged kidney

Which of the cystic renal diseases is associated with an increased risk of renal cell carcinoma (RCC)?

Dialysis-associated cystic disease

Nephrotic and Nephritic Syndromes

What are the classic features of the following:

Nephrotic syndrome

Massive proteinuria (>3.5 g/d), hypoalbuminemia, hyperlipidemia, edema

Nephritic syndrome

Hypertension, azotemia, RBC casts, oliguria, hematuria

What term describes the type of immune deposits found outside of the glomerular BM (GBM) but within the podocytes?

Subepithelial

What term describes the type of immune deposits found outside the endothelium but inside the GBM?

Subendothelial

Name the immunofluorescence pattern of deposition of immunoglobulins and/or complement associated with the following diseases:

Membranous glomerulonephritis (GN)

Granular or "starry-sky"

Goodpasture syndrome

Linear

IgA nephropathy (Berger disease)

Mesangial

Poststreptococcal

Granular or "starry-sky"

Name the electron microscopic (EM) appearance of the immunoglobulin and/or complement deposits in the following diseases:

Membranous GN

"Spike and dome" subepithelial deposits

Membranoproliferative GN (MPGN)

Subendothelial humps, "tram track"

Poststreptococcal GN

Subepithelial humps

Name the glomerulopathy most closely associated with each of the following statements:

X-linked syndrome of GN, lens dislocation, nerve deafness, and posterior cataracts	Alport syndrome
Nodular glomerulosclerosis, glomerular capillary basement membrane thickening	Diabetic glomerulosclerosis (Kimmelstiel-Wilson disease)
Commonly associated with HIV infection, heroin abuse, sickle cell disease, and obesity	Focal-segmental glomerulosclerosis (FSGS)
Diffuse loss of foot processes of the visceral epithelial cells on EM, but normal appearance on light microscopy	Minimal change disease (lipoid nephrosis)
Apple green birefringence on Congo red stain	Amyloidosis
C-ANCA	Granulomatosis with polyangiitis (GPA) (formerly known as Wegener granulomatosis)
Most common cause of nephrotic syndrome in kids	Minimal change disease (lipoid nephrosis)
Most common cause of nephrotic syndrome in Caucasian adults	Membranous nephropathy
Most common cause of nephrotic syndrome in AA adults	FSGS
Electron dense deposits in the GBM proper and autoantibody to C3 nephritic factor	MPGN type II (aka dense deposit disease)
Crescents seen in glomeruli on light microscopy	Rapidly progressive glomerulonephritis (RPGN)
Most common cause of end-stage renal disease	Diabetic glomerulosclerosis
Basement membrane thickening and splitting (*train tracks*)	MPGN type I
Syndrome of hematuria and hemoptysis caused by anti-GBM antibodies	Goodpasture syndrome
Mesangial widening, recurrent hematuria, and proteinuria	IgA nephropathy
Associated with hepatitis C	MPGN
Associated with solid tumors, systemic lupus erythematosus (SLE)	Membranous nephropathy

Responds well to steroids	Minimal change disease (aka steroid responsive nephropathy)
X-linked recessive defect in collagen type IV	Alport syndrome
Asymptomatic familial hematuria	Thin membrane disease (GBM is only 50%–60% of normal thickness)
"Wire loop lesions"	SLE—lupus nephropathy (diffuse proliferative pattern)
Henoch-Schönlein purpura	IgA nephropathy
Irregularly thick GBM with splitting of lamina densa seen on EM	Alport syndrome
Upper respiratory vasculitis and granulomas	GPA (formerly known as Wegener granulomatosis)

Renal Tubular Acidosis

Name the type of renal tubular acidosis (RTA) associated with the following statements:

Decreased bicarbonate reabsorption	Type II (proximal)
Dysfunction of principal cells	Type IV
Decreased acidification and acid excretion	Type I (distal)
Hyperkalemia	Type IV
Nongap metabolic acidosis	Types I, II, IV
Fanconi syndrome	Type II (proximal)
Aldosterone deficiency/resistance	Type IV
Most common RTA	Type IV

Acid-Base Disturbance

Name the simple acid-base disturbance and the associated compensatory response:

pH >7.4, P_{CO_2} >40 mm Hg	Metabolic alkalosis → hypoventilation
pH <7.4, P_{CO_2} >40 mm Hg	Respiratory acidosis → renal HCO_3^- reabsorption
pH >7.4, P_{CO_2} <40 mm Hg	Respiratory alkalosis → renal HCO_3^- secretion
pH <7.4, P_{CO_2} <40 mm Hg	Metabolic acidosis → hyperventilation

What is the formula for calculating anion gap?	$Na^+ - (Cl^- + HCO_3^-)$
What is a normal anion gap range?	8 to 12 mEq/L
List three common causes of nongap metabolic acidosis:	1. Diarrhea 2. RTA 3. Hyperchloremia
Name the most common cause of respiratory acidosis:	Hypoventilation (which can be caused by acute/chronic lung disease, sedatives, weakening of respiratory muscles)
List three common causes of respiratory alkalosis:	1. Hyperventilation 2. Early aspirin ingestion 3. Gram-negative sepsis
List five common causes of metabolic alkalosis:	1. Excessive vomiting 2. Diuretic abuse 3. Antacid use 4. Hyperaldosteronism 5. Cushing syndrome
List nine possible causes of anion gap metabolic acidosis:	"MUD PILERS" 1. Methanol 2. Uremia 3. Diabetic ketoacidosis 4. Paraldehyde 5. Isoniazid (INH) or Iron tablet overdose 6. Lactic acidosis 7. Ethylene glycol or Ethanol 8. Rhabdomyolysis (massive) 9. Salicylate toxicity

Acute Kidney Injury

List the three main types of acute kidney injury (AKI)	1. Prerenal 2. Intrinsic renal 3. Postrenal
List four common prerenal causes of AKI:	1. Hypovolemia 2. Decreased RBF (eg, decreased cardiac output, renal artery stenosis [RAS]) 3. High peripheral vascular resistance 4. Drugs (eg, diuretics, NSAIDs)

List five common causes of intrinsic AKI:

1. Acute tubular necrosis (ischemic, nephrotoxic, sepsis)
2. Acute GN
3. Autoimmune vasculitis (eg, lupus, scleroderma)
4. Interstitial nephritis
5. Hemolytic uremic syndrome (children)

What is the general mechanism for the development of postrenal AKI?

Any outflow obstruction (benign prostatic hyperplasia [BPH], bladder-neck, stones, prior gynecologic surgery, bilateral ureteric)
Note: postrenal AKI accounts for <5% of all causes of AKI

Name the type of AKI associated with each of the following:

Oliguria and Fe_{Na} <1%

Prerenal

Oliguria and Fe_{Na} >1%

Intrinsic

Hyaline urine casts

Prerenal

Muddy brown/granular casts

Intrinsic (muddy brown casts are particularly associated with ATN)

Blood urea nitrogen (BUN): creatinine ratio >20

Prerenal

Urine osmolality >500 mOsm

Prerenal

List the effects of uremia on each of the following organs or systems:

Nervous system

Asterixis, confusion, seizures, coma

Cardiovascular system

Fibrinous pericarditis

Hematologic system

Coagulopathy (due to platelet dysfunction), immunosuppression

Gastrointestinal system

Nausea, vomiting, gastritis

Skin

Pruritis

Endocrine system

Glucose intolerance

List six nonuremic complications of renal failure:

1. Metabolic acidosis
2. Hyperkalemia → arrhythmias
3. Na^+ and H_2O excess → pulmonary edema and congestive heart failure (CHF)
4. Hypocalcemia → osteodystrophy (from failure to secrete active vitamin D)
5. Anemia (↓ EPO secretion)
6. Hypertension (from renin hypersecretion)

What substances cause direct injury to the proximal tubules?	Nephrotoxins: drugs (aminoglycosides), toxins, and massive amounts of myoglobin (typically in the setting of a crush injury or strenuous exercise)

Renal Infections

What infection commonly presents with flank pain, costovertebral angle tenderness, fever, dysuria, pyuria, bacteriuria?	Acute pyelonephritis
What are the two major causes of pyelonephritis?	1. Ascending infection (from UTI) 2. Hematogenous seeding
What are the most common organisms responsible for acute pyelonephritis?	*Escherichia coli* (most common), *Proteus*, *Klebsiella*, *Enterobacter*, *Pseudomonas* (think enteric gram-negative rods)
What is the greatest risk factor for pyelonephritis?	Vesicoureteral reflux (or incompetence)
List five possible sequelae of acute pyelonephritis:	1. Abscess 2. Necrotizing papillitis 3. Renal scars 4. Perinephric abscess 5. Pyonephrosis
What condition is characterized by broad renal scarring, deformed calyces, progressive loss of renal parenchyma, and thyroidization of kidneys?	Chronic pyelonephritis
What finding on microscopic examination of urine is pathognomonic for pyelonephritis?	WBC casts

Tubulointerstitial Diseases

Name the tubulointerstitial disease associated with each of the following clinical scenarios:	
Abuse of phenacetin-containing compounds	Renal papillary necrosis
Penicillin and NSAID use; associated with eosinophilia	Interstitial nephritis

AR syndrome characterized by dysfunction of proximal tubules, leading to impaired reabsorption of amino acids, glucose, phosphate, and bicarbonate

Fanconi syndrome

AR disease characterized by impaired tryptophan reabsorption; clinically resembles pellagra

Hartnup disease

AR syndrome characterized by impaired active chloride reabsorption in the loop of Henle; clinically mimics the actions of loop diuretics

Bartter syndrome

AR syndrome characterized by reabsorptive defect of NaCl in the DCT; clinically mimics the actions of thiazide diuretics

Gitelman syndrome

AD syndrome characterized by increased reabsorption of Na^+ in the distal and collecting tubules due to increased activity of the epithelial sodium channels (ENaC); treat with amiloride

Liddle syndrome

Name the five diseases associated with renal papillary necrosis:

1. Diabetes mellitus
2. Acute pyelonephritis
3. Analgesic nephropathy
4. Sickle cell disease
5. Urinary tract obstruction

Renal Vascular Disease

Name the renal vascular pathology associated with each of the following statements:

Macroscopically, kidneys have a fine granular surface; hyaline arteriolosclerosis, interstitial fibrosis, glomerular sclerosis

Benign nephrosclerosis

Hyperplastic arteriolitis (onion-skinning); presents with diastolic BP >130, encephalopathy, proteinuria, hematuria, and papilledema

Malignant nephrosclerosis

Pediatric syndrome characterized by ARF, microangiopathic hemolytic anemia, thrombocytopenia, and hypertension

Classic hemolytic-uremic syndrome (HUS)

Syndrome characterized by ARF, microangiopathic hemolytic anemia, hypertension, fever, and mental status changes; associated with ADAMTS-13 defect	Thrombotic thrombocytopenic purpura (TTP)
What is the most common cause of HUS?	*Escherichia coli* O157:H7 (75% of cases)
What three groups of patients are at increased risk of developing renal failure from benign nephrosclerosis?	1. African Americans 2. Diabetics 3. Patients with hypertension
What type of infarction typically occurs in the kidneys?	"White," due to end-organ type arterial supply of kidneys
What conditions are associated with diffuse cortical necrosis?	Obstetric catastrophes (eg, severe placental abruption) and septic shock
Name two major causes of RAS:	1. Atherosclerosis (70%) 2. Fibromuscular dysplasia (30%)
What group of people is most likely to have secondary hypertension due to fibromuscular dysplasia-induced RAS?	Women in their 20s and 30s

Urolithiasis

Name the type of renal calculi associated with each of the following statements:	
Radiopaque (two types)	1. Calcium stones 2. Struvite stones
Staghorn calculi	Struvite (aka ammonium magnesium phosphate)
Infection with urease-positive bacteria	Struvite (think *Proteus*)
Most common type of calculus	Calcium
Gout (or any other hyperuricemic condition)	Calcium
Elevated PTH	Calcium
Secondary to inherited defect of amino acid transporter	Cystine (due to cystinuria)
"Envelope-shaped" crystals	Calcium
"Coffin lid" crystals	Struvite (ammonium magnesium phosphate)

| Rhomboid crystals | Uric acid |
| Hexagonal crystals | Cystine |

| What are the signs and symptoms associated with urinary stone disease? | Renal colic (flank pain radiating to groin), hematuria, and pyelonephritis |

Renal and Urinary Tract Tumors

| What must be ruled out in an older adult with hematuria? | Urinary tract malignancies (renal and bladder) |

Name the renal or urinary neoplasm associated with each of the following statements:

Large, palpable flank mass in a toddler	Wilms tumor (aka nephroblastoma) or neuroblastoma
Most common tumor of the renal pelvis	Transitional cell carcinoma
Benign tumor of kidney often associated with tuberous sclerosis	Angiomyolipoma
Most common renal malignancy	Renal cell carcinoma (RCC)
Clear cells	RCC
Associated with phenacetin abuse, cigarette smoking, cyclophosphamide, and aniline dyes	Transitional cell carcinoma
Large, benign tumor of kidney, composed of eosinophilic cells; arises from the intercalated cells of collecting duct	Oncocytoma
Secondary polycythemia	RCC
Associated with *Schistosoma haematobium*	Squamous cell carcinoma of the bladder
Invades renal vein and sometimes IVC	RCC
Painless hematuria in an older patient who smokes	Transitional cell carcinoma of the bladder
Classically manifests clinically with hematuria, flank pain, and a flank mass	RCC

| Which gene is most commonly altered in clear cell carcinomas? | *VHL* (*von Hippel-Lindau*) gene (mutated or hypermethylated) |

| Which gene is most commonly altered in papillary RCCs? | *MET* |

Which hormone is secreted by 5% to 10% of all RCCs?	Erythropoietin
RCCs are associated with ectopic production of which other hormones?	ACTH, renin, parathyroid hormone receptor protein (PTHrp), prolactin

Name the syndrome characterized by Wilms tumor plus each of the following findings:

Gonadal dysgenesis, nephropathy associated with *WT1* gene mutations	Denys-Drash syndrome
WT1 gene mutation, aniridia, GU malformations, and mental/motor retardation	**WAGR** complex
Organomegaly, hemihypertrophy, macroglossia, gigantism, neonatal hypoglycemia associated with the *WT2* gene	Beckwith-Wiedemann syndrome

Name the most common genetic defect associated with each of the following:

Transitional cell carcinoma	Chromosome 9p and 9q alterations
RCC	Alterations of chromosome 3 affecting the *VHL* gene
Wilms tumor	Deletion of *WT1* gene (tumor suppressor gene on 11p13)
Beckwith-Wiedemann syndrome	*WT2* gene deletion (11p15.5)
What is the inheritance pattern of Beckwith-Wiedemann syndrome?	Genomic (paternal) imprinting

Urinary System

Name the urinary disease associated with each of the following statements:

Fibrous masses over the sacrum and lower aorta that encroach on the ureters causing obstruction and hydronephrosis	Sclerosing retroperitonitis
How does chronic urinary outlet obstruction affect the bladder wall?	Chronic obstruction causes bladder wall hypertrophy
What are the common symptoms of lower urinary tract infection (cystitis)?	Dysuria, frequency, urgency
What is the most common source of bacteria that causes cystitis?	Colon (*E. coli* = 80%)

Why are women at 10 times the risk of men for developing a urinary tract infection (UTI)?

The female urethra is shorter and more likely to be colonized with fecal flora

List the most common UTI organisms:

"SEEKS PP"
Serratia marcescens
Escherichia coli
Enterobacter cloacae
Klebsiella pneumoniae
Staphylococcus saprophyticus
Proteus mirabilis
Pseudomonas aeruginosa

Which UTI-causing bacterium is frequently nosocomial, drug-resistant, and may produce a red pigment?

Serratia marcescens

Which UTI-causing bacterium is most common in young, sexually active women?

S. saprophyticus

Isomorphic red cells in the urine suggest bleeding from what portion of the urinary tract?

Lower urinary tract (ie, nonglomerlular bleeding)

What type of trauma commonly causes extravasation of urine into the superficial perineal space?

Straddle injury (rupture of urethra below urogenital diaphragm)

Name the four types of urinary incontinence:

1. Stress
2. Urge
3. Overflow
4. Total

Name the type of voiding dysfunction or incontinence associated with the following characteristics:

A small urinary bladder and detrusor overactivity resulting in bladder wall thickening

Hypertonic neurogenic bladder

A large urinary bladder and detrusor areflexia that may result in overflow incontinence

Atonic neurogenic bladder

Small amounts of urine leakage associated with coughing, laughing, or straining

Stress incontinence

Leakage of urine associated with sudden, strong need to urinate

Urge incontinence

PHARMACOLOGY

Renal

For each of the following drugs, provide:
1. The mechanism and location of action (MLOA)
2. Indication(s) (IND)
3. Significant side effects and unique toxicity (TOX) (if any)

Furosemide, ethacrynic acid	**MLOA:** inhibitor of $Na^+/K^+/2Cl^-$ cotransporter in thick ascending loop of Henle **IND:** diuresis, hypertension, CHF, and other edematous states (ascites, nephrotic syndrome, etc.) **TOX: "CHIA DOG"** Calciuria Hypokalemic metabolic alkalosis Interstitial nephritis Allergy to sulfa Dehydration Ototoxicity Gout
Spironolactone	**MLOA:** competitive aldosterone receptor antagonist; acts in collecting duct (CD) **IND:** diuresis, CHF **TOX:** hyperkalemic metabolic acidosis, gynecomastia, antiandrogen effects
Triamterene and amiloride	**MLOA:** block epithelial Na^+ channels (ENaC) in collecting duct **IND:** used in combination with other diuretics (especially loop and thiazide diuretics) for their K^+-sparing properties **TOX:** leg cramps (triamterene)
Acetazolamide	**MLOA:** carbonic anhydrase inhibitor (CAI) $\rightarrow\downarrow HCO_3^-$ reabsorption in PCT $\rightarrow\uparrow$ urine osmolarity **IND:** diuresis, glaucoma, altitude sickness **TOX:** metabolic acidosis, ammonia toxicity, neuropathy **Note:** sulfa allergy

Mannitol	**MLOA:** $\uparrow$ tubular fluid osmolarity $\rightarrow\uparrow$ urine flow; acts in PCT, thin descending limb, and CD **IND:** diuresis, elevated intracranial pressure (ICP) **TOX:** pulmonary edema, dehydration
Thiazides—chlorothiazide, hydrochlorothiazide	MLOA: inhibitor of NaCl reabsorption in early DCT $\rightarrow\uparrow$ urine osmolarity **LOA**: DCT **IND**: hypertension, CHF **TOX**: may cause hyperglycemia, hyperlipidemia, hypercalcemia, and allergic response in patients sensitive to sulfa drugs
ACE inhibitors (eg, lisinopril)	**MLOA:** inhibitor of ACE $\rightarrow\downarrow$ levels of AT II ($\rightarrow\uparrow$); prevents inactivation of bradykinin (potent vasodilator) **IND**: hypertension, renal protective effects in diabetics, CHF **TOX: "CAPTOPRIL"** Cough Angioedema Proteinuria Taste changes HypOtension Pregnancy issues (fetal renal toxicity) Rash Increased renin and K^+ Lowers AT II **Contraindicated in bilateral RAS**
Angiotensin receptor blockers (eg, losartan)	**MLOA:** AT II receptor antagonist **IND:** hypertension **TOX**: dizziness, headache; teratogenic
Demeclocycline	**MLOA:** ADH antagonist in CD **IND:** SIADH

Name the diuretic of choice in the following situations:

Diuresis in sulfa-allergic patient	Ethacrynic acid (a loop diuretic)
Hypercalcemia	Loop diuretics (eg, furosemide)—decrease positive luminal potential that aids in paracellular reabsorption of Ca^{2+}
Hyperaldosteronism	Spironolactone
Nephrogenic DI	Thiazide diuretics (eg, chlorothiazide)
Severe edematous states	Loop diuretics (eg, furosemide)
Elevated ICP	Mannitol

Altitude sickness   Acetazolamide

Calcium stones   Thiazide diuretics (eg, chlorothiazide)
                                      —reduce urinary excretion of Ca^{2+} by
                                      increasing Na^+/Ca^{2+} exchange

Which diuretics decrease blood pH?   CAIs and K^+-sparing diuretics

Which diuretics increase blood pH?   Loop and thiazide diuretics

Which diuretics increase urinary Ca^{2+}?   Loop diuretics and spironolactone

Which diuretics decrease urinary Ca^{2+}?   Thiazide diuretics and amiloride

Which diuretics increase urinary NaCl?   All classes

CHAPTER 10

Hematology-Oncology

EMBRYOLOGY

Name the site(s) of red blood cell
(RBC) production during each of the
following developmental phases:

First trimester	Yolk sac
Second trimester	Liver and spleen
Third trimester	Central and peripheral skeleton
Postpartum	Axial skeleton

PATHOLOGY

Coagulopathy

What is the most common inherited hypercoagulable state?	Factor V Leiden
The factor V Leiden mutation inhibits factor V cleavage by which protein?	Protein C
What is the effect of estrogen, endogenous or exogenous, on thrombosis?	Estrogen induces a hypercoagulable state
What clotting factors require vitamin K for their synthesis?	Factors II, VII, IX, X, and proteins C and S
What common laboratory test is used to assess the intrinsic coagulation system?	Partial thromboplastin time (PTT)
What common laboratory test is used to assess the extrinsic coagulation pathway?	Prothrombin time (PT)

What commonly used anticoagulant interferes with the intrinsic pathway?	Heparin
What commonly used anticoagulant interferes with the extrinsic pathway?	Warfarin **Remember: "WEPT"**—Warfarin affects the Extrinsic pathway and is monitored by PT
The use of the chelator, ethylene diamine tetra acetate (EDTA), as an anticoagulant in tubes is designed to inactivate what factor in the blood?	Calcium
What inhibitor of the coagulation cascade inactivates factors Va and VIIIa?	Protein C
What are the two major functions of von Willebrand factor?	1. Transport of factor VIII 2. Linkage of platelets and collagen
Dysfunction of what clotting component results in mucous membrane hemorrhage, petechiae, purpura, and prolonged bleeding time?	Platelet abnormalities
Dysfunction of what clotting component results in hemarthroses, purpura, and prolonged PT and/ or PTT?	Coagulation factor abnormalities

Name the coagulopathy associated with the following clinical and pathologic features:

Most common hereditary bleeding disorder	von Willebrand disease
Most common type of hemophilia	Hemophilia A (factor VIII deficiency)
Most common cause of acquired platelet dysfunction	Aspirin use
Autosomal dominant (AD) disorder causing increased bleeding time	von Willebrand disease
Autosomal recessive (AR) defect in platelet adhesion caused by lack of GpIIb/IX	Bernard-Soulier disease
AR defect in platelet aggregation caused by deficiency of GpIIb/ GpIIIa, a membrane receptor responsible for binding fibrinogen	Glanzmann thrombasthenia

Common presentation includes hemarthroses and easy bruising, ↑ PTT, normal PT	Hemophilia (A and B)
Prolonged bleeding time with normal platelet count, normal PT, and ↑ PTT	von Willebrand disease
Prolonged PT, PTT, ↑ bleeding time, thrombocytopenia, presence of fibrin split products	Disseminated intravascular coagulation (DIC)
Normal PT, PTT, normal platelet count, ↑ bleeding time	Aspirin use
Syndrome characterized by antiplatelet antibodies (commonly anti-Ib-IX or IIb-IIIa), often post-viral infections	Idiopathic thrombocytopenia (ITP)
Syndrome characterized by thrombocytopenia, microangiopathic hemolytic anemia, renal failure following *Shigella* or *E. coli* O157:H7 infection	Hemolytic uremic syndrome
Syndrome characterized by thrombocytopenia, microangiopathic hemolytic anemia, fever, and neurologic symptoms	Thrombotic thrombocytopenic purpura (TTP)
Widespread hyaline microthrombi in arterioles and capillaries causing schistocytes and helmet cells	Microangiopathic hemolytic anemia
Splenomegaly, epistaxis, petechiae, generalized tender lymphadenopathy, serum antibodies (+)	SLE-autoimmune thrombocytopenia

Anemia

List five of the most common causes of microcytic anemia:	1. Iron deficiency 2. Lead poisoning 3. Chronic disease (sometimes normocytic) 4. Sideroblastic 5. Thalassemia
List four of the most common causes of normocytic anemia:	1. Sickle cell anemia 2. Aplastic anemia 3. Acute blood loss 4. Hemolytic anemia

List five of the most common causes of macrocytic anemia:	1. Liver disease 2. Vitamin B_{12} deficiency 3. Folate deficiency 4. Alcoholism 5. Hypothyroidism
What is the primary site of iron absorption? Vitamin B_{12}? Folate?	Duodenum; terminal ileum (need intrinsic factor); jejunum (respectively)
What is the major cause of iron deficiency anemia in adults?	Menorrhagia or gastrointestinal (GI) bleeding (ie, colon cancer, ulcers)
What are two common clinical complaints in an anemic patient?	1. Dyspnea on exertion 2. Fatigue
Which amino acid substitution in the *β-globin* gene is most commonly seen in sickle cell anemia?	Glu6 $\rightarrow$ Val
What is the major type of hemoglobin in homozygous sickle cell anemia?	HbS
In sickle cell disease, what is the mechanism of ischemic necrosis of the bones, lungs, liver, brain, spleen, or penis?	$\downarrow O_2$ tension $\rightarrow$ abnormal RBCs sickle $\rightarrow$ microvascular occlusions
What is the major regulatory enzyme in heme biosynthesis?	Aminolevulinate (ALA) synthase
What two common enzyme deficiencies can cause hemolytic anemia?	1. Glucose-6-phosphate dehydrogenase (G6PD) 2. Pyruvate kinase
What hemolytic anemia is associated with exposure to oxidant stress?	G6PD deficiency
What two common RBC membrane defects can cause hemolytic anemia?	1. Hereditary spherocytosis 2. Paroxysmal nocturnal hematuria (PNH)
What common cause of atypical pneumonia is associated with cold autoimmune hemolytic anemia?	*Mycoplasma pneumoniae*
What viral illness is associated with cold autoimmune hemolytic anemia?	Infectious mononucleosis
What type of anemia is caused by lack of intrinsic factor (IF) secretion by gastric parietal cells?	Pernicious anemia (vitamin B_{12} deficiency)

What two autoimmune diseases of the GI tract can cause megaloblastic anemia?	1. Pernicious anemia (due to lack of IF production) 2. Crohn disease of the distal ileum (due to lack of IF-B12 complex reabsorption)
What parasites are capable of causing megaloblastic anemia?	*Diphyllobothrium latum* (by depleting B_{12}) and *Giardia lamblia* (by depleting folate)
How does gastric resection cause megaloblastic anemia?	Parietal cells, which are responsible for IF production may be removed when the gastric fundus is resected
What type of malignancy is associated with pernicious anemia?	Gastric carcinoma
Name three medications capable of causing autoimmune hemolytic anemia:	1. Penicillin 2. Cephalosporins 3. Quinidine
What types of malignancies are associated with autoimmune hemolytic anemia?	Leukemias and lymphomas
What laboratory tests are seen in hemolytic anemia?	↑ Unconjugated bilirubin, ↑ urine urobilinogen, ↓ hemoglobin, hemoglobinuria, ↓ haptoglobin, hemosiderosis
Name two commonly used medications that can cause aplastic anemia:	1. Nonsteroidal anti-inflammatory drugs (NSAIDs) 2. Chloramphenicol
What happens to the total iron binding capacity (TIBC), serum iron concentration, and percent saturation of transferrin in each of the following diseases?	
Iron deficiency anemia	↑ TIBC, ↓ serum iron, ↓ % saturation, ↓ ferritin
Anemia of chronic disease	↓ TIBC, ↓ serum iron, normal saturation, ↑ ferritin
Iron overload	TIBC down, ↑ serum iron, maximal saturation, ↑ ferritin
Name the type(s) of anemia associated with the following clinical and pathologic features:	
Most common type of anemia	Iron deficiency anemia
Abnormal Schilling test	Pernicious anemia

ABO incompatibility, lymphoid neoplasm, Raynaud phenomena, anti-i antibodies	Cold autoimmune hemolytic anemia
Atrophic glossitis	Pernicious anemia
Autosplenectomy	Sickle cell anemia
Basophilic stippling of erythrocytes, blue/gray discoloration at gumline, wrist/foot drop	Anemia from lead poisoning
Celiac sprue	Folate deficiency anemia (megaloblastic)
Chronic atrophic gastritis	Pernicious anemia
Colon cancer	Iron deficiency anemia (early) and anemia of chronic disease (late)
Crescent-shaped erythrocytes and Howell-Jolly bodies	Sickle cell anemia
Deficiency of α- or β-globin gene synthesis	Thalassemia
Deficiency of decay accelerating factor	Paroxysmal nocturnal hemoglobinuria
Demyelination of the dorsal and lateral tracts of the spinal cord	Pernicious anemia
End-stage liver disease	Macrocytic anemia
Helmet cells, burr cells, triangular cells	Microangiopathic anemia (2° to DIC, thrombotic thrombocytopenic purpura-hemolytic-uremic syndrome [TTP-HUS], or mechanical heart valves)
Hypersegmented polymorphonuclear neutrophils (PMNs)	Vitamin B_{12} or folate deficiency
Increased serum lactate dehydrogenase (LDH), increased reticulocyte count, and low haptoglobin	Hemolytic anemia
Microcytosis, atrophic glossitis, esophageal webs (Plummer-Vinson syndrome)	Iron deficiency anemia
Pancytopenia and fatty infiltration of bone marrow	Aplastic anemia
CLL, infectious mononucleosis, M. pneumoniae infections	Cold autoimmune hemolytic anemia

Systemic lupus erythematosus (SLE), chronic lymphocytic leukemia (CLL), lymphomas, drugs; + direct Coombs test (due to IgG autoantibodies)	Warm autoimmune hemolytic anemia
AD deficiency of spectrin, positive osmotic fragility test	Hereditary spherocytosis
Reduced erythropoietin	Anemia of chronic disease
Ringed sideroblasts	Sideroblastic anemia, seen in bone marrow
Basophilic stippling	Lead poisoning, seen in peripheral smear
Susceptibility to infection by encapsulated organisms	Sickle cell anemia (from splenic autoinfarction)
Transient normocytic anemia	Anemia of acute blood loss
What is the genetic defect in thalassemias?	Splicing defect, causing decreased α or β sub-chain production
Name the type of thalassemia responsible for each of the following findings:	
β-Thalassemia associated with growth retardation, frontal bossing, and hepatosplenomegaly (HSM) (from extramedullary hematopoiesis), jaundice, and iron overload (2° to transfusions), and ↑ Hgb F	β-Thalassemia major (β−/β−) **Note:** β-thalassemia minor (β+/β−), typically asymptomatic
α-Thalassemia associated with mild microcytic anemia, usually asymptomatic	α-Thalassemia minor (two alleles affected) **Note:** when only one allele involved (carrier state) → no anemia
α-Thalassemia associated with pallor, splenomegaly, chronic hemolytic anemia, and intraerythrocytic inclusions	Hgb H disease (three alleles affected)
α-Thalassemia associated with stillborn fetus	Hydrops fetalis (all four alleles affected)

White Blood Cell (WBC) Neoplasms

What are the two major categories of lymphoma?	1. Hodgkin disease (HD) 2. Non-Hodgkin lymphoma (NHL)

Name the general type of lymphoma (HD or NHL) associated with the following clinical and pathologic features:

Interleukin (IL)-5 secreting Reed-Sternberg (RS) cells	HD
Commonly arises from B cells	NHL
Constitutional symptoms including fever, night sweats, weight loss	Both
Mediastinal lymphadenopathy, contiguous spread	HD
Many cases associated with Epstein-Barr virus (EBV)	HD
Peripheral lymphadenopathy, noncontiguous spread	NHL
Bimodal age distribution, but most common in young men	HD
Peak incidence from 20 to 40 years of age	NHL
Associated with immunosuppression including AIDS	NHL
Painful lymphadenopathy with alcohol consumption	HD

Name the type of HD associated with each of the following clinical and pathologic findings:

Most common type	Nodular sclerosis
Abundance of RS cells	Mixed cellularity
Commonly seen in older patients with HD	Mixed cellularity
Widely disseminated disease with poor prognosis	Lymphocyte depletion
Abundance of lymphocytes	Lymphocyte predominance
Commonly seen in men <35 years presenting with cervical or axillary lymphadenopathy	Lymphocyte predominance
High proportion of RS cells relative to lymphocytes	Lymphocyte depletion

Name the type of NHL associated with each of the following clinical and pathologic findings:

Overexpression of cyclin D1	Mantle cell lymphoma
Starry-sky appearance on histopathology	Burkitt lymphoma
Clinically similar to CLL; characterized by nodules of small lymphocytes	Small cell lymphocytic lymphoma
Older adults with *BCL2* gene mutations	Follicular lymphoma
Often appears at extranodal sites and can cause small bowel obstruction	Diffuse large cell lymphoma
Child presenting with enlarging mandibular mass	Burkitt lymphoma **Note:** presents as abdominal/pelvic mass in sporadic form
Common in children who present with a mediastinal mass and a syndrome similar to that of acute lymphocytic leukemia (ALL)	Lymphoblastic lymphoma
TdT+ lymphocytes	Precursor B- or T-cell acute lymphoblastic leukemia/lymphoma
Endemic in Africa and associated with EBV	Burkitt lymphoma

Name the specific leukemia associated with the following age brackets:

0 to 14 years old	ALL
15 to 39 years old	AML
40 to 59 years old	AML and CML
>60 years old	CLL

Name the specific leukemia associated with each of the following findings:

Very high white cell counts, often >200,000	Chronic myelogenous leukemia (CML)
Isolated lymphocytosis	CLL
TdT+ lymphoblasts	ALL
Large, immature myeloblasts predominate	Acute myelogenous leukemia (AML)
Neoplastic pre-T or pre-B lymphocytes, CD10 ⊕	ALL

CD19/CD20 and CD5 ⊕ malignant cells	CLL
Bone marrow is replaced with myeloblasts	AML
Philadelphia chromosome t(9:22)	CML
Auer rods	AML
Low leukocytic alkaline phosphatase	CML (also seen in PNH) **Note:** this distinguishes CML from a benign leukemoid reaction, which has a high leukocyte alkaline phosphatase
Associated with fatigue, thrombocytopenia, signs of anemia, frequent infections, leukemia cutis, and DIC	AML (M3)
Bone pain, fever, generalized lymphadenopathy, HSM, and signs of central nervous system (CNS) spread	ALL
"Dry tap" on bone marrow biopsy and splenomegaly	Hairy cell leukemia
Excellent prognosis if treated early	ALL
May progress to AML	CML
Most responsive to therapy	ALL
Associated with prior exposure to radiation	CML
Peripheral leukocytes containing tartrate-resistant acid phosphatase (TRAP) and cytoplasmic projections	Hairy cell leukemia **Remember:** *"TRAP the Hairy beast"*

Myeloproliferative Disorders

Name the four chronic myeloproliferative disorders:	1. CML 2. Polycythemia vera 3. Essential thrombocytosis 4. Myelofibrosis with myeloid metaplasia
Name the myeloproliferative disorder associated with each of the following clinical and pathologic findings:	
↑ RBC mass and low/normal erythropoietin	Polycythemia vera **Note:** compare with hypoxic state or exogenous EPO or EPO-secreting tumor, where RBC mass is increased with elevated EPO

Tear drop deformity of erythrocytes, bone marrow hypercellularity	Myelofibrosis with myeloid metaplasia
Plethoric complexion, pruritus after showering, blurred vision, splenomegaly, and epistaxis	Polycythemia vera
Erythromelalgia (throbbing or burning of hands and feet)	Essential thrombocytosis
Basophilia	Polycythemia vera
Widespread extramedullary hematopoiesis with megakaryocytic proliferation in the bone marrow	Myelofibrosis with myeloid metaplasia
Hyperviscosity syndrome	Polycythemia vera and essential thrombocytosis
Peripheral thrombocytosis, bone marrow megakaryocytosis, and splenomegaly	Essential thrombocytosis

Name the plasma cell disorder associated with the following clinical and pathologic findings:

Bone pain, osteopenia, pathologic fractures, and "punched-out" lytic lesions on x-ray	Multiple myeloma
Russel bodies and "plymphocytes" (plasmacytoid lymphocytes)	Waldenstrom macroglobulinemia
Bence-Jones proteinuria	Multiple myeloma and Waldenstrom macroglobulinemia
Small M-spike on plasma electrophoresis in an otherwise healthy patient	Monoclonal gammopathy of undetermined significance (MGUS)
Hypercalcemia; renal insufficiency	Multiple myeloma
Hyperviscosity syndrome	Waldenstrom macroglobulinemia
Large M-spike on plasma electrophoresis	Multiple myeloma (IgG, IgA) and Waldenstrom macroglobulinemia (IgM)
Primary amyloidosis	Multiple myeloma (Ig light chains)

Peripheral Blood Smear

Name the condition associated with each of the following peripheral blood smear findings:

Defective PMN degranulation → accumulation of giant granules in PMNs and other leukocytes	Chediak-Higashi anomaly

Atypical lymphocytes	Infectious mononucleosis
Large numbers of Auer rods	AML (M3 subtype)
Basophilic stippling	Lead poisoning
Burr cells (echinocytes)	Burns, uremia
Dumbbell-shaped bilobed nuclei	Pelger-Huet anomaly
Giant platelets	Bernard-Soulier disease, May-Hegglin anomaly
Heinz bodies, bite cells	G6PD deficiency
Helmet cells, schistocytes	Microangiopathic hemolytic anemia (DIC, TTP, HUS)
Howell-Jolly bodies	Asplenia
Hypersegmented PMN nuclei	Megaloblastic anemia
Intracytoplasmic rings	Malaria, babesiosis
Lymphocytic cerebriform nuclei	Sézary syndrome
Nucleated erythrocytes	Hemolytic anemia
Rouleau formation	Multiple myeloma and Waldenstrom macroglobulinemia
Small platelets	Wiskott-Aldrich syndrome
Smudge cells	CLL
Spherocytes	Hereditary spherocytosis
Spur cells (acanthocytes)	Abetalipoproteinemia, liver disease
Target cells (codocytes)	Thalassemias, iron deficiency anemia, liver disease, sickle cell anemia
Teardrop cells (dacryocytes)	Myelofibrosis
Toxic granulations in leukocytes (Dohle bodies)	Sepsis

Chromosomal Translocation

Name the neoplasm associated with the following chromosomal translocations and genes/gene products:	
t(11:14) protooncogene under Ig promoter	Mantle cell lymphoma
t(11:22) EWS (EWS-FLI1 fusion protein)	Ewing sarcoma
t(14:18) BCL2	Follicular lymphoma

t(15:17) (PML/RAR-β [retinoic acid receptor alpha])	AML (M3 subtype, treated with retinoic acid)
t(3:6) VHL	von Hippel-Lindau syndrome (t[3:8] and t[3:11] are two common variants seen in VHL)
t(8:14) c-myc and IgH	Burkitt lymphoma (t[8:22] and t[2:8] are two common variants seen in Burkitt lymphoma)
t(9:22) bcr-abl fusion protein	CML (treated with imatinib)

Tumor Markers

Name the neoplasm associated with the following tumor markers:

α_1-AT	Liver cancer, yolk-sac tumors
α-Fetoprotein (AFP)	Germ cell tumors, hepatocellular carcinoma
Alkaline phosphatase	Metastatic bone involvement, Paget disease
β-HCG	**H**ydatiform moles, **C**horiocarcinoma, **G**estational trophoblastic tumors
CA-125	Ovarian cancers
Carcinoembryonic antigen (CEA)	Colon, pancreatic, and other cancers of the GI tract
Prostate-specific antigen (PSA)	Prostate cancer
S-100	Melanoma, neural tumors

Cancer Genetics

For each of the following tumor suppressor genes, state the function and the malignancy/malignancies they are associated with:

| *APC* | **Function:** regulation of β-catenin in the Wnt/β-catenin signaling pathway—promotes cell adhesion and regulates cell proliferation |
| | **Associated malignancies:** familial adenomatosis polyposis (FAP) and many GI cancers |

BRCA1 and *BRCA2*

Function: DNA repair and transcriptional regulation

Associated malignancies: breast and ovarian cancers

NF1 and *NF2*

Function: regulates signal transduction through the ras pathway

Associated malignancies: neurofibromas, optic gliomas, pheochromocytoma (NF1), schwannomas, ependymoma/meningioma (NF2)

p16

Function: regulates cell cycle by inhibiting cyclin-dependent kinases

Associated malignancies: pancreatic and esophageal carcinomas and malignant melanoma

p53

Function: regulates cell death and proliferation in response to DNA damage

Associated malignancies: most human cancers, Li-Fraumeni syndrome

Rb

Function: regulates transition from G1 to S in the cell cycle by sequestering E2Fs, a family of transcription factors

Associated malignancies: retinoblastoma, osteosarcoma

WT1

Function: inhibits transcription of genes promoting cell proliferation

Associated malignancies: Wilms tumor

For each of the following oncogenes, state the function and the malignancy/malignancies they are associated with:

abl

Function: promotes cell proliferation through tyrosine kinase activity

Associated malignancies: CML, ALL

BCL2

Function: overexpression prolongs cell survival by inhibiting apoptosis through sequestration of cytochrome c within mitochondria

Associated malignancies: follicular and undifferentiated lymphomas

cyclin D	**Function:** promotes cell proliferation by stimulating the phosphorylation of pRb
	Associated malignancies: lymphoma, breast, liver, and esophageal cancers
CDK4	**Function:** promotes cell proliferation by phosphorylating pRb
	Associated malignancies: sarcoma, glioblastoma multiforme, malignant melanoma
HER2/neu	**Function:** amplification promotes cell proliferation by enhancing growth factor signal transduction
	Associated malignancies: breast, ovarian, lung, stomach cancers
myc	**Function:** promotes cell proliferation by transcriptional activation of specific genes
	Associated malignancies: Burkitt lymphoma, small cell carcinoma of the lung, neuroblastoma
ras	**Function:** signal transduction through the MAP kinase pathway
	Associated malignancies: colon cancer and many other human cancers
ret	**Function:** receptor tyrosine kinase that promotes cell proliferation in response to growth factors
	Associated malignancies: multiple endocrine neoplasia 2A and 2B; familial medullary thyroid carcinoma
sis	**Function:** β-chain of PDGF which promotes cell proliferation
	Associated malignancies: astrocytomas, osteosarcomas

Miscellaneous Oncology

Name the type of neoplasm associated with the following diseases:

Actinic keratosis	Squamous cell carcinomas of skin
AIDS	Aggressive malignant lymphomas, Kaposi sarcoma, brain lymphomas

Barrett esophagitis	Esophageal adenocarcinoma
Chronic atrophic gastritis	Gastric adenocarcinoma
Cirrhosis	Hepatocellular carcinoma
Down syndrome	ALL
Dysplastic nevus	Malignant melanoma
Immunodeficiency states	NHL
Myasthenia gravis	Thymoma
Paget disease of bone	Secondary osteosarcoma and fibrosarcoma
Plummer-Vinson syndrome, achalasia	Squamous cell carcinomas of esophagus
Tuberous sclerosis	Astrocytoma and cardiac rhabdomyosarcoma
Ulcerative colitis	Colonic adenocarcinoma
Xeroderma pigmentosum	Squamous and basal cell carcinomas of skin

List the four major differences between benign and malignant neoplasms:	1. Differentiation and anaplasia 2. Rate of growth 3. Local invasion 4. Metastases (most important difference)
What are the three ways a tumor can spread?	1. Invasion of lymphatic system (eg, carcinoma of the breast) 2. Hematogenous (typical of sarcomas) 3. Seeding of body cavity (eg, ovarian cancer)
Which four carcinomas characteristically spread hematogenously?	Follicular thyroid carcinoma, HCC, Choriocarcinoma, RCC
What four classes of genes are the primary targets for genetic mutation leading to cancer?	1. Protooncogenes (promote cellular growth) 2. Tumor suppressor genes (inhibit cellular growth) 3. Genes that regulate and mediate apoptosis 4. Genes that regulate and mediate DNA repair
What three genetic mechanisms can lead to the activation of protooncogenes?	1. Point mutations 2. Chromosomal rearrangements 3. Amplification

What three chromosomal abnormalities are characteristic of tumor cells?	1. Amplification 2. Deletion 3. Translocation
What three factors influence tumor growth?	1. Doubling time of tumor cells 2. Cell proliferation 3. Cell death (apoptosis)
Name the six small, round, blue cell tumors of childhood:	1. Ewing sarcoma 2. Lymphoma 3. Neuroblastoma 4. Medulloblastoma 5. Rhabdomyosarcoma 6. Primitive neuroectodermal tumors

Chemical Carcinogens

What are the two steps in the process of chemical carcinogenesis?	1. Initiation: cells undergo irreversible genetic mutation 2. Promotion: chemicals promote growth of initiated cells

Name the neoplasm associated with each of the following chemical, viral, and microbial carcinogens and types of radiant energy:

Aflatoxin	Hepatocellular carcinoma
Aniline dyes	Bladder cancer
Aromatic hydrocarbons	Lung cancer (aromatic hydrocarbons found in cigarettes)
Asbestos	Malignant mesothelioma **Note:** lung cancer is still most common
EBV	Burkitt lymphoma, nasopharyngeal cancer, B-cell lymphoma in AIDS patients, some types of HD
Estrogen	Breast carcinoma and endometrial carcinoma
Helicobacter pylori	Gastric adenocarcinoma and marginal zone lymphoma (MALToma)
Hepatitis B and C virus	Hepatocellular carcinoma
Human papilloma virus	Cervical squamous cell carcinoma and genital warts
Human T-cell lymphocytic virus-1 (HTLV-1)	T-cell leukemia/lymphoma
Ionizing radiation	Myeloid leukemias and thyroid cancers

Nitrosamines	Gastric cancer
Polyvinylchloride (PVC) assembly	Hepatic hemangiosarcoma
Ultraviolet radiation	Skin cancers
Clonorchis sinensis	Cholangiocarcinoma
Schistosoma haematobium	Squamous cell carcinoma of the urinary bladder

Paraneoplastic Syndromes

Name the process of profound weight loss and weakness due to muscle and fat loss in a patient with an advanced neoplasm:	Cancer cachexia

Name the tumor associated with the following paraneoplastic syndromes:

Acanthosis nigricans	Many types of visceral malignancies
Carcinoid syndrome	Carcinoid and neuroendocrine carcinomas of the bronchi or GI tract
Clubbing of fingers	Pulmonary or thoracic malignancies
Cushing syndrome	Adrenocorticotropic hormone (ACTH)-secreting pituitary adenoma or a cortisol-secreting adrenal adenoma
DIC	AML (M3)
Hypercalcemia	Parathyroid hormone (PTH)-secreting squamous cell carcinoma of the lung
Lambert-Eaton myasthenic syndrome	Small cell carcinoma of the lung
Thrombophlebitis	Pancreatic or lung adenocarcinoma
Syndrome of inappropriate antidiuretic hormone (SIADH)	Antidiuretic hormone (ADH)-secreting small cell carcinoma of the lung

PHARMACOLOGY

Medication for Anemia

Name the drug of choice for each of the following groups of anemic patients:

Adolescent girls with heavy periods and pregnant women	Iron
Patients on methotrexate who develop megaloblastic anemia	Folate

Elderly patients with atrophic gastritis who develop megaloblastic anemia	Cyanocobalamin (vitamin B_{12})
Patients with anemia secondary to end-stage renal disease	Erythropoietin
Patients with extremely low WBC count and prone to infection	G-CSF, GM-CSF (eg, Filgrastim)

Chemotherapeutic Agents

For each of the following drugs, provide:
1. The mechanism of action (MOA)
2. Indication(s) (IND)
3. Significant side effects and unique toxicity (TOX) (if any)

Methotrexate	**MOA:** folate analog that inhibits dihydrofolate reductase and, consequently, S phase of the cell cycle
	IND: leukemia, lymphoma, carcinoma, sarcoma
	TOX: myelosuppression (reversible with leucovorin)
5-Fluorouracil	**MOA:** inhibits pyrimidine synthesis which inhibits S phase progression
	IND: colon cancer and other solid tumors
	TOX: myelosuppression and phototoxicity
Cytarabine	**MOA:** inhibits pyrimidine synthesis which inhibits S phase progression
	IND: acute leukemias
	TOX: neurotoxicity
6-Mercaptopurine or 6-thioguanine	**MOA:** inhibits purine synthesis which inhibits S phase progression
	IND: leukemia, lymphoma
	TOX: myelosuppression, hepatotoxicity
Busulfan	**MOA:** DNA alkylating agent
	IND: palliative role in CML treatment
	TOX: pulmonary fibrosis, hyperpigmentation

Cyclophosphamide	**MOA:** DNA alkylating agent **IND:** NHL, breast and ovarian carcinomas **TOX:** hemorrhagic cystitis (prevented with mesna), myelosuppression, SIADH
Nitrosoureas (carmustine, lomustine, streptozocin)	**MOA:** DNA alkylating agent capable of crossing the blood-brain barrier **IND:** brain tumors **TOX:** CNS toxicity including dizziness and ataxia
Cisplatin	**MOA:** DNA alkylating agent **IND:** testicular cancer, female reproductive tract cancers, bladder and testicular cancers **TOX:** nephrotoxicity (prevent with amifostine) and acoustic nerve damage
Doxorubicin/adriamycin	**MOA:** intercalates into DNA and inhibits DNA replication **IND:** Hodgkin disease, myeloma, sarcoma, solid tumors **TOX:** cardiotoxicity, alopecia, myelosuppression
Bleomycin	**MOA:** intercalates into DNA and causes DNA strand breaks **IND:** testicular cancer, lymphomas **TOX:** pulmonary fibrosis, myelosuppression
Etoposide	**MOA:** inhibits topoisomerase, causing double-stranded breaks in DNA **IND:** small cell carcinoma of lung, prostate cancer, testicular cancer **TOX:** bone marrow suppression, hypotension
Prednisone	**MOA:** may trigger apoptosis **IND:** CLL, HD, lymphomas **TOX:** cushingoid reaction, immunosuppression, cataracts, acne, osteoporosis, hypertension (HTN), peptic ulcers, hyperglycemia
Tamoxifen/raloxifene	**MOA:** estrogen receptor agonist/antagonist **IND:** breast cancer **TOX:** increased risk of endometrial cancer

Vinblastine/vincristine	**MOA:** binds tubulin to inhibit formation of the mitotic spindle **IND:** HD, lymphoma, Wilms tumor, choriocarcinoma **TOX:** vincristine: peripheral neuropathy and paralytic ileus; vinblastine: myelosuppression
Paclitaxel	**MOA:** binds tubulin and prevents disassembly of the mitotic spindle **IND:** ovarian and breast cancers **TOX:** myelosuppression, hypersensitivity, neuropathy

Anticoagulants

What test is used to monitor anticoagulation in a patient treated with heparin?	PTT
What test is used to monitor anticoagulation in a patient treated with warfarin?	PT (used to calculate INR)
Warfarin	**MOA:** causes synthesis of dysfunctional vitamin K-dependent clotting factors (II, VII, IX, X) **IND:** chronic treatment and prophylaxis of venous thromboembolism, thromboprophylaxis in atrial fibrillation **TOX:** hemorrhage, teratogenic, skin/tissue necrosis
Heparin	**MOA:** increases PTT by activating antithrombin III **IND:** acute treatment of DVT, pulmonary embolus, angina, myocardial infarction (MI), ischemic stroke **TOX:** hemorrhage, heparin-induced thrombocytopenia (HIT), osteoporosis
Low-molecular-weight heparin (LMWH) (eg, enoxaparin)	**MOA:** similar to heparin **IND:** anticoagulation outside of the hospital, commonly for DVT
Thrombolytics (streptokinase, urokinase, tissue plasminogen activator, anistreplase)	**MOA:** facilitate the conversion of plasminogen to plasmin, which cleaves thrombin and fibrin clots **IND:** acute therapy for MI, ischemic stroke, hemodynamically significant pulmonary embolism **TOX:** hemorrhage

Clopidogrel and ticlopidine

MOA: antiplatelet agent that blocks adenosine diphosphate (ADP) receptors to inhibit platelet aggregation

IND: acute coronary syndrome, percutaneous coronary intervention, transient ischemic attacks, and stroke

TOX: hemorrhage, leukopenia, diarrhea

Eptifibatide and tirofiban

MOA: prevent platelet aggregation by blocking glycoprotein IIb/IIIa receptors

IND: acute coronary syndromes

TOX: hemorrhage

CHAPTER 11

Skin and Connective Tissue

EMBRYOLOGY/ANATOMY/HISTOLOGY

Name the embryonic structures that
give rise to each of the following:

    Epidermis

    Ectoderm

    Melanocytes

    Neural crest cells

Name the layers of the epidermis:

"Californians Like Girls in String
Bikinis" (from surface → base)

Stratum **C**orneum

Stratum **L**ucidum (lacking in thin skin
of face and genitalia)

Stratum **G**ranulosum

Stratum **S**pinosum

Stratum **B**asalis

What epidermal dendritic cells are
responsible for antigen presentation?

Langerhans cells

Name the type of collagen described
by the following statements:

    Found in *B*one, tendons, skin,
fascia, cornea, and dentin; replaces
reticulin later in wound repair

Type I
Remember: b**ONE**

    Found in *C*artilage, nucleus
pulposus, and ocular vitreous body

Type II
Remember: car**TWO**lage

Found in skin, blood vessels, uterus, fetal tissues, and involved in early wound repair (granulation tissue)	Type III (Reticulin)
Component of Basement membrane or basal lamina	Type IV **Remember:** type IV, under the floor/ basement membrane
Found at epiphyseal plates	Type X
Accounts for ~90% of collagen in the body	Type I
Mnemonic for collagen types I to IV	"Be Cool, Read Books"

Name the epithelial cell specialization described by the following statements:

Allows adjacent cells to communicate via connexons	Gap junction **Note:** missing in cancer cells
Connects cells to underlying extracellular matrix	Hemidesmosomes
Extends around entire perimeter; contains E-cadherin and actin filaments	Zona adherens
Prevents diffusion across intracellular space; extends around entire perimeter	Zona occludens (tight junction)
Small, discrete sites of attachment; contains desmoplakin and keratin	Macula adherens (desmosome)

Helical array of polymerized dimers of α and β tubulin	Microtubules
How are the internal structures of cilia organized?	9 + 2 arrangement of microtubules (nine doublets around two central microtubules)
Which enzyme causes bending of cilia and how does it work?	Dynein is an adenosine triphosphatase (ATPase) that links the nine doublets and causes bending by differential sliding

Name the cytoskeletal elements that perform the following functions:

Microvilli, muscular contraction, cytokinesis, adhering junction	Actin and myosin

Cilia, flagella, mitotic spindle, neurons, centrioles	Microtubules
Vimentin, desmin, cytokeratin, glial fibrillary acid protein, neurofilaments	Intermediate filaments
Where are apocrine sweat glands found?	Axilla, mons pubis, and anal regions

PATHOLOGY

Skin

Give the dermatologic term for each of the following descriptions:	
Flat, nonpalpable, circumscribed lesion <1 cm in diameter; different color than surrounding skin	Macule (eg, freckle)
Flat, nonpalpable lesion >1 cm in diameter	Patch (eg, vitiligo)
Palpable, solid, elevated skin lesion <1 cm in diameter	Papule (eg, mole)
Raised, flat-topped lesion >1 cm in diameter	Plaque (eg, psoriasis)
Fluid-containing lesion <1 cm in diameter	Vesicle (eg, herpes)
Fluid-containing lesion >1 cm in diameter	Bulla (eg, pemphigus)
Pus-filled, raised area	Pustule (eg, acne)
Palpable, solid, elevated lesion >1 cm in diameter	Nodule (eg, squamous cell carcinoma)
Name the dermatologic disorder characterized by the following descriptions:	
Autosomal recessive (AR) defect in melanin synthesis → predisposition to multiple skin disorders	Albinism (oculocutaneous)

Acquired loss of epidermal melanocytes → depigmented white patches	Vitiligo
Masklike facial hyperpigmentation associated with pregnancy	Melasma
Tan-brown, evenly pigmented, localized overgrowth of melanin-forming cells of the skin present at birth with benign behavior and variable histology	Nevocellular nevus (mole)
Often multiple, atypical, irregularly pigmented lesions and on non-sun-exposed skin that have the potential to transform into malignant melanoma	Dysplastic nevus
Eruption of comedones and pustules; ↑ during puberty and adolescence; associated with proliferation of *Propionibacterium*	Acne vulgaris
Umbilicated, pearly, dome-shaped papules typically occurring in the genitals; caused by poxvirus infection	Molluscum contagiosum
Benign papilloma caused by HPV infection, most commonly found on dorsum of hand; koilocytes are characteristic	Verruca vulgaris (common wart)
Common benign neoplasm of older adults; sharply demarcated, tan-brown plaques with a "pasted on" appearance	Seborrheic keratosis (senile keratosis)
Benign, flesh-colored, dome-shaped, nodule with central keratin-filled plug that resembles squamous cell carcinoma; may resolve without treatment	Keratoacanthoma
Yellowish papules or nodules that tend to occur on the eyelids; associated with hypercholesterolemia	Xanthoma (on the eyelids = xanthelasma)
Accumulation of excessive dermal collagen that can occur following skin trauma; results in large, raised tumorlike scar	Keloid

Proliferation of Langerhans cells; electron microscopy (EM) shows Birbeck granules	Histiocytosis X
A T-cell lymphoproliferative disease arising in the skin; initially simulates eczema or other inflammatory dermatoses	Mycosis fungoides (cutaneous T-cell lymphoma)
Rough, scaling epidermal lesion, usually <1 cm, due to chronic sunlight exposure; may be a precursor for squamous cell carcinoma	Actinic keratosis
Thickened, "velvety," hyperpigmented skin in the flexural areas; may be suggestive of visceral malignancy or insulin resistance	Acanthosis nigricans
Capillary hemangioma appearing as a purple-red area on the face or neck	Port-wine stain
Multiple painful, red nodules on the anterior shins; can be associated with drugs, infection, or inflammatory diseases	Erythema nodosum
"Herald patch" followed by the appearance of scaly lesions in a "christmas-tree" like distribution	Pityriasis rosea
Diffuse, sloughing, erythematous, non-scarring rash accompanied by fever seen in infants and children; caused by exfoliative toxin	Staphylococcal scalded skin syndrome

Name the inflammatory skin lesion associated with each of the following findings:

Characteristic "target" macule or papule; associated with infections, drugs, cancers, and autoimmune disease	Erythema multiforme
Silvery scaling plaques over the knees, elbows, and scalp	Psoriasis
"Saw toothing" of rete ridges	Lichen planus
Munro microabscesses in the stratum corneum	Psoriasis

Pruritic eruption commonly on flexor surfaces; associated with asthma and allergic rhinitis	Atopic dermatitis (eczema)
Wickham stria	Lichen planus
Purple, pruritic, polygonal, papules	Lichen planus
Characteristic rete elongation and parakeratosis	Psoriasis
Fever combined with erosions and hemorrhagic crusting of mucosal surfaces	Stevens-Johnson syndrome
Type IV hypersensitivity reaction following exposure to allergens such as poison ivy or poison oak	Allergic contact dermatitis
Sometimes associated with severe destructive rheumatoid arthritis-like lesions of the fingers	Psoriasis (psoriatic arthritis)

Name the blistering skin disease associated with each of the following descriptions:

Subepidermal bullae causing detachment of the entire thickness of the epidermis	Bullous pemphigoid
Pruritic subepidermal blisters occurring in groups; eosinophils and IgA deposits at tips of dermal papillae; seen in patients with celiac disease	Dermatitis herpetiformis
Intraepidermal/suprabasal blisters that often rupture; may be fatal	Pemphigus vulgaris
Immunofluorescence demonstrates linear deposition of complement and antibodies to hemidesmosome proteins BPAG1 and BPAG2	Bullous pemphigoid
IgA and IgG antibodies to gluten	Dermatitis herpetiformis
Antibodies (Abs) to the desmosomal protein desmoglein 3 in the macula adherens	Pemphigus vulgaris

Name the neurocutaneous syndrome characterized by each of the following features:

Port-wine stains of the face, ipsilateral glaucoma, retinal lesions, and hemangiomas of the meninges

Sturge-Weber syndrome

Hypopigmented macules (ash-leaf spots), adenoma sebaceum, seizures, and mental retardation

Tuberous sclerosis

Multiple organ hemangioblastomas, cysts, and paragangliomas throughout the body

von Hippel-Lindau disease

Café au lait spots, acoustic neuromas, and meningiomas

Neurofibromatosis

Which syndrome is characterized by erythroderma, pruritus, lymphadenopathy, and blood involvement of malignant T cells?

Sézary syndrome (leukemic form of cutaneous T-cell lymphoma)

Connective Tissue Diseases

Name the connective tissue disorder characterized by each of the following descriptions:

Immune complex deposition in almost any organ, characteristic butterfly malar rash, wire loop lesions in kidney, Libman-Sacks endocarditis, ANA, anti-dsDNA, anti-Smith antibodies

Systemic lupus erythematous

Calcinosis, Raynaud phenomenon, esophageal dysfunction, sclerodactyly, telangiectasias; anticentromere antibodies

CREST syndrome (limited cutaneous systemic sclerosis)

Autosomal dominant (AD) mutation in the *fibrillin-1* gene (*FBN1*) on chromosome 15q

Marfan syndrome

Most common form is an AD defect in collagen type I synthesis; may be confused with child abuse

Osteogenesis imperfecta

Proximal muscle weakness, elevated serum creatine kinase, less often associated with malignancy	Polymyositis
Abnormal collagen synthesis causing bleeding tendency, hypermobile joints, and hyperextensible skin	Ehlers-Danlos syndrome
Blue sclera and brittle bones	Osteogenesis imperfecta
Proximal muscle weakness, heliotrope rash, more often associated with malignancy	Dermatomyositis
Anti-Jo-1, anti-SRP, anti-Mi-2 antibodies	Dermatomyositis/polymyositis
Antinuclear ribonucleoprotein (anti-nRNP) antibodies	Mixed connective tissue disease
Widespread visceral involvement; anti-Scl-70 antibodies	Diffuse scleroderma
Triad of xeropthalmia (dry eyes), xerostomia (dry mouth), arthritis; anti-Ro, anti-La antibodies	Sjögren syndrome

Skin Cancer

Name the skin malignancy associated with each of the following statements:

The most common skin malignancy	Basal cell carcinoma
Associated with excessive sunlight exposure; may arise from dysplastic nevus cells	Malignant melanoma
Actinic keratosis is a precursor lesion	Squamous cell carcinoma
Locally aggressive, ulcerating, and hemorrhagic; almost never metastasizes	Basal cell carcinoma
Occurs in sun-exposed areas and tends to involve the *lower* part of the face	Squamous cell carcinoma
Occurs in sun-exposed areas and tends to involve the *upper* part of the face	Basal cell carcinoma

Histopathology characterized by "keratin pearls"	Squamous cell carcinoma
Histopathology shows darkly staining cells with palisading nuclei	Basal cell carcinoma
Associated with arsenic and radiation exposure	Squamous cell carcinoma
What are the characteristics worrisome for malignant melanoma?	ABCDE's Asymmetry Border (irregular) Color Diameter Evolving
What is the most important prognostic factor in malignant melanoma?	Depth of invasion (Breslow thickness)
What clinical variant of malignant melanoma has the poorest prognosis?	Nodular melanoma
What clinical variant of malignant melanoma often appears on the hands and feet of dark-skinned people?	Acral-lentiginous melanoma

Miscellaneous Skin Disorders

Name the dermatologic finding(s) associated with each of the following diseases:

Gastric adenocarcinoma	Acanthosis nigricans
Addison disease	Hyperpigmentation and striae
Rheumatic fever	Erythema marginatum
Kawasaki syndrome	Erythematous palms and soles; dry, red lips; desquamation of fingertips
Insulin resistance, diabetes mellitus type 2	Acanthosis nigricans
Sézary syndrome	Mycosis fungoides (lymphoma of the skin-simulating eczema)
Severe chronic renal failure	Uremic frost

Bacterial endocarditis	Osler nodes (tender, raised lesions on pads of fingers or toes) and Janeway lesions (small, erythematous lesions on palms or soles)
Xeroderma pigmentosum	Dry skin and melanoma
Henoch-Schönlein purpura	Purpuric lesions on extensor surfaces of arms, legs, buttock
Hypothyroidism	Cool, dry skin with coarse brittle hair
Graves' disease	Warm, moist skin with fine hair; pretibial myxedema
Graft-versus-host disease	Maculopapular rash
von Recklinghausen disease (NF-1)	Multiple café au lait spots
Familial hypercholesterolemia	Xanthomas (particularly on the tendons)
Systemic lupus erythematosus	Malar rash and photosensitivity
Pellagra	Dermatitis (particularly a scaling, red rash in sun-exposed areas)
Amyloidosis	Purpura, petechiae, and ecchymoses ("pinch purpura"); macroglossia
Inflammatory bowel disease	Erythema nodosum

Name the dermatologic finding(s) associated with each of the following infectious diseases:

Streptococcus pyogenes	Impetigo (honey-colored crust)
Pseudomonas aeruginosa	Ecthyma gangrenosum
Anthrax	Vesicular papules covered by black eschar
Parvovirus B19	Erythema infectiosum (*slapped cheek* appearance)
Lyme disease	Erythema chronicum migrans
Primary syphilis	Painless chancre
Secondary syphilis	Rash over palms and soles, condyloma latum
Rocky Mountain spotted fever	Rash over palms and soles (migrates centrally)

Congenital cytomegalovirus   Pinpoint petechial "blueberry muffin" rash

HPV (in genital region)   Condylomata acuminata

Herpes simplex virus (type 1)   Painful vesicles (at border of lips)

Leprosy   Hypopigmented, anesthetic skin patches

CHAPTER 12

Musculoskeletal

ANATOMY

Name the peripheral nerve or region of the brachial plexus injured in each of the following scenarios:

Erb-Duchenne or Waiter's tip palsy	Upper trunk of the brachial plexus (C5, C6)
Klumpke injury due to sudden upward jerk of the arm; associated with Horner syndrome	Lower trunk of the brachial plexus (C8, T1)
Claw hand (impaired wrist flexion and adduction)	Ulnar nerve
Wrist drop	Radial nerve
Vague pain in wrist with tingling, burning sensation in hand (carpal tunnel syndrome)	Median nerve
Deltoid paralysis	Axillary nerve
Winged scapula after mastectomy (paralyzed serratus anterior)	Long thoracic nerve
Foot drop	Common peroneal nerve
Loss of ability to plantarflex	Tibial nerve
Anterior shoulder dislocation	Axillary nerve
Positive distal tingling on percussion of anterior wrist (Tinel) and tingling on forced flexion (Phalen) tests	Median nerve (at wrist)
Anterior hip dislocation resulting in loss of adduction of the thigh	Obturator nerve
Loss of ability to rise from a seated position or climb stairs due to loss of gluteus maximus function	Inferior gluteal nerve

Positive Trendenlenburg sign (when contralateral leg is raised, contralateral hip falls secondary to ipsilateral gluteus medius weakness)	Superior gluteal nerve

Name the fracture associated with the following statements:

Laceration of the deep brachial artery and/or radial nerve	Midshaft fracture of the humerus
Greatest risk of upper extremity compartment syndrome in children (Volkman contracture)	Supracondylar fracture of the humerus
Young person with fall on outstretched hand, tenderness in the anatomic snuffbox	Scaphoid fracture
Caused by closed fist striking a hard object	Boxer's fracture or fracture of the fifth metacarpal
Elderly woman falling on an outstretched hand with the wrist extended	Colles fracture (fracture of the distal radius with dorsal displacement of hand)
Associated with foot drop due to injury of common peroneal nerve	Fracture of fibular neck
Lower extremity fracture caused by landing on foot from a large vertical drop	Calcaneal fracture (must check lumbar spine x-rays for associated fracture)

List the muscles that make up the hypothenar eminence:	Opponens digiti minimi, Abductor digiti minimi, Flexor digiti minimi (**OAF**)
List the muscles that make up the thenar eminence:	Opponens pollicis, Abductor pollicis brevis, Flexor pollicis brevis
What are the functions of the thenar and hypothenar muscles?	Oppose, Abduct, and Flex
What muscles ADduct at the metacarpophalangeal (MCP) joints?	Palmar interosseous muscles (**PAD**)
What muscles ABduct at the MCP joints?	Dorsal interosseous muscles (**DAB**)
What ligaments make up the borders of the anatomic snuffbox?	Extensor pollicis longus, extensor pollicis brevis, abductor pollicis longus

What artery passes through the anatomic snuffbox?	Radial artery
How can one test for radial or ulnar artery patency?	Allen test (used before arterial blood sampling from the radial artery)
What structures are damaged by lateral impact to the knee/twisting injury?	The terrible triad: anterior cruciate ligament (ACL), medial collateral ligament (MCL), and medial meniscus
What does a positive anterior drawer/ Lachman sign suggest?	Torn ACL
What does abnormal passive abduction (valgus instability) of the leg suggest?	Torn MCL
What is the most common site for a clavicular fracture?	Middle one-third
What is the term for increased pressure within a fascial compartment that causes damage to muscles and neurovascular structures?	Compartment syndrome
What are the six P's of compartment syndrome?	1. Pain out of proportion/pain with passive stretch 2. Parasthesias 3. Paralysis 4. Pallor 5. Pulselessness 6. Poikilothermia (cold)
What ligaments can be stretched or torn by inversion of the ankle?	Anterior talofibular ligament (most common, "Always Tears First"), calcaneofibular (second most common), posterior talofibular ligament (least common)
What common carpal bone fracture can lead to avascular necrosis?	Scaphoid fracture
What are the muscles of the rotator cuff?	Supraspinatus, Infraspinatus, Teres minor, Subscapularis (**SITS**) muscles
What term is used to describe the syndrome of pain on extension of the wrist and fingers?	Lateral epicondylitis (tennis elbow)

Name the syndrome characterized by sensory loss of the medial forearm and hand, disappearance of radial pulse on turning head away from affected side, with atrophy of thenar, hypothenar, and interosseous muscles:	Thoracic outlet syndrome (often due to cervical accessory rib)
Fracture that presents with leg in abduction, external rotation, and appearing shorter than the contralateral leg	Femoral neck fracture
Injury that presents with an internally rotated and adducted leg appearing shorter than the contralateral leg?	Posterior dislocation of the hip
Most common site of avascular necrosis	Medial circumflex femoral artery (femoral head)

PHYSIOLOGY

State the key cellular events in excitation-contraction coupling in skeletal muscle:	1. Action potentials cause depolarization of T tubules 2. Ca^{2+} release from sarcoplasmic reticulum 3. Ca^{2+} binds troponin C, causes conformational change 4. Tropomyosin moves to expose actin-binding site 5. Actin and myosin interact to generate contractile force 6. Ca^{2+} reuptake by sarcoplasmic reticulum
How does Ca^{2+} activate contraction in smooth muscle cells?	By binding to calmodulin, activating myosin light-chain kinase (MLCK)
Name the type(s) of muscle fiber associated with each of the following cellular or histologic features:	
Peripherally located nucleus	Skeletal muscle fibers
Centrally located nucleus	Smooth and cardiac muscle fibers
Distinct banding pattern	Cardiac and skeletal muscle fibers; bands are appearance of sarcomeres
Capacity to regenerate	Smooth muscle fibers

Z-lines	Cardiac and skeletal muscle fibers; Z-lines are borders that separate sarcomeres
Gap junctions	Smooth muscle fibers
Intercalated disks	Cardiac muscle fibers
Synapse with peripheral nerves	Skeletal muscle fibers
Inositol triphosphate (IP_3)-mediated calcium release	Smooth muscle fibers
Ca^{2+}-mediated calcium release	Cardiac muscle fibers
Voltage-mediated, T-tubule-mediated calcium release	Skeletal muscle fibers
Troponin is the major calcium-binding protein	Cardiac and skeletal muscle fibers
Name the type of skeletal muscle fiber associated with each of the following features:	
Slow twitch	Type 1—*one slow*
Fast twitch	Type 2
Abundant lipid stores	Type 1—*fat*
Red color	Type 1—*red*
White color	Type 2
Primarily uses anaerobic metabolism, few mitochondria	Type 2
Primarily uses aerobic metabolism, many mitochondria	Type 1—*ox*
Abundant glycogen stores	Type 2
Generation of a sustained force	Type 1
Generation of a sudden movement	Type 2
Mnemonic for type 1 fibers	**Remember: "One Slow, Fat, Red Ox"**
Effect of estrogen on osteoblast and osteoclasts	Inhibits apoptosis of osteoblasts, induces apoptosis of osteoclasts
Method of bone formation of axial and appendicular skeleton	Endochondral ossification

PATHOLOGY

Non-neoplastic Bone Disorders

Name the bone disease associated with
the following clinical and pathologic
features:

AD disorder characterized by short limbs due to narrow epiphyseal plates, normal torso, enlarged head, frontal bossing, and bow legs	Achondroplasia, most common cause of dwarfism
A group of disorders characterized by abnormalities of type 1 collagen	Osteogenesis imperfecta
Inadequate proline and lysine hydroxylation of procollagen	Scurvy
Vitamin D deficiency → failure of bone mineralization	Rickets (children) or osteomalacia (adults)
Vitamin C deficiency → bone lesions, bleeding from gums. and petechial hemorrhages	Scurvy
Associated with blue sclera and multiple fractures	Osteogenesis imperfecta
↑Parathyroid hormone (PTH) → "Brown tumor" of bone (fibrosis, giant cells, osteoclasts hemorrhagic debris, and cyst formation)	Osteitis fibrosa cystica (von Recklinghausen disease of bone)
Disorder of increased osteoclastic activity followed by increased osteoblastic activity that results in multiple fractures and increased serum alkaline phosphatase	Paget disease of bone (osteitis deformans)
Marrow fibrosis, moth-eaten bones on x-ray (XR), and metastatic calcifications	Osteitis fibrosa cystica (von Recklinghausen disease of bone), caused by hyperparathyroidism
Multiple lytic lesions of spine and skull	Multiple myeloma
Progressive decrease in bone mass most pronounced in menopausal women	Osteoporosis
Hereditary disorder of increased bone density caused by defective osteoclast function and bone overgrowth	Osteopetrosis

Lateral curvature of spine, usually with rotational component; most common in adolescent females	Scoliosis
Subperiosteal hemorrhage, failure of ephiphyseal cartilage replacement by osteoid, osteoporosis, corkscrew hair	Scurvy (vitamin C deficiency)
Delayed fontanelle closure, "Rachitic rosary" (thickening of costochondral junction), and Harrison groove	Rickets (vitamin D deficiency)
Marked cortical thinning and attenuation of bone trabeculae	Osteogenesis imperfecta
Poor calcification of bone leading to skeletal abnormalities, including bowing of legs, craniotabes, and pigeon breast deformity in children	Rickets
Mosaic pattern of lamellar bone, increased serum alkaline phosphatase	Paget disease of bone (osteitis deformans)
Bone infection → sequestrum and involucrum around the inflammatory focus	Pyogenic osteomyelitis
Infarction of osteocytes leading to joint pain and osteoarthritis	Avascular necrosis
Avascular necrosis of the head of the femur; typically presents with painless limp in obese adolescent	Legg-Calve-Perthés disease
Partial avulsion of tibial tuberosity; typically presents as knee pain in an active adolescent	Osgood-Schlatter disease
Granulomatous disease caused by spread of tuberculosis to spine	Pott disease
Vertebral compression fractures causing pain, kyphosis, and loss of height in the elderly	Osteoporosis
What is the most likely etiology of Paget disease?	Slow reaction to paramyxovirus infection of osteoblasts
What are the three phases of Paget disease of bone?	1. Osteolytic phase: bone reabsorption by large osteoclasts 2. Mixed phase: osteoblastic and osteoclastic activity results in mosaic pattern of bone 3. Burnt-out phase: osteoblastic activity predominates

Name six complications of Paget disease of bone:	1. High-output cardiac failure due to intraosseous atrioventricular (AV) shunting 2. Hearing loss 3. Leontiasis ossea 4. Osteosarcoma 5. Osteoarthritis 6. Bone pain from fractures
What is the name of a fluid collection in popliteal fossa that usually communicates with synovial space?	Baker cyst

Osteomyelitis

Name the most common organism(s) responsible for pyogenic osteomyelitis in each of the following patients:

Otherwise healthy adult	*Staphylococcus aureus*
Intravenous drug user	*Pseudomonas* spp.
Sickle cell anemia patient	*Salmonella*
Newborn	*Streptococci* spp. or *Escherichia coli*
Child	*S. aureus*
Most common mechanism of seeding for adults	*Traumatic*
Most common mechanism of seeding for children	*Hematogenous*

Neoplasia of Bone

Name the bone tumor associated with the following clinical and pathologic findings:

Most common bone tumor	Metastatic tumors to bone
Most common primary bone tumor	Multiple myeloma
Most common benign tumor of bone	Osteochondroma or exostosis
Most common primary malignant tumor of bone	Osteosarcoma
Benign sessile tumor attached to the bone surface, usually affecting skull and facial bones	Osteoma

Benign tumor (<2 cm) that is painful at night (due to excess PGE_2), relieved with aspirin and common in males <25 years old (y/o)	Osteoid osteoma
Malignant tumor typically occurring in the metaphyseal region prior to epiphyseal closure in patients <25 y/o	Osteosarcoma
Mushroom-shaped, laterally protruding tumor that may result from lateral displacement of the growth plate	Osteochondroma or exostosis
Benign tumor composed primarily of mature hyaline cartilage	Chondroma
Benign tumor composed of fibrous trabeculae of woven bone resembling Chinese characters	Fibrous dysplasia
Nodule of hyaline cartilage encased in reactive bone	Enchondroma
Malignant, painful, *small round blue cell tumor of childhood* occurring typically in the appendicular skeleton (may also affect ribs)	Ewing sarcoma/primitive neuroectodermal tumor (PNET)
Malignant tumor composed of multinucleated giant cells within a fibrous stroma, occurring in the epiphyses of long bones	Giant cell tumor of bone
Homer-Wright pseudorosettes, onion skin appearance on x-ray	Ewing sarcoma/PNET
Malignant tumor of cartilage found in the central skeleton	Chondrosarcoma
Double bubble or soap bubble appearance on XR	Giant cell tumor of bone
Benign but painful bone tumor that appears as a radiolucent nidus surrounded by dense bone	Osteoid osteoma or osteoblastoma
Codman triangle on x-ray forms as tumor, causing periosteal elevation	Osteosarcoma
What is the most common genetic defect associated with Ewing sarcoma/PNET?	t(11;22)(q24;q12) translocation (85%) associated with an *EWS-FLI1* fusion gene product
Mutation of what gene increases the risk of osteosarcoma by 1000×?	*Rb* gene

What malignancies are most likely to metastasize to bone?	Breast, lung, thyroid, kidney, and prostate (BLT with a Kosher pickle)
What pediatric disease is characterized by the triad of skull lesions, diabetes insipidus, and exophthalmos?	Hand-Schüller-Christian disease or histiocytosis X
What pediatric disease is characterized by polyostotic fibrous dysplasia, café au lait spots, precocious puberty, and other endocrine disorders?	McCune-Albright syndrome

Arthritis

Name the arthritic joint disease associated with the following clinical and pathologic findings:

Most common type of arthritis	Osteoarthritis
Most common type of infective arthritis and most common cause of arthritis in sexually active adults	Gonococcal arthritis
Anti-IgG Fc antibodies	Rheumatoid arthritis (RA); anti-IgG Fc antibodies are called rheumatoid factor
Subcutaneous rheumatoid nodules	RA
Heberden (DIP) and Bouchard (PIP) nodes	Osteoarthritis
PIP and MCP involvement	RA **Note:** RA almost never affects DIP
Most commonly affects great toe (podagra)	Gout
Presents as pain in weight-bearing joints after use, improves with rest	Osteoarthritis
Infrequent complication of psoriasis asymmetrically affecting DIP and PIP joints in the lower extremities	Psoriatic arthritis
Swan-neck and boutonniere deformity	RA
Chronic low back pain, rigidity, fixation of spine causing a condition referred to as bamboo spine	Ankylosing spondylitis

Infection causing migratory polyarthritis and erythema chronicum migrans; may lead to pericarditis and aseptic meningitis	Lyme disease
Arthritic joint disease associated with inflammatory bowel disease	Ankylosing spondylitis
Presents as morning stiffness improving with use, symmetric joint involvement, systemic symptoms	RA
Arthritis in the absence of systemic symptoms	Osteoarthritis
Triad of conjunctivitis or anterior uveitis, urethritis, and arthritis	Reactive arthritis, previously known as Reiter syndrome **Remember:** *can't see, can't pee, can't bend a knee*
Tophi (nodules of fibrous tissue) and crystals may be found on Achilles tendon or at external ear	Gout
Osteophyte formation at edge of articular surface and at sites of ligamentous attachment	Osteoarthritis
Filling of the joint space by granulation tissue (ie, a pannus)	RA
Frayed fragments of cartilage and osteophytes released into synovium forming "joint mice"	Osteoarthritis
Associated with hyperuricemia, thiazide diuretic use, and urate kidney stones	Gout
Eburnation of bone due to cartilage erosion	Osteoarthritis
Marginal erosion of subchondral bone	RA
Precipitation of urate crystals in joints resulting in an inflammatory response	Gout
Precipitation of calcium pyrophosphate dihydrate crystals in joints → inflammatory response	Pseudogout (aka calcium pyrophosphate deposition disease [CPPD])
Associated with deficiency of hypoxanthine guanine phosphoribosyl transferase (HGPRT)	Lesch-Nyhan syndrome (X-linked disease which may include gout as one of its manifestations)

Positively birefringent, rhomboid-shaped crystals	Pseudogout = Positively birefringent
Negatively birefringent, needle-shaped crystals in synovial fluid	Gout
Infective monoarticular arthritis typically causing knee pain and a pustular rash	Gonococcal arthritis
Infective polyarticular arthritis caused by *Borrelia burgdorferi*	Lyme disease
Stress, alcohol binge, or a large meal may precipitate an attack of this type of arthritis	Gout
Treatment for acute gout attack	Indomethacin (NSAID), colchicine (use limited by GI side effects), prednisone
Treatment for chronic gout	Allopurinol (inhibits xanthine oxidase), probenecid (inhibits reabsorption of uric acid)
Anticytokine therapy for RA is directed at which two cytokines?	1. Interleukin (IL)-1 2. Tumor necrosis factor (TNF)
What is the factor produced by activated T cells and fibroblasts that promotes bone destruction by osteoclasts?	Receptor activator of nuclear factor κ B ligand (RANKL), also known as TNF-related activation-induced cytokine (TRANCE)
What group of diseases is associated with high incidence (90%) in HLA-B27-positive patients?	Seronegative spondyloarthropathies (ankylosing spondylitis, reactive arthritis, arthritis associated with inflammatory bowel disease [IBD])
Name four extra-articular manifestations of RA:	1. Pleural and pericardial effusions 2. Acute vasculitis 3. Inflammatory lesions of lungs, pleura, myocardium, pericardium, peripheral nerves, and eyes 4. Amyloidosis (in severe, long-term disease)
What chemotactic factors are generated by urate crystal activation of complement?	C3a and C5a
How is tissue injury mediated in gout?	Release of lysosomal enzymes from neutrophils
Why are leukemia, multiple myeloma, and other neoplastic processes associated with gout?	High cell turnover releases uric acid and predisposes to an attack of gout

What is the renal complication of long-standing gout?

Urate nephropathy

Which syndrome is characterized by cutaneous pigmentation, leg ulcerations, splenomegaly, neutropenia, and RA?

Felty syndrome

What two bacteria most commonly cause nongonococcal septic arthritis?

S. aureus and *Streptococcus* spp.

Calcium and phosphate lab values in osteoporosis

Both calcium and phosphate levels are normal

CHAPTER 13

Behavioral Science

LIFE CYCLE

Development

At what age is an average child expected to do each of the following:

Hold his/her head up	3 months
Sit up without support	6 months
Crawl	9 months
Walk	12 months
Ride a tricycle	36 months (tricycle at 3 years)
Display stranger anxiety	7 months
Use a pincer grasp	9 months **Remember:** an upside-down pincer grasp forms the number "**9**"
Say their first word	12 months (**1** word at **1** year)
Use two-word combinations	24 months (**2** words at **2** years)
Use three-word sentences	36 months (**3** words at **3** years)
Understand object permanence	12 to 24 months
Toilet training	30 to 36 months
"No" phase, repeated temper tantrums	24 months (address tantrums by ignoring behavior)
Show abstract reasoning (formal operations)	Adolescence/puberty

At what age are the following reflexes considered normal:

Babinski	0 to 12 months
Palmar	0 to 2 months
Rooting	0 to 3 months

Name the components of the Apgar score:	**APGAR** (0, 1, or 2 in each category) **A**ppearance/color (blue/pale, trunk pink, all pink) **P**ulse (0, <100, >100) **G**rimace (0, grimace, grimace + cough) **A**ctivity/muscle tone (limp, some, active) **R**espiratory effort (0, irregular, regular)
Determine the Apgar score for these patients:	
Newborn with a pink trunk, heart rate (HR) = 50, a grimace and cough when stimulated, strong muscle tone, and an irregular respiratory effort	7
A blue newborn, HR = 30, a grimace when stimulated, appears limp, and has no respiratory effort	2
What is the definition of low birth weight?	Less than 2500 g
Name four sequelae of low birth weight:	1. Infections 2. Respiratory distress syndrome 3. Persistent fetal circulation 4. Necrotizing enterocolitis
What term describes the act of a child reverting to a more primitive mode of behavior due to stress?	Regression
Name three findings that are suggestive of each type of abuse listed below:	
Physical child abuse	1. Fractures at different stages of healing 2. Cigarette burns 3. Retinal hemorrhage/detachment (32% of kids <5 years old are physically abused)
Sexual child abuse	1. Genital/anal trauma 2. STDs 3. UTIs (25% of kids <8 y/o are sexually abused)
Elder abuse	1. Evidence of depleted finances 2. Poor hygiene 3. Spiral fractures

Name the changes found in the elderly in each of the following categories:

Psychiatric	Depression and anxiety more common; ↑ suicide rate
Sexual	**Men**: slower erection/ejaculation, ↑ refractory period **Women**: vaginal shortening, thinning, and dryness **Note**: sexual interest does not decrease
Sleep patterns	↓ Rapid eye movement (REM), slow-wave sleep; ↑ sleep latency, awakenings
Cognitive	↓ Learning speed; intelligence stays the same

Name three conditions that would qualify normal bereavement as pathologic grief:	1. Prolonged grief (>1 year) 2. Excessively intense grief (sleep disturbances, significant weight loss, suicidal ideations) 3. Grief that is delayed, inhibited, or denied
Name the Kübler-Ross stages of dying:	Denial, anger, bargaining, depression, acceptance **Note**: one or more stages can occur at once and not necessarily in this order

PHYSIOLOGY

Sleep

Name the sleep stage associated with each of the following descriptions:

Light sleep, peacefulness, ↓ HR and BP	Stage 1
Deepest non-REM sleep; sleepwalking, bedwetting	Stages 3 and 4
Deeper sleep; EEG shows sleep spindles and K-complexes; occupies ~half of total sleep time in young adults	Stage 2
Beta waves (↑ frequency, ↓ amplitude) only	Awake (eyes open) and alert
Beta, alpha, and theta waves → "sawtoothing"	REM

Alpha waves	Awake (eyes closed)
Dreaming, loss of motor tone, ↑ brain O_2 use, erections; occurs every 90 minutes	REM
Delta (slow) waves (↓ frequency, ↑ amplitude)	Stages 3 and 4

Name the sleep disorder described in each of the following statements:

Abnormal behavior associated with sleep or sleep-wake transitions (eg, sleep terrors, enuresis, somnambulism)	Parasomnia
Disturbance in amount, quality, or timing of sleep (eg, insomnia, narcolepsy)	Dyssomnia
Nighttime respiratory effort against an impeded airway, resulting in lapses in breathing and chronic fatigue	Obstructive sleep apnea

What is a useful drug for night terrors and sleepwalking?	Benzodiazepines (shortens stage 4 sleep)
Which drug treats enuresis in children by decreasing stage 4 sleep?	Imipramine
What is the main neurotransmitter involved in REM sleep?	Acetylcholine (ACh)

Name four physiologic changes that occur in REM sleep:

1. Increased and variable pulse
2. Increased and variable BP
3. Penile/clitoral tumescence
4. REMs

Name four clinical findings of narcolepsy:

1. Sleep paralysis (brief paralysis upon awakening)
2. Hypnagogic (**go**ing to sleep) and hypnopompic (waking) hallucinations
3. REM latency (sleep episodes all start in REM)
4. Cataplexy (sudden loss of muscle tone, especially with extreme emotion)

How is narcolepsy treated?

Stimulants (eg, amphetamines), scheduled naps

| What three sleep pattern changes are typical of depressed patients? | 1. Reduced slow-wave sleep
2. REM latency
3. "Terminal insomnia" (early-morning awakenings) |

Excitement

Name three possible etiologies of sexual dysfunction:	1. Drugs (eg, selective serotonin reuptake inhibitors [SSRIs], ethanol [EtOH], antihypertensives) 2. Disease (eg, depression, diabetes, myocardial infarction [MI]) 3. Psychologic (eg, aversion, hypoactive desire, premature ejaculation)
What disorder of sexual function is characterized by painful spasm of the outer one-third of the vagina during intercourse or pelvic examination?	Vaginismus
What is a paraphilia?	Unusual sexual activities or sexual desire for unusual objects (eg, pedophilia, voyeurism, and so forth)

Behavioral Neurochemistry

For each of the following diseases, describe the associated neurotransmitter activity:	
Schizophrenia	↑ Dopamine (DA)
Depression	↓ Norepinephrine (NE) and 5-HT
Alzheimer dementia	↓ ACh in Alzheimer dementia
Parkinson disease	↓ DA
Huntington disease	↓ GABA and ACh

SUBSTANCE ABUSE

| What is the lifetime prevalence of substance abuse/dependence? | 13% |
| How is "dependence" defined? | Withdrawal occurs if substance is stopped and patient has tolerance to substance |

Excluding tobacco and caffeine, what is the most commonly abused substance?	Alcohol
What is a short, useful alcoholism screening tool?	"CAGE" questions Have you felt the need to Cut down? Have you ever felt Annoyed by criticism of your drinking? Have you ever felt Guilty about drinking? Have you ever had an Eye opener?
What is the most serious complication of alcohol withdrawal and when is it most likely to occur?	Delirium tremens (DTs); peak occurrence is 2 to 7 days **Note:** DTs are a medical emergency
What is the mortality rate of DTs?	15% to 20%
Name three gastrointestinal (GI) complications of alcoholism:	1. GI bleeding (from ulcers, gastritis, esophageal varices, or Mallory-Weiss tears) 2. Pancreatitis 3. Liver disease
Which syndrome of anterograde amnesia, confabulations, ataxia, and nystagmus results from thiamine deficiency in chronic alcoholics?	Wernicke-Korsakoff syndrome **Remember:** Wobbly—Konfabulations (associated with bilateral mammillary body necrosis)
Identify the drug responsible for these intoxication syndromes:	
Central nervous system (CNS) and respiratory depression, euphoria, pinpoint pupils, nausea, and ↓ GI motility	Opioids; inspect for track marks along veins
Psychomotor agitation, dilated pupils, euphoria, ↑ HR and BP, prolonged wakefulness and attention, delusions, ↑ pain threshold	Amphetamines
All of the above, plus tactile hallucinations, angina, and sudden cardiac death	Cocaine
Belligerence, psychomotor agitation, nystagmus, ataxia, homicidality, psychosis, delirium, ↑ HR, and fever	Phencyclidine hydrochloride (PCP)
Delusions, visual hallucinations, postuse "flashbacks"	Lysergic acid diethylamide (LSD)

Euphoria, ↑ appetite, dry mouth, paranoid delusions, erythematous conjunctiva	Marijuana
Disinhibition, emotional lability, slurred speech, ataxia, blackouts, coma	Alcohol
What is the drug of choice for opioid overdose?	Naloxone (competitively inhibit opioid receptors)
Which drugs can be used to help maintain abstinence in opiate use disorder?	Methadone and buprenorphine (long-acting oral opioids)

PSYCHOLOGY

What are the three parts of Freud's structural theory of the mind?	1. Id 2. Superego 3. Ego
Which of these parts is described by the following statements:	
Represents conscience and moral values	Superego
Controlled by primitive wishes and pleasures; represents instinctive sexual and aggressive drives	Id
Bridges unconscious mind and external world	Ego
What Freudian term encompasses repressed sexual feelings of a child for the opposite-sex parent, plus a rivalry with the same-sex parent?	Oedipus complex
What type of insight therapy, developed by Freud, may be useful for chronic personality problems?	Psychoanalysis
What describes a scenario in which a patient's unconscious feelings from past relationships are experienced in the present relationship with the physician?	Transference reaction

What reaction occurs when the physician unconsciously reexperiences feelings about his/her parents (or other important persons) with the patient?

Countertransference reaction

Name the four mature ego defense mechanisms:

1. Suppression
2. Altruism
3. Sublimation
4. Humor

Note: defense mechanisms are automatic and unconscious

Name the type of learning that is described by each of the following statements:

Reflexive response is elicited by a learned stimulus

Classical conditioning

Tendency of an organism to follow the first thing they see after birth

Imprinting

Behavior is eliminated when not reinforced

Extinction

Behavior is determined by its consequences

Operant conditioning

Unwanted behavior is paired with painful stimulus

Aversive conditioning

Type of classical conditioning where the subject learns that it cannot escape a painful stimulus

Learned helplessness

In what type of reinforcement schedule is a reward presented after a random, unpredictable number of responses?

Variable ratio (slowest extinction when not rewarded); example = slot machine

In what type of reinforcement schedule is a reward presented after every response?

Continuous (rapid extinction when not rewarded); example = vending machine

Criteria for mental retardation begin below what IQ level?

Less than 70 (2 SD below the mean of 100)

PSYCHIATRY

Name the type of amnesia described below:

Inability to remember things that occurred before insult to CNS

Retrograde amnesia

Inability to remember things that occurred after a CNS injury → no new memory formation	Anterograde amnesia
Complication of electroconvulsive therapy (ECT)	Retrograde amnesia
Thiamine deficiency causing bilateral mammillary body necrosis; seen in alcoholics	Korsakoff (anterograde) amnesia

Delirium or dementia?

Waxing and waning level of consciousness	Delirium
Rapid onset; transient	Delirium
Characterized by memory loss	Dementia (think deMEMtia)
Associated with disturbances in sleep-wake cycle	Delirium
Often irreversible	Dementia
Associated with changes in sensorium (hallucinations and illusions)	Delirium

Name four major causes of delirium:	"HIDE": 1. Hypoxia 2. Infection (often UTIs) 3. Drugs 4. Electrolyte abnormalities
What is the most common etiology for dementia?	Dementia of Alzheimer type (DAT) = 70% to 80% of cases
Name some other etiologies for dementia:	"DEMENTIASS" Degenerative diseases (Parkinson, Huntington) Endocrine (thyroid, pituitary, parathyroid) Metabolic (electrolytes, glucose, hepatorenal dysfunction, EtOH) Exogenous (CO poisoning, drugs, heavy metals) Neoplasia Trauma Infection (encephalitis, meningitis, cerebral abscess, syphilis, prion diseases, HIV, Lyme disease) Affective disorders (depression may mimic dementia)

Stroke (multi-infarct dementia, ischemia, vasculitis)

Note: vascular causes ~10% of dementias

Structure (normal-pressure hydrocephalus [NPH])

Note: NPH is one of the few reversible causes of dementia

Mood Disorders

Name the nine key features of major depressive disorder (MDD):

"SIG E CAPSS"
1. Sleep changes (insomnia/hypersomnia)
2. Inability to experience pleasure, interest decreases
3. Guilt or feelings of worthlessness
4. Energy ↓ (fatigue)
5. Concentration ↓, indecisiveness increases
6. Appetite disturbance with weight change (>5% body weight in 1 month)
7. Psychomotor changes (agitation or retardation)
8. Suicidal ideations
9. Sadness (depressed mood for most of the day)

What features are required to make the diagnosis of MDD?

Two episodes (involving five of the above nine including #1 or 2) of impaired functioning for 2 weeks, separated by 2 months

What is the suicide rate in MDD?

Approximately 15% to 30%

Name the risk factors for suicide:

"SAD PERSONS"
Sex—male (women > attempts; men > actual suicides)
Age (↓ 15–24 and the elderly), Access to weapons
Depression
Previous attempts = #1 risk factor
Ethanol
Rational thought
Sickness
Organized plan
No spouse
Social support lacking

What is the first-line pharmacotherapy for MDD?	SSRIs
Name two other alternate pharmacotherapies:	1. Tricyclic antidepressants (TCAs) 2. Monoamine oxidase inhibitors (MAOIs)
What is a safe, effective treatment for refractory MDD?	ECT
What is the distinctively abnormal, elevated, expansive mood that lasts >1 week *or* is severely impairing (eg, requiring hospitalization)?	Manic episode

What are the seven key features of mania?

"DIG FAST" (at least three of the following for diagnosis):

1. **D**istractibility
2. **I**nsomnia
3. **G**randiosity
4. **F**light of ideas or racing thoughts
5. **P**sychomotor Agitation
6. **S**peech that is pressured (hyperverbal)
7. **T**houghtlessness (↑ pleasurable activities with ↑ consequences)

Name the following mood disorders:

Chronic disorder >2 years (alternating hypomania and mild depression); no period of euthymia >2 months and *no* significant impairment	Cyclothymia
Less severe features for several days that are *not* impairing; no psychotic features	Hypomania
History of major depressive episodes and at least one hypomanic episode	Bipolar II disorder
Manic episodes that often alternate with depressive episodes	Bipolar I disorder

Somatoform Disorders

Name the somatoform disorder associated with each of the following descriptions:

Preoccupation with an imagined physical defect, causing significantly impaired social and occupational functioning	Body dysmorphic disorder

Multiple, unrelated physical complaints leading to excessive medical attention seeking and severely impaired functioning	Somatization disorder (requires four pain, two GI, one sexual/GU, and one pseudoneurologic complaints) **Note:** cannot be intentional or fake
Prolonged preoccupation with concerns of having a serious illness (despite negative medical workups) and exaggerated attention to bodily or mental sensations	Hypochondriasis
Conscious simulation of physical or psychologic illness solely to receive attention from medical personnel	Factitious disorder (Munchausen syndrome) **Note:** technically *not* a somatoform disorder because it is intentional
Intentionally simulating illness for personal gain (usually financial)	Malingering **Note:** also *not* a somatoform disorder; suspect in cases involving litigation
Sudden onset of motor/sensory neurologic disorder following traumatic emotional event	Conversion disorder

Name the type of gain associated with each of the following descriptions:

Interpersonal or social advantages gained indirectly from illness	Secondary gain
Benefits of illness on the patient's internal psychic economy	Primary gain
Advantage gained by the caretaker	Tertiary gain

Name the type of anxiety disorder associated with each of the following:

Maladaptive reaction to environmental or psychologic stress that interferes with functioning and does not remit after the stress ends	Adjustment disorder
Marked, persistent fear of an object/situation that is excessive and unreasonable → stimulus is avoided; patient has insight (treat by exposure therapy)	Specific phobia
Occurs after a person is subjected to a traumatic event; lasts >1 month; may be debilitating	Posttraumatic stress disorder (PTSD)
Symptoms of PTSD that occur within 4 weeks of the stressor and last <4 weeks	Acute stress disorder

Moments of intense fear characterized by palpitations, choking sensation, GI upset, perspiration, chest pain, and chills	Panic disorder
Excessive worrying for the majority of days over the past 6 months that causes significant impairment	Generalized anxiety disorder
Recurrent, intrusive, senseless thoughts and impulses; plus the repetitive behaviors driven by the will to decrease the anxiety caused by them	Obsessive-compulsive disorder (OCD)

Name the dissociative disorder characterized by the following statements:

Two or more separate personalities in one individual; ↑ in women and sexually abused	Dissociative identity disorder (formerly multiple personality disorder)
A complete, often transient, inability to remember important personal information	Dissociative amnesia
Amnesia plus sudden wandering from home and taking on a different identity	Dissociative fugue

Psychoses

Give the appropriate term for each of the following psychotic symptoms:

	Delusion
False belief or wrong judgment held with conviction despite incontrovertible evidence to the contrary	
	Illusion
False perception of an actual external stimulus	
	Loose association
Thought disorder whereby ideas are not logically connected to those that occur before or after	
	Ideas of reference
Misinterpreting others' actions or environmental cues as being directed toward one's self when, in fact, they are not	

Subjective perception of an object or event when no such external stimulus exists	Hallucination

Name the psychotic disorder characterized by each of the following findings:

Two or more psychotic symptoms and disturbed behavior for >6 months; results in impaired functioning	Schizophrenia
Psychotic symptoms lasting 1 to 6 months	Schizophreniform disorder
Psychotic symptoms lasting >1 day, but <1 month (often with obvious precipitating psychosocial stressor)	Brief psychotic disorder
Fixed, nonbizarre delusional system; without other thought disorders or impaired functioning	Delusional disorder
Symptoms of major mood disorder as well as of schizophrenia (with psychotic features occurring before mood disturbance); chronic social and occupational impairment	Schizoaffective disorder
Clouded consciousness, predominantly visual hallucinations, often occurring in inpatient setting	Psychotic disorder due to a general medical condition
Adopting the delusional system of a psychotic person	Shared psychotic disorder (Folie-à-deux)

Name the five subtypes of schizophrenia:	1. Disorganized 2. Catatonic 3. Paranoid 4. Undifferentiated 5. Residual
Give two examples of positive symptoms of schizophrenia:	1. Hallucinations 2. Delusions
Positive symptoms respond best to what type of drugs?	Typical antipsychotics
Give four examples of negative symptoms that are characteristic of schizophrenia:	The 4 A's: 1. Affect flat 2. Alogia 3. Anhedonia 4. Avolition

| Negative symptoms respond best to what type of drugs? | Atypical antipsychotics |
| | **Note:** worse prognosis if negative symptoms predominate |

Childhood Disorders

Name the disorder of childhood described by each of the following statements:

Repetitive behaviors (in patient <18 y/o) that violate social norms; may exhibit physical aggression, cruelty to animals, vandalism, and robbery, along with truancy, cheating, and lying	Conduct disorder (predominantly **actions**)
Recurrent pattern of negativistic, hostile, and disobedient behavior toward authority figures; loss of temper and defiance (but not theft or lying)	Oppositional defiant disorder (predominantly **words**)
Developmentally inappropriate degrees of inattention, impulsiveness, and hyperactivity at home, in school, and in social situations	Attention deficit hyperactivity disorder (ADHD)
Developmental disorder with stereotyped movements and nonprogressive impairments in social interactions, communication, and behavior	Autism spectrum disorder
Progressive syndrome of autism, dementia, ataxia, and purposeless hand movements; regression of development; mainly in girls	Rett syndrome

Personality Disorders

List the three cluster A personality disorders:	"Weird"
	1. Paranoid
	2. Schizoid
	3. Schizotypal

List the four cluster B personality disorders:	"Wild"
	1. Histrionic
	2. Borderline
	3. Antisocial
	4. Narcissistic

List the three cluster C personality disorders:	"Worried"
	1. Avoidant
	2. Obsessive-compulsive
	3. Dependent

Name the personality disorder characterized by each of the following statements:

Socially inhibited, sensitive to rejection, feels inferior	Avoidant (C)
Peculiar appearance, interpersonal awkwardness, "magical" or odd thought patterns, no psychosis	Schizotypal (A)
Impulsive, unstable mood, chaotic relationships, feels empty and alone, self-mutilation, females >> males	Borderline (B)
Sense of entitlement, grandiosity, lacks empathy for others, insists on special treatment when ill	Narcissistic (B)
Suspicious and distrustful, uses projection as primary defense mechanism	Paranoid (A)
Lacks self-confidence, submissive, and clingy	Dependent (C)
Unable to maintain intimate relationships, extroverted, melodramatic, sexually provocative	Histrionic (B)
Disregards and violates rights of others, criminality, males > females; if <18 y/o = conduct disorder	Antisocial (B)
Lifelong pattern of voluntary social withdrawal, no psychosis, shows minimal emotions	Schizoid (A)

PHARMACOLOGY

Antidepressants

For each of the following drugs, provide:

1. The mechanism of action (MOA)
2. Indication(s) (IND)
3. Significant side effects and unique toxicity (TOX) (if any)

TCAs (imipramine, clomipramine, amitriptyline, desipramine, nortriptyline, doxepin, amoxapine)

MOA: prevents reuptake of NE and 5-HT

IND: depression, enuresis (imipramine), depression in elderly (nortriptyline), OCD (clomipramine), depression with psychotic features (amoxapine), neurologic pain

TOX: sedation (desipramine is least sedating), anticholinergic effects, lethal in overdose → respiratory depression, hyperpyrexia, and Tri-C's: Cardiac arrhythmia, Convulsions, Coma

SSRIs (fluoxetine, paroxetine, sertraline, citalopram, fluvoxamine, escitalopram)

MOA: selectively blocks reuptake of 5-HT (usually requires 2–3 weeks to take effect)

IND: depression, premenstrual syndrome (fluoxetine), OCD (fluvoxamine)

TOX: agitation, insomnia, sexual dysfunction, "serotonin syndrome" with MAOIs (muscle rigidity, hyperthermia, cardiovascular collapse)

Bupropion

MOA: heterocyclic agent, mechanism not well known

IND: depression, smoking cessation

TOX: agitation, seizures, insomnia ($\downarrow$ sexual side effects)

Trazodone

MOA: mainly inhibits serotonin reuptake

IND: depression, insomnia, PTSD

TOX: postural hypotension, sedation, priapism

Venlafaxine

MOA: inhibits 5-HT and NE reuptake

IND: depression, generalized anxiety disorder

TOX: stimulant effects, minimal effects on P-450

Mirtazapine

MOA: 5-HT2 receptor antagonist and α_2-antagonist → $\uparrow$ NE and 5-HT release

IND: depression

TOX: sedation, $\uparrow$ appetite, $\uparrow$ cholesterol

MAOIs (TIP: Tranylcypromine, Isocarboxazid, Phenelzine)	**MOA**: nonselective MAOIs
	IND: atypical depressions, anxiety disorders, pain disorders, eating disorder
	TOX: hypertensive crisis with tyramine or meperidine ingestion, "serotonin syndrome" with SSRIs
Lithium	**MOA**: prevents generation of inositol triphosphate (IP3) and diacylglycerol (DAG) 2° messenger systems
	IND: bipolar disorder (prevents and treats acute mania)
	TOX: hypothyroidism, nephrogenic DI, teratogenesis (Ebstein anomaly)
Carbamazepine	**MOA**: blocks sodium channels and inhibits action potentials
	IND: bipolar disorder, mixed episodes, and rapid cycling form
	TOX: agranulocytosis, elevated LFTs, teratogenesis (neural tube defects), Stevens-Johnson syndrome
Valproic acid	**MOA**: increases CNS levels of GABA
	IND: bipolar disorder, mixed manic episodes, and rapid cycling form
	TOX: hepatotoxicity, thrombocytopenia, teratogenesis (neural tube defects)

Antipsychotics

What is the name for the stereotyped oral-facial movements that occur as a result of long-term antipsychotic use?	Tardive dyskinesia
Describe the chronology of extrapyramidal side effects from neuroleptic medications:	Rule of 4's: 4 hours—acute dystonia 4 days—akinesia 4 weeks—akathisia 4 months—tardive dyskinesia (usually irreversible)
What is the characteristic triad of neuroleptic malignant syndrome (NMS)?	Muscle rigidity, autonomic instability, and hyperpyrexia
What is the treatment for NMS?	Dantrolene and DA agonists

For each of the following drugs, provide:

1. The mechanism of action (MOA)
2. Indication(s) (IND)
3. Significant side effects and unique toxicity (TOX) (if any)

Typical antipsychotics—high potency (haloperidol, perphenazine, trifluoperazine)	**MOA**: block D_2 DA receptors (less blockade of α_2, muscarinic, and histaminic receptors)
	IND: schizophrenia, psychosis (especially positive symptoms)
	TOX: ↑ neurologic (eg, extrapyramidal) SEs, NMS, tardive dyskinesia, Parkinsonism, hyperprolactinemia
Typical antipsychotics—low potency (chlorpromazine, thioridazine)	**MOA**: block D_2 DA receptors (more blockade of α_2, muscarinic, and histaminic receptors)
	IND: schizophrenia, psychosis
	TOX: ↓ neurologic SEs, ↑ anticholinergic and endocrine SEs; cardiac conduction defects and retinal pigmentation (thioridazine), corneal and lenticular deposits (chlorpromazine)
Atypical antipsychotics (clozapine, risperidone, olanzapine, quetiapine)	**MOA**: block $5\text{-}HT_2$; block D_4 and $D_1 > D_2$ receptors
	IND: schizophrenia, psychosis (especially negative symptoms); OCD/ anxiety disorder (olanzapine)
	TOX: ↓ anticholinergic and extrapyramidal symptoms (EPS); metabolic syndrome (hyperlipidemia, glucose intolerance), agranulocytosis (clozapine)

MEDICAL ETHICS

What are four key components to informed consent?	The patient must:
	1. Understand the health implications of their diagnosis
	2. Be informed of risks, benefits, and alternatives to treatment
	3. Be aware of outcome if they do not give their consent
	4. Have the right to withdraw consent at any time

Name four exceptions to informed consent:

1. Patient not legally competent to make decisions
2. In an emergency (implied consent)
3. Patient waives the right to informed consent
4. Therapeutic privilege—withholding info that would severely harm the patient or undermine decision-making capacity if revealed

What are five situations in which parent/legal guardian consent is not required to treat a minor?

1. Emergencies
2. STDs
3. Prescription of contraceptives
4. Treatment of EtOH/drug treatment
5. Care during pregnancy

What four criteria qualify a minor as emancipated?

1. Self-supporting
2. In the military
3. Being married
4. Having children that they support

What type of directive is based on the incapacitated patient's prior statements and decisions?

Oral advance directive (substituted judgment standard)

What type of written advance directive gives instructions for the patient's future health care should he/she become incompetent to make decisions?

Living will

What type of document allows the patient to designate a surrogate to make medical decisions in case the patient loses decision-making capacity?

Durable power of attorney

Name the ethical responsibility of the physician described by each of the following statements:

Requires physicians to "do no harm"

Nonmaleficence

Requires physicians to act in the best interests of the patient

Beneficence (may conflict with patient autonomy)

Demands respect for patient privacy and autonomy

Confidentiality

Name five exceptions to confidentiality:	1. Suspected child and/or elder abuse 2. Suicidal/homicidal patient 3. Impaired automobile driver 4. Specific infectious diseases—physician duty to report to public officials or individuals at risk 5. Tarasoff decision—law requiring physician to directly inform/protect potential victim from harm
What elements are required in order to prove a malpractice claim?	The **"4 D's"**: must prove that the physician showed **D**ereliction (deviation from standard of care) of a **D**uty that caused **D**amages **D**irectly to the patient
What is the legal standard of death?	Failure to meet cardiorespiratory criteria and irreversible cessation of all brain functions (including brainstem)

Biostatistics

For each description, name the proper term and the equation used to calculate the value described below:

Probability that a person without the disease will be correctly identified	Specificity $TN/(TN + FP)$
Probability that a person who tests positive actually has the disease	Positive predictive value $TP/(TP + FP)$
Probability that a person who has a disease will be correctly identified	Sensitivity $TP/(TP + FN)$
Total number of cases in a population at any given time	Prevalence $TP + FN/(\text{entire population})$
Number of new cases that arise in a population over a given time interval	Incidence Prevalence $\times$ duration of disease (approximately)
Used in case-control studies to approximate the relative risk if the disease prevalence is too high	Odds ratio $TP \times TN/FP \times FN$
Used in cohort studies to compare incidence rate in exposed group to that in unexposed group	Relative risk $(TP/[TP + FP])/(FN/[FN + TN])$
Probability that patient with a negative test actually has no disease	Negative predictive value $TN/(FN + TN)$

How are incidence and prevalence related?	Incidence × disease duration = prevalence
	Prevalence > incidence for chronic diseases; prevalence = incidence for acute diseases
What quality is desirable for a screening tool?	High sensitivity (**SNOUT**—**SeN**sitivity rules **OUT**)
What quality is desirable for a confirmatory test?	High specificity (**SPIN**—**S**pecificity rules **IN**)
Name four ways to reduce bias:	1. Use of placebo 2. Blinded studies (single, double) 3. Crossover studies (each subject is own control) 4. Randomization

Name the type of statistical distribution described below:

Asymmetry with tail to the right	Positive skew
Two peaks	Bimodal
Scores cluster in the high end	Negative skew
Bell-shaped	Normal (Gaussian)

What percent of the area under a normal curve falls within 1, 2, and 3 standard deviations (SD) of the mean?	68% (1 SD), 95% (2 SD), 99.7% (3 SD)
How is standard error of the mean (SEM) calculated?	Square root of SD/square root of sample size

Name the term for each of the following descriptions:

Refers to the reproducibility of a test	Reliability
Refers to the appropriateness of a test (whether the test measures what it is supposed to)	Validity
Absence of random variation in a test; consistency and reproducibility of a test	Precision
Closeness of a measurement to the truth	Accuracy
Test that compares the difference between two means	*t*-test

Test that analyzes the variance of three or more variables	Analysis of variance (ANOVA)
Test that compares percentages or proportions	χ^2 (chi-squared test)
Absolute value that indicates the strength of a relationship	r (always between -1 and 1)
Observational study where the sample is chosen based on presence/absence of risk factors	Cohort study (eg, prospective, historical)
Experimental study comparing benefits of *two* or more alternative treatments	Clinical trial
Observational study where the sample is chosen based on disease presence/absence	Case-control study (usually retrospective)
Assembling data from multiple studies to achieve great statistical power	Meta-analysis
Hypothesis postulating that there is no difference between groups	Null hypothesis (H_0)
Error of mistakenly rejecting H_0 (stating that there is a difference when there really is not)	Type I error (α)
Error of failing to reject H_0 (stating there is no difference when there really is)	Type II error (β)
Probability of rejecting H_0 when it is in fact false	Power ($1-\beta$)
Probability of making an α error	P value

PUBLIC HEALTH/EPIDEMIOLOGY

Name four reportable STDs:	1. Gonorrhea 2. Syphilis 3. Hepatitis B 4. Acquired immunodeficiency syndrome (AIDS) (nonreportable = HIV, chlamydia, genital herpes)
What is the leading cause of mortality in each of the following age groups:	
<1 y/o	Congenital anomalies
1 to 14 y/o	Unintentional injuries

15 to 24 y/o	Unintentional injuries (mostly car accidents)
25 to 64 y/o	Cancer (#1 lung, #2 breast/prostate, #3 colon)
65 years and older	Heart disease
What is 1° disease prevention?	Aims to prevent disease occurrence (eg, vaccination, education)
What is 2° disease prevention?	Early detection of disease; screening programs
What is 3° disease prevention?	Reduces disability resulting from disease (eg, physical therapy for stroke)
What is the current definition of "obese"?	BMI >30, BMI >25 is overweight
Approximately what percentage of the US population is obese?	~30%, >50% overweight
What is the divorce rate in the United States?	~50%
Name three risk factors for divorce:	1. Teenage marriage 2. Mixed religions 3. Low SES **Note:** peaks during second and third years
What is the criterion to qualify for hospice care?	Medically anticipated death within 6 months
What federal program addresses health care needs of the elderly?	MedicarE (**Elderly**)
What federal and state program addresses health care needs of the underprivileged?	MedicaiD (**Destitute**)
What 1996 law helps to protect rights to health coverage during events such as changing or losing jobs, pregnancy, moving, or divorce?	Health Insurance Portability and Accountability Act (HIPAA)

CHAPTER 14

Make the Diagnosis

NUTRITION

1-year-old (y/o) impoverished child presents with lethargy and poor wound healing; physical examination (PE): low-grade fever, pallor, oral mucosal petechiae, and bleeding gums	Scurvy
50-y/o with a history of (h/o) long-term treatment of psoriasis with methotrexate presents with nausea and fatigue; PE: within normal limits (WNL); workup (W/U): MCV >100, hypersegmented neutrophils, and normal vitamin B_{12} levels	Folic acid deficiency
42-y/o alcoholic presents with ataxia and shortness of breath (SOB); PE: nystagmus, cardiomegaly with flow murmur, ↓ DTRs, ↓ peripheral sensation, and hepatomegaly	Beriberi
48-y/o Scandinavian woman presents with weakness, ataxia, and SOB; PE: ↓ balance and vibratory sensation in lower extremities; W/U: MCV >100, hypersegmented PMNs, and positive Schilling test	Pernicious anemia

MICROBIOLOGY AND INFECTIOUS DISEASES

4-y/o with a superficial skin infection consisting of erythematous pustules with honey-colored crust	Impetigo, most commonly due to *Staphylococcus aureus*

6-y/o child with poor hygiene presents with complaints of severe perianal itching that is worse at night; W/U: a "scotch tape test" reveals eggs visualized under the microscope

Pinworm infection (*Enterobius vermicularis*)

36-y/o man presents with flu-like symptoms since moving to a farm in Ohio 2 months ago; PE: fever and generalized lymphadenopathy; chest x-ray (CXR): bilateral hilar adenopathy

Histoplasmosis

Patient with recent h/o antibiotic use presents with fever, bloody diarrhea, and abdominal pain; PE: tender abdominal examination, guaiac + stool; complete blood count (CBC): leukocytosis; colonoscopy: tan nodules seen attached to erythematous bowel wall with superficial erosions

Pseudomembranous colitis (*Clostridium difficile* colitis)

18-y/o student returns to clinic with a rash after being treated with ampicillin for fever and sore throat; PE: tonsillar exudates and enlarged posterior cervical lymph nodes; W/U: ↑ lymphocytes and ⊕ heterophile antibody test

Infectious mononucleosis due to Epstein-Barr virus (EBV)

28-y/o with h/o treatment for 2° syphilis 5 hours ago with intramuscular (IM) penicillin presents with fever, chills, muscle pain (myalgias), and headache

Jarisch-Herxheimer reaction

6-month-old boy presents with a 10-day history of sneezing, runny nose, and congestion and is now developing a worsening cough; PE: severe, paroxysmal cough followed by a high-pitched inspiratory "whoop"; CBC: marked lymphocytosis

"Whooping cough" due to *Bordetella pertussis*

33-y/o northern European with h/o eating raw fish presents with SOB and weakness; W/U: megaloblastic anemia, operculated eggs on stool examination

Diphyllobothrium latum infection (with vitamin B_{12} deficiency)

17-y/o swimmer presents with pain and discharge from the left ear; PE: movement of tragus is extremely painful; Gram stain shows gram-negative rods

Otitis externa (most likely due to *Pseudomonas aeruginosa*)

10-y/o with sickle cell disease and recent h/o prodromal illness presents with sudden-onset pallor, fatigue, and tachycardia; CBC: pancytopenia with reticulocytes <1%	Parvovirus B19 aplastic crisis
44-y/o parrot owner presents with fever, chills, headache, and cough; PE: Horder spots on abdomen and splenomegaly; CXR: bilateral, interstitial infiltrates	Psittacosis
33-y/o epileptic with recent loss of consciousness presents with fever and cough with purulent, putrid sputum; W/U: Gram stain reveals mixed oral flora; CXR: consolidation of right lower lobe	Aspiration pneumonia
50-y/o man presents with a fever of unknown origin; 1 month ago he had a dental procedure; He has a history of rheumatic heart disease; PE: significant for a heart murmur, splinter hemorrhages, Janeway lesions, Roth spots, and Osler nodes	Subacute bacterial endocarditis due to *Streptococcus viridans*
9-y/o with recent viral prodromal illness presents to ER vomiting and lethargic after being given aspirin for fever; W/U: impaired liver function; computed tomography (CT): cerebral edema	Reye syndrome
15-y/o new pet owner presents with painful axillary lumps and fever; PE: cervical lymphadenopathy	Catscratch disease
2-month-old with maternal h/o rash and flu in first trimester presents with a rash and failure to attain milestones; PE: microcephaly, cataracts, jaundice, continuous machinery-like murmur at left upper sternal border, and hepatosplenomegaly (HSM)	Congenital rubella
8-y/o from Connecticut presents with fever, rash, headache, and joint pain after playing in the woods; PE: distinctive macule with surrounding 6 cm target-shaped lesion	Lyme disease

35-y/o man with h/o urinary catheterization presents with fever, chills, dysuria, and perineal pain; PE: swollen, tender, hot prostate; urinalysis (UA): WBCs and culture ⊕ for *Escherichia coli*

Acute bacterial prostatitis

38-y/o man with a h/o asthma presents with recurrent fever, wheezing, and cough productive of brown mucous plugs; CBC: eosinophilia, high IgE titers; CXR: mucoid impaction of dilated central bronchi

Allergic bronchopulmonary aspergillosis

6-y/o unvaccinated child presents with rhinorrhea, cough, conjunctivitis; PE: oral lesions are noted which are bluish with an erythematous border

Measles

37-y/o man with a recent h/o upper respiratory infection (URI) presents with fever and severe chest pain; PE: friction rub and Kussmaul sign; W/U: ↑ ESR, normal cardiac enzymes, and diffuse ST elevations on ECG

Acute pericarditis

4-y/o presents with barking cough, fever, and rhinorrhea; PE: respiratory distress and tachypnea; x-ray of soft tissues of neck reveals "steeple sign"

Croup

18-y/o sexually active woman with h/o treatment for purulent vaginitis presents with a fever and tenderness, warmth, and swelling of her right knee

Gonococcal arthritis

Newborn presents with rash and maternal h/o intrauterine growth retardation (IUGR) and flu during first trimester; PE: petechial rash, chorioretinitis, microcephaly, ↓ hearing, and HSM; W/U: ↓ platelets and periventricular calcifications on head CT

Congenital cytomegalovirus (CMV)

25-y/o West Virginian man presents with fever, headache, myalgia, and a petechial rash that began peripherally but now involves his whole body, even his palms and soles; W/U: shows +OX19 and OX2 Weil-Felix reaction

Rocky Mountain spotted fever

10-y/o presents with fevers and a pruritic rash spreading from the trunk to the arms; PE: vesicles of varying stages	Varicella
29-y/o athlete presents with a red, pruritic skin eruption with an advancing peripheral, creeping border on the forearm; W/U shows septate hyphae in KOH scraping	Tinea corporis (ringworm)
8-y/o presents with fever, photophobia, stiff neck, and headache; PE: ⊕ Kernig and Brudzinski signs; lumbar puncture shows normal glucose and ↓ WBCs	Viral meningitis
21-y/o presents with nausea, vomiting, bloating, and foul-smelling stools on returning from a camping trip; W/U: binucleate, flagellated trophozoites in stool	Giardiasis
14-y/o adolescent boy with a h/o recent travel to Mexico now presents with jaundice and dark yellow urine; PE: icterus and firm hepatomegaly; W/U: ↑ bilirubin (BR), ↑ LFTs with alanine transaminase (ALT) > aspartate transaminase (AST)	Hepatitis A infection
26-y/o sexually active, native Caribbean presents with painless, beefy-red ulcers of the genitalia and inguinal swelling; W/U: Donovan bodies on Giemsa-stained smear	Granuloma inguinale
Patient presents with sudden onset of severe watery diarrhea, vomiting, and abdominal discomfort 4 hours after eating potato salad at a picnic; the symptoms resolve spontaneously within 24 hours	*Staphylococcus aureus*-induced food poisoning
6-y/o with recent h/o sore throat presents with multiple joint pain and swelling, fever, and SOB; PE: erythema marginatum, subcutaneous nodules, and apical systolic murmur; W/U: ↑ ESR and CRP	Acute rheumatic fever (sequela of streptococcal infection)

25-y/o woman presents with malodor-
ous vaginal discharge; W/U: visual-
ization of the discharge under the
microscope demonstrates multiple
vaginal epithelial cells covered in
bacteria

Bacterial vaginosis due to *Gardenella vaginalis*

73-y/o presents with a painful, unilateral, vesicular rash in the distribution
of the CN V_1; cornea shows diminished
sensation and stains with fluorescein

Herpes zoster ophthalmicus

29-y/o missionary with h/o travel to
rural India presents with high fever
and right upper quadrant (RUQ) pain;
PE: severe hepatomegaly and dullness
over right lower lung; abdominal CT:
large, cavitating lesion in liver

Amebic liver abscess

25-y/o sexually active man presents
with dysuria, irritation, and cloudy
discharge; W/U: a Gram stain of the
discharge reveals neutrophils, but no
organisms are visualized

Nongonococcal urethritis, most likely
due to *Chlamydia trachomatis*

31-y/o obese woman presents with
pruritis in her skin fold beneath her
pannus; PE: whitish curd-like concre-
tions beneath the abdominal panniculus; W/U shows budding yeast on 10%
KOH preparation

Cutaneous candidiasis

20-y/o college student presents with
acute onset of altered mental status,
fever, malaise, nausea/vomiting,
and headache; PE: photophobia and
nuchal rigidity; lumbar puncture w/
gram stain: numerous gram-negative
diplococci

Meningitis due to *Neisseria meningitidis*

27-y/o HIV-positive man presents with
a several week h/o worsening SOB,
chest pain, dry cough, and a low-grade
fever; chest x-ray: bilateral interstitial
infiltrates; CD4 count: 124 cells/mm^3

Pneumocystis pneumonia due to
Pneumocystis jirovecii

NEUROSCIENCE

55-y/o man presents with lower extremity weakness and muscle atrophy; PE: positive Babinski reflex, upper extremity hyperreflexia, and spasticity	Amyotrophic lateral sclerosis (ALS)
65-y/o presents with a gradual decline in memory and inability to complete activities of daily living; W/U: CT shows marked enlargement of ventricles and temporal lobe atrophy	Alzheimer disease
65-y/o woman with a h/o spinal metastases from breast cancer presents with pain radiating down the back of her leg, saddle anesthesia, urinary retention; PE: absent ankle jerk reflexes; W/U: CT shows large bony fragment in lumbar spinal canal	Cauda equina syndrome
65-y/o man with a h/o carotid atherosclerosis presents with aphasia and right-sided weakness; PE: dense right-hemiparesis, positive Babinski on right; W/U: CT shows left middle cerebral artery (MCA) territory infarction and edema	Left MCA cerebrovascular accident
20-y/o presents with nausea, vomiting, and headache 2 hours after being hit in the temple with a baseball; patient lost consciousness initially but recovered quickly; W/U: CT shows lens-shaped, right-sided hyperdense mass adjacent to temporal bone that does not cross suture lines	Epidural hematoma
40-y/o with a h/o *Campylobacter* enteritis 1 week ago presents with ascending symmetric muscle weakness; CSF shows ↑ protein, normal cellularity (albuminocytologic dissociation)	Guillain-Barré syndrome
37-y/o man with family history (FH) of a father who died at 45 with worsening tremor and dementia presents with poor memory, depression, choreiform movements, and hypotonia; W/U: MRI demonstrates marked atrophy of the caudate nucleus	Huntington disease

25-y/o with a h/o bilateral temporal lobe contusions 1 week ago presents with a sudden increase in appetite, sexual desire, and hyperorality	Klüver-Bucy syndrome
30-y/o woman with insidious onset of diplopia, scanning speech, paresthesias, and numbness of right upper extremity and urinary incontinence; W/U: MRI shows discrete areas of periventricular white matter lesions and CSF analysis is positive for oligoclonal bands	Multiple sclerosis
65-y/o woman with a h/o neurofibromatosis type 2 presents with headache, right-sided leg jerking, and worsening mental status; PE: papilledema and right-sided pronator drift; W/U: CT scan shows dural-based, enhancing, left-sided softball-sized tumor	Meningioma
55-y/o with a h/o squamous cell carcinoma of the lung presents with nausea, vomiting, headache, and diplopia; PE: papilledema, left oculomotor palsy, right pronator drift; MRI: multiple round, hyperintense cortical and cerebellar lesions	Metastases to brain
30-y/o woman presents with unilateral throbbing headache, nausea, photophobia, scotoma; similar symptoms occur monthly at the same time of her menstrual cycle	Migraine
65-y/o with urinary incontinence, loss of short-term memory, and dementia; PE: wide based, magnetic gate; W/U: CT scan shows massively dilated ventricular system	Normal pressure hydrocephalus
60-y/o presents with gradual onset of pill-rolling tremor; PE: masked facies, stooped posture, festinating gait, cogwheel muscle rigidity, coarse resting tremor	Parkinson disease

65-y/o presenting with visual hallucinations and cognitive decline followed
by motor problems; PE: masked facies,
stooped posture, festinating gait, cogwheel muscle rigidity, coarse resting
tremor

Lewy body dementia

30-y/o presents with loss of libido,
galactorrhea, and irregular menses; PE:
bitemporal hemianopia; W/U: negative
beta human chorionic gonadotropin
(β-hCG)

Prolactinoma (prolactin-secreting
pituitary adenoma)

45-y/o presents with the gradual onset
of sharp pain radiating from his but-
tocks down his leg that began 2 weeks
ago when he began to lift a heavy box;
PE: positive straight leg raise test

Sciatica from acute herniation of a
lumbar disc

50-y/o with a h/o polycystic kidney
disease presents with "worst headache
of life," photophobia, nausea; PE: right
eye deviated down and out; W/U: CSF
is xanthochromic

Subarachnoid hemorrhage from
ruptured berry aneurysm

32-y/o man with a h/o Arnold-Chiari
malformation presents with bilateral
upper extremity muscle weakness; PE:
loss of pain and temperature sensation,
↓ DTR in upper extremities and scolio-
sis; MRI shows central cavitation of the
thoracic spinal cord

Syringomyelia

75-y/o alcoholic man on warfarin for
h/o atrial fibrillation presents with
declining mental status, headache,
and papilledema; CT shows crescentic,
hypodense, 2 cm fluid collection along
convexity

Chronic subdural hematoma

36-y/o woman with family h/o renal
cell carcinoma presents with gait disturbance and blurred vision; PE: retinal
hemangiomas, nystagmus, cerebellar ataxia, dysdiadochokinesia; MRI
shows two cerebellar cystic lesions

von Hippel-Lindau disease

50-y/o woman with sudden onset of
severe unilateral eye pain beginning
while at movie theater; PE: decreased
visual acuity, shallow anterior chamber
with dilated and fixed pupil

Acute angle closure glaucoma

A 50-y/o with a h/o alcoholism presents with psychosis, opthalmoplegia, and ataxia; MRI: mammillary body atrophy and diffuse cortical atrophy

Wernicke encephalopathy

62 y/o woman with difficulty climbing stairs; PE: proximal muscle weakness that improves with muscle use, dry oral mucosa; W/U: autoantibodies to calcium channel

Lambert-Eaton myasthenic syndrome

CARDIOVASCULAR

56-y/o woman presents with dyspnea on exertion (DOE); PE: loud S_1, delayed P_2, and a diastolic rumble; W/U: trans-esophageal echocardiogram shows mobile, pedunculated left atrial mass

Atrial myxoma

60-y/o presents with chest pain relieved by sitting up and leaning forward; PE: pericardial friction rub; ECG: diffuse ST segment elevation; echocardiogram: pericardial effusion with thickening of the pericardium

Acute pericarditis

65-y/o man presents with 1-week h/o fever, DOE, and orthopnea; PE: new, blowing holosystolic murmur at apex radiating into left axilla; W/U: blood cultures show *Viridans* spp. strepto-cocci; echocardiogram: oscillating mass attached to mitral valve

Acute infective endocarditis

60-y/o presents with dyspnea and palpitations; PE: 20 mm Hg decline in systolic BP with inspiration (pulsus paradoxus), ↓ BP, jugular venous dis-tention, diminished S_1 and S_2; echocar-diogram: large pericardial effusion

Tamponade

58-y/o man with Marfan syndrome presents with the abrupt onset of "tearing" chest pain radiating to the back; PE: ↓ BP, asymmetric pulses, declining mental status; CXR: widened mediastinum

Aortic dissection

70-y/o diabetic with hypercholesterolemia presents with angina, syncope, DOE, and orthopnea; PE: diminished, slowly rising carotid pulses, crescendo-decrescendo systolic murmur at second interspace at the right upper sternal border	Aortic stenosis
80-y/o diabetic with HTN and a h/o rheumatic heart disease presents with left-sided weakness; PE: pulses are irregularly irregular; ECG: absence of P waves and irregularly irregular QRS complexes	Atrial fibrillation (leading to embolic stroke)
70-y/o with a h/o coronary artery disease (CAD) presents with worsening DOE, orthopnea, and paroxysmal nocturnal dyspnea; PE: jugular venous distention, S_3 gallop, positive hepatojugular reflex, bibasilar rales, and peripheral edema; CXR: cardiomegaly, bilateral pleural effusions	Congestive heart failure (CHF)
50-y/o alcoholic presents with worsening DOE, orthopnea, and paroxysmal nocturnal dyspnea; PE: laterally displaced apical impulse; ECG: four-chamber dilation, mitral and tricuspid regurgitation	Alcoholic dilated cardiomyopathy
35-y/o man with FH of sudden cardiac death presents with DOE and syncope; PE: double apical impulse, S_4 gallop, holosystolic murmur at apex and axilla; ECG: left ventricular hypertrophy and mitral regurgitation	Hypertrophic cardiomyopathy
40-y/o black man with a h/o HTN presents with chest pain, dyspnea, and severe headache; PE: BP = 210/130 mm Hg in all four extremities, flame-shaped retinal hemorrhages, papilledema; W/U: negative vanillylmandelic acid (VMA), urine catecholamines, and cardiac enzymes	Malignant hypertension
35-y/o woman with a h/o rheumatic fever presents with worsening DOE and orthopnea; PE: loud S_1, opening snap and low-pitched diastolic murmur at the apex; CXR: left atrial enlargement	Mitral stenosis

65-y/o man presents with substernal pressure for the past hour with radiation of the pain into the jaw and left arm, nausea, diaphoresis, and dyspnea; PE: S$_4$ gallop; W/U: ↑ serum troponin and CK-MB; ECG: ST segment elevation in leads aVL, V$_1$ to V$_6$	Anterior myocardial infarction

PULMONARY

7-y/o with a h/o environmental allergies presents in acute respiratory distress; PE: tachypnea, expiratory wheezes, intercostal retractions, accessory muscle usage during respiration; CXR: hyperinflation; CBC: eosinophilia	Bronchial asthma
60-y/o with a 50 pack-year h/o smoking presents with fever and cough productive of thick sputum for the past 4 months; PE: cyanosis, crackles, wheezes; W/U: Hct = 48, WBC = 12,000; CXR: no infiltrates	Chronic bronchitis
60-y/o with a 50 pack-year h/o smoking presents with DOE and dry cough, but no chest pain; PE: ↓ breath sounds, ↑ heart rate (HR), hyperresonant chest, distant S$_1$ and S$_2$; CXR: hyperlucent lung fields	Emphysema
60-y/o with 50 pack-year h/o smoking presents with fatigue, DOE, hoarseness, anorexia; PE: miosis, ptosis, anhydrosis, dullness to percussion at right apex; CXR: large, hilar mass extending into the right superior pulmonary sulcus	Pancoast tumor (most likely bronchogenic squamous cell carcinoma, causing Horner syndrome)
60-y/o 4 days s/p total knee replacement has a sudden onset of tachycardia, tachypnea, sharp chest pain, hypotension; W/U: arterial blood gas (ABG) shows respiratory alkalosis; ECG: sinus tachycardia; lower extremity venous duplex ultrasound (U/S): clot in right femoral vein	Pulmonary embolism (most likely from DVT)

30-y/o black woman presents with DOE, fever, arthralgia; PE: iritis, erythema nodosum; W/U: eosinophilia, ↑ serum ACE levels; PFT: restrictive pattern; CXR: bilateral hilar lymphadenopathy, interstitial infiltrates; lymph node biopsy: noncaseating granulomas	Sarcoidosis
40-y/o white man presents with chronic rhinosinusitis, ear pain, cough, dyspnea; PE: ulcerations of nasal mucosa, perforation of nasal septum; W/U: ↑ C-ANCA; U/A: red cell casts; biopsy of nasal lesions: necrotizing vasculitis and granulomas	Granulomatosis with polyangiitis (formerly Wegener syndrome)
45 y/o inmate with cough, hemoptysis night sweats, fever; PE: unilateral crackles; W/U: acid fast bacilli smear +; CXR: cavitary lesion in upper lobe, hilar lymphadenopathy	Pulmonary tuberculosis
20 y/o male with abrupt onset dyspnea; PE: absent breath sound on right, right side hyperresonant to percussion, trachea deviation to left	Tension pneumothorax

GASTROENTEROLOGY

20-y/o woman presents with bloody diarrhea and joint pain; PE: abdominal tenderness, guaiac ⊕ stool; laboratory values: ↑ ESR and CRP, HLA-B27 +; colonoscopy: granular, friable mucosa with pseudopolyps throughout the colon	Ulcerative colitis (UC)
28-y/o patient with a h/o of UC presents with severe abdominal pain, distention, and high fever; PE: severe abdominal tenderness; CBC: leukocytosis; abdominal x-ray (AXR): dilated (>6 cm) transverse colon with "lead pipe" appearance	Toxic megacolon
Cirrhotic patient presents with massive hematemesis; PE: jaundice, ↓ BP, ↑ HR, ascites; W/U: stems pancytopenia, ↑ ALT and AST; EGD: actively bleeding vessel with numerous cherry red spots	Esophageal varices

38-y/o man with recent h/o fatigue, excessive thirst, and impotence presents with hyperpigmentation of his skin; PE: cardiomegaly, HSM; W/U: ↑ glucose, ferritin, transferrin, and serum iron	Hemochromatosis (hereditary)
19-y/o woman with recent h/o behavioral disturbance presents with jaundice and resting tremor; PE: pigmented granules in cornea and HSM; W/U: ↓ serum ceruloplasmin	Wilson disease
29-y/o with a h/o intermittent jaundice since receiving blood transfusion after motor vehicle accident (MVA) 2 years ago; PE: RUQ tenderness, hepatomegaly; W/U: negative HBV serology	Hepatitis C infection
31-y/o woman presents with 10-month h/o foul-smelling, greasy diarrhea; PE: pallor, hyperkeratosis, multiple ecchymoses, and abdominal distention; W/U: abnormal D-xylose test	Celiac disease
60-y/o white man presents with steatorrhea, weight loss, arthritis, and fever; small bowel biopsy shows PAS ⊕ macrophages and gram-positive bacilli	Whipple disease
19-y/o Jewish woman with h/o chronic abdominal pain presents with recurrent UTIs and pneumaturia; PE: diffuse abdominal pain; CT: enterovesical fistula; colonoscopy: skip lesions of linear ulcers and transverse fissures giving cobblestone appearance to mucosa	Crohn disease
21-y/o man presents with hematemesis after ingestion of aspirin and seven shots of whiskey; PE: diaphoretic, ↑ HR, epigastric tenderness; EGD: edematous, friable, reddened gastric mucosa	Acute gastritis
Patient with a h/o peptic ulcer disease (PUD) presents with melena; PE: ↑ HR, diaphoretic, diffuse abdominal pain; W/U: nasogastric tube (NGT) aspirate is bloody; EGD: visible bleeding vessel distal to the pylorus	Bleeding duodenal ulcer

40-y/o obese, mother of four children presents with constant RUQ pain radiating to right scapula, N/V; PE: fever, tenderness, and respiratory pause induced by RUQ palpation, painful palpable gallbladder; W/U: ↑ WBC, ↑ ALP; U/S: thickened gallbladder wall, pericholecystic fluid with gallstones present	Acute cholecystitis
39-y/o man presents with dull, steady epigastric pain radiating to the back after an alcohol binge, N/V; PE: fever, ↑ BP, epigastric tenderness, guarding, and distention; W/U: ↑↑ amylase/lipase, ↑ WBC; AXR: ⊕ sentinel loop and colon cutoff sign	Acute pancreatitis
65-y/o black man with a h/o smoking presents with anorexia, weight loss, pruritis, and painless jaundice; PE: palpable, nontender, distended gallbladder, migratory thrombophlebitis; W/U: ↑ direct BR, ALP, carcinoembryonic antigen (CEA), and CA 19-9	Pancreatic adenocarcinoma
60-y/o black man with a h/o gastroesophageal reflux disease (GERD) presents with weight loss and dysphagia; EGD: partially obstructing mass near GE junction	Esophageal adenocarcinoma
65-y/o presents with severe worsening left lower quadrant (LLQ) pain, N/V, and diarrhea; PE: fever, LLQ tenderness, local guarding, and rebound tenderness; W/U: ↑ WBC; abdominal CT: edematous colonic wall with localized fluid collection	Diverticulitis
30-y/o woman presents with periumbilical pain which has now migrated to the RLQ followed by anorexia, N/V; PE: low-grade fever, local RLQ guarding, rebound tenderness, RLQ tenderness on LLQ palpation; W/U: β-hCG negative, ↑ WBC with left shift	Appendicitis

55-y/o presents with colicky abdominal pain, small-caliber stools, and occasional melena; PE: cachexia, abdominal discomfort, guaiac ⊕ colonoscopy shows obstructing mass seen in ascending colon	Right-sided colon carcinoma
80-y/o woman presents with halitosis, dysphagia, and regurgitation of undigested foods; W/U: barium swallow shows posterior midline pouch greater than 2 cm in diameter arising just above the cricopharyngeus muscle	Zenker diverticulum
55-y/o Asian woman with a h/o HBV presents with dull RUQ pain; PE: weight loss, painful hepatomegaly, ascites, jaundice; W/U: ↑ ALT/AST, ↑ α-fetoprotein; abdominal CT: mass seen in right lobe of liver	Hepatocellular carcinoma
55-y/o with a h/o choledocholithiasis presents with fever, chills, and RUQ pain; PE: jaundice; W/U: ↑ WBC, BR, and ALP; U/S: stone in common bile duct	Cholangitis
43-y/o man presents with epigastric pain, diarrhea, and recurrent peptic ulcers; PE: epigastric tenderness; W/U: ↑ fasting gastrin levels, paradoxic ↑ in gastrin with secretin challenge; octreotide scan: detects lesion in pancreas	Zollinger-Ellison syndrome
72-y/o presents with recurrent, low-grade, painless hematochezia; PE: guaiac ⊕ stool; colonoscopy reveals slightly raised, discrete, scalloped lesion with visible draining vein in right colon	Angiodysplasia
63-y/o Japanese man with a h/o atrophic gastritis presents with weight loss, indigestion, epigastric pain, and vomiting; PE: supraclavicular lymph node; W/U: anemia, ⊕ fecal occult blood	Gastric carcinoma

48-y/o with chronic watery diarrhea, hot flashes, and facial redness; PE: shows II/VI right-sided ejection murmur; W/U: ↑ 5-hydroxyindoleacetic acid (5-HIAA) in urine	Carcinoid syndrome
40-y/o presents with dysphagia, regurgitation, and weight loss; W/U: barium swallow demonstrates dilated esophagus with distal narrowing (*bird beak* appearance)	Achalasia
16-y/o with strong FH of colorectal CA presents with rectal bleeding and abdominal pain; W/U: anemia; flexible sigmoidoscopy: >100 adenomatous polyps visualized	Familial adenomatous polyposis (FAP)
47-y/o man with a h/o EtOH abuse presents with several episodes of vomiting followed by hematemesis; endoscopy shows longitudinal mucosal tear at GE junction	Mallory-Weiss syndrome
34-y/o bulimic presents with sudden-onset retrosternal pain after vigorous vomiting; upper GI series shows extravasation of contrast into mediastinum	Boerhaave syndrome
44-y/o heavy smoker presents with heartburn and regurgitation that is worse when lying down and is relieved with antacids; upper GI series reveals mild hiatal hernia	GERD
5-day-old infant presents with abdominal distention and failure to pass meconium until after a rectal examination; XR shows massively dilated colon	Hirschsprung disease
43-y/o man with a h/o ulcerative colitis with W/U notable for elevated ALP and positive P-ANCA; MRCP shows "beading" (alternating dilation and stricturing) of intra and extrahepatic bile ducts	Primary sclerosing cholangitis

39-y/o woman with a h/o rheumatoid arthritis presents with fatigue and pruritus; PE: jaundice and HSM; W/U reveals ↑↑ ALP and γ-glutamyl transpeptidase (GGT) and presence of antimitochondrial antibodies	Primary biliary cirrhosis
2-week-old first-born male infant presents with projectile nonbilious vomiting and dehydration; PE: visible peristalsis and palpable "olive-like" mass in epigastrum	Hypertrophic pyloric stenosis
50-y/o with long h/o retrosternal pain drinks and smokes despite undergoing treatment for GERD; biopsy of distal esophagus shows nonciliated columnar epithelial cells with goblet cells	Barrett's esophagus
34-y/o woman with factor V Leiden deficiency presents with abdominal distention and jaundice; PE: pitting pedal edema, markedly visible leg veins, HSM, and absent hepatojugular reflex; U/S shows obstruction of hepatic veins	Budd-Chiari syndrome
7-month-old infant presents with vomiting and currant jelly-appearing stools; PE: right-sided, sausage-shaped, palpable mass in abdomen; barium enema (BE) shows telescoping of intestines	Intussusception

REPRODUCTIVE-ENDOCRINE

31-y/o presents with loss of libido, galactorrhea, and irregular menses; PE: bitemporal hemianopia; W/U: negative β-hCG	Prolactinoma
7-month-old with history of multiple infections turns cyanotic when aggravated; PE: abnormal facies, cleft palate, heart murmur; W/U: hypocalcemia, tetralogy of Fallot	DiGeorge syndrome (22qll)

Patient presents to clinic with polyuria and polydipsia; W/U: urine specific gravity <1.005, urine osmolality <200 mOsm/kg, hypernatremia	Diabetes insipidus
30-y/o white woman presents with weight loss, tremor, and palpitations; PE: brisk DTRs, ophthalmopathy, pretibial myxedema; W/U: $\downarrow$ TSH, $\uparrow$ T_4, $\uparrow$ T_3 index	Graves' disease
40-y/o woman presents with fatigue, constipation, and weight loss; PE: puffy face, cold dry hands, coarse hair, and enlargement of thyroid gland; W/U: $\uparrow$ TSH, $\downarrow$ T_3 and T_4, $\oplus$ antimicrosomal and antithyroglobulin AB	Hashimoto disease
32-y/o woman with a h/o recurrent PUD presents with episodes of hypocalcemia and nephrolithiasis; W/U: fasting hypoglycemia, $\uparrow$ gastrin levels, and hypercalcemia	Multiple endocrine neoplasia (MEN) 1
70-y/o presents with episodal hypertension, nephrolithiasis, and diarrhea; PE: $\uparrow$ BP, thyroid nodule; W/U: $\uparrow$ calcitonin levels, $\uparrow$ urinary catecholamines	MEN 2
Female patient presents with bone pain, kidney stones, depression, and recurrent ulcers; W/U: hypercalcemia, hypophosphatemia, and hypercalciuria	Hyperparathyroidism
35-y/o woman presents with weight gain, irregular menses, and HTN; PE: $\uparrow$ BP, $\uparrow$ weight in face and upper back, hirsutism, multiple ecchymoses; W/U: $\uparrow$ ACTH levels and suppression with high-dose dexamethasone suppression test	Cushing disease
50-y/o woman presents with HTN, muscle weakness, and fatigue; W/U: hypokalemia, hypernatremia, and metabolic alkalosis	Conn syndrome
30-y/o woman presents with progressive weakness, weight loss, N/V; PE: hyperpigmentation of skin, $\downarrow$ BP; W/U: hyperkalemia, hyponatremia, and eosinophilia	Addison disease

40-y/o presents with episodes of HA, diaphoresis, palpitations, and tremor; PE: ↑ BP, ↑ HR; W/U: ↑ in urinary VMA and homovanillic acid	Pheochromocytoma
17-y/o white adolescent with a h/o diabetes mellitus (DM) presents with diffuse abdominal pain, N/V, and slight confusion; PE: ↓ BP, shallow, rapid breathing pattern; W/U: glucose = 300, hypokalemia, hypophosphatemia, and metabolic acidosis	Diabetic ketoacidosis (DKA)-DM type 1
60-y/o diabetic obese patient found at home confused and disoriented; PE: ↓ BP, ↑ HR; W/U: glucose >1000	Hyperosmolar hyperglycemic non-ketotic (HHNK)-DM type 2
50-y/o woman presents with a h/o weakness, blurred vision, and confusion several hours after meals, which improves with eating; W/U: ↑ fasting levels of insulin and hypoglycemia	Insulinoma (with Whipple triad)
Newborn presents with ambiguous genitalia; PE: lethargy and ↓ BP; W/U: ↓ Na$^+$, ↑ K$^+$, ↑ 17 α-OH-progesterone, ↑ ACTH, and karyotype of 46,XX	Congenital adrenal hyperplasia (21α-hydroxylase deficiency)
7-y/o girl presents with breast buds and monthly vaginal bleeding; PE: height and weight >>95 percentile, full pubic and axillary hair; hand x-ray shows advanced bone age	Precocious puberty
21-y/o woman presents with no h/o menarche; PE: normal breast tissue, no axillary or pubic hair, vagina ending in blind pouch, no palpable cervix or uterus; karyotype shows 46,XY	Androgen insensitivity (testicular feminization) syndrome
45-y/o with recent h/o coarsening of facial features presents with headaches and states that his shoes no longer fit; PE: enlarged jaw, tongue, hands, and feet, and bitemporal hemianopia	Acromegaly
65-y/o smoker with a h/o lung cancer presents with fatigue and oliguria; W/U: ↓ Na$^+$, ↓ serum osmolarity, ↑↑ urine osmolarity	Syndrome of inappropriate antidiuretic hormone (SIADH)

20-y/o sexually active woman presents with crampy abdominal pain and purulent vaginal discharge; PE: fever and adnexal tenderness; W/U: ↑ WBCs, ↑ ESR, and combined infection with *Chlamydia trachomatis* and *Neisseria gonorrhoeae*	Pelvic inflammatory disease (PID)
18-y/o woman with 3 days of vaginal pruritis; PE: thick, white discharge; W/U: budding yeast on KOH preparation	Vaginal candidiasis
28-y/o woman postpartum day 1 with excessive hemorrhage in labor becomes weak and loses consciousness; PE: hypotension; W/U: ↓ cortisol, ↓ TSH, ↓ fT_4, ↓ LH, ↓ FSH	Sheehan syndrome (pituitary apoplexy)
31-y/o woman with a h/o PID presents with sudden-onset nausea and LLQ pain; PE: ↓ BP, ↑ HR, rebound tenderness in LLQ; W/U shows ⊕ β-hCG and fluid in cul-de-sac on U/S	Ruptured ectopic pregnancy
28-y/o man presents with gynecomastia and painless lump in his left testicle for 3 months; PE: firm 4 cm mass on left testis; W/U: ↑↑ serum hCG and AFP	Testicular carcinoma
35-y/o man with sensation of heaviness in left scrotum; appears like a "bag of worms" on examination	Varicocele
62-y/o obese nun with a h/o menopause at age 57 presents with vaginal bleeding for the past 4 months; PE shows normal-sized uterus; Pap smear reveals abnormal endometrial cells	Endometrial carcinoma
52-y/o obese patient presents with numbness in hands and feet; PE: ↑ BP and retinopathy; W/U: ↑ HbA_{1c} and glycosuria	DM type 2
55-y/o woman presents with an itching, scaling, oozing rash over her left nipple; PE: serosanguinous discharge and eczematous redness of left nipple with axillary lymphadenopathy	Paget disease of the breast

4-y/o girl presents with a "bunch of grapes" protruding from her vagina; W/U: desmin positive	Sarcoma botryoides
37-y/o woman presents with dysmenor-rhea, dyspareunia, menorrhagia, and pain coinciding with her menstrual cycle; PE: nodularity of uterosacral ligaments and cul-de-sac	Endometriosis
22-y/o woman with 6-month h/o amen-orrhea presents for infertility evalu-ation; PE: obesity, hirsutism; W/U: ↑ LH:FSH ratio, ↑ testosterone, and enlarged ovaries on U/S	Polycystic ovarian syndrome (Stein-Leventhal syndrome)
44-y/o with recent h/o thyroidectomy presents with muscle cramping; PE: cir-cumoral numbness, positive Trousseau and Chvostek signs	Hypoparathyroidism
23-y/o woman marathon runner pres-ents with lack of menses for 5 months; PE shows no signs of pregnancy; W/U: negative β-hCG, normal prolactin and thyroid hormones	Secondary amenorrhea
28-y/o black woman at 35 weeks gesta-tion in her first pregnancy presents with swollen legs; PE: ↑ BP and pitting pedal edema; W/U: 3+ proteinuria	Preeclampsia
2-y/o child presents with developmen-tal delay; PE: macroglossia, short stat-ure, and protuberant abdomen; W/U: ↑ TSH, ↑ T_3 and T_4	Congenital hypothyroidism (cretinism)
51-y/o woman with 9-month h/o amenorrhea presents with fatigue and flushing of skin; PE: atrophic vaginal mucosa; W/U: ↑ FSH and LH	Menopause
24-y/o woman presents with painless lump in her left breast; PE: small, firm, palpable, and freely mobile, rubbery mass in the upper-outer quadrant of the breast	Fibroadenoma

19-y/o man is brought to you for failure of pubertal maturation; PE: anosmia, ↓ muscle mass, no axillary or pubic hair, and hypogonadism; W/U: ↓ LH and FSH	Kallmann syndrome
9-y/o girl presents with muscle cramps; PE: rounded face with flat nasal bridge, abnormal dentition, positive Trousseau and Chvostek sign, and shortened third and fourth metacarpals	Albright hereditary osteodystrophy (pseudohypoparathyroidism)
22-y/o pregnant woman at 27 weeks with painless vaginal bleeding that stopped after an hour; W/U: placenta overlying the cervical os on U/S	Placenta previa
19-y/o woman with a h/o recent hydatidiform mole presents with vaginal bleeding, nausea, and vomiting; PE: vascular growth at cervical os and enlarged uterus; W/U: ↑↑ β-hCG	Choriocarcinoma
35-y/o man presents for sterility evaluation; PE: eunuchoid body habitus, small testicles, and gynecomastia; karyotype reveals 47,XXY	Klinefelter syndrome
35-y/o African American female with heavy menstrual bleeding and pelvic pressure; PE: irregularly shaped uterus; W/U: anemia	Leiomyoma (fibroid)
6-y/o boy with intellectual disability; PE: microcephaly, smooth philtrum, thin vermillion border, small palpebral fissures, micrognathia	Fetal alcohol syndrome

RENAL AND GENITOURINARY

Patient hospitalized for CHF is started on an aminoglycoside for a UTI and develops oliguria, N/V, and malaise; PE: ↑ BP and asterixis; serum electrolytes: ↑ creatinine (Cr), K+; UA: "muddy brown" casts, FeNa+ >3%	Acute kidney injury (drug-induced ATN)

70-y/o black man with a h/o of life-long DM presents with peripheral edema, SOB, and oliguria; PE: auscultatory rales, pitting edema, myoclonus, and uremic frost; serum electrolytes: ↑ Cr, hyperkalemia, hypocalcemia, hyperphosphatemia	Chronic renal failure
Teenage female presents with fever, chills, and flank pain; PE: costovertebral angle (CVA) tenderness; UA: leukocyte esterase ⊕, 30 WBC/hpf with WBC casts	Pyelonephritis
32-y/o man presents with pain and hematuria; PE: ↑ BP, palpable kidney, and midsystolic ejection click; abdominal U/S: multiple cysts of renal parenchyma; cerebral angiogram: unruptured berry aneurysm	Autosomal dominant (adult) polycystic kidney disease
20-y/o man presents with significant blood loss following a trauma and begins to have decreased urine output; W/U: oliguria, FeNa <1%, and BUN:Cr >20	Acute renal failure—prerenal
12-y/o girl with recent h/o sore throat 10 days ago presents with low urine output and dark urine; PE: periorbital edema; W/U: hematuria, ↑ BUN and Cr, ↑ antistreptolysin O (ASO) titer	Poststreptococcal glomerulonephritis
45-y/o Asian man with a h/o hepatitis B presents with malaise, edema, and foamy urine; PE: anasarca; W/U: proteinuria (>3.5 g/day), hyperlipiduria, hyperlipidemia and hypoalbuminemia	Membranous glomerulonephritis
Male infant is born with flattened facies, joint position abnormalities, and hypoplastic lungs; oligohydramnios was noted prior to delivery	Potter sequence—secondary to renal agenesis
80-y/o man presents with urinary hesitancy, nocturia, and weak urinary stream; PE: diffusely enlarged rubbery prostate; serum electrolytes: ↑ Cr, UA is WNL	Benign prostatic hyperplasia (BPH)

68-y/o man, who is a smoker, presents with flank pain and hematuria; PE: fever, palpable kidney mass; W/U: hypercalcemia, polycythemia	Renal cell carcinoma
20 y/o man presents with acute onset of left testicular pain and N/V; PE: swollen, tender testicle in transverse position, absent cremasteric reflex on left side; Doppler: no flow detected in left testicle	Testicular torsion
65-y/o man, who is a smoker, presents with painless hematuria and occasional urinary urgency and frequency; PE: unremarkable; urine cytology positive for malignant cells	Bladder—urothelial carcinoma
85-y/o man presents with back pain, weight loss, and weak urinary stream; PE: palpable firm nodule on digital rectal examination (DRE); W/U: ↑ PSA	Prostate cancer
25-y/o Asian man presents with N/V and colicky right flank pain; PE: acute distress and CVA tenderness; W/U: hematuria and discrete radiopacities on abdominal XR	Renal stones
45-y/o with documented h/o aortic atheromatous plaques presents with recent-onset, severe left flank pain, and hematuria; abdominal CT: wedge-shaped lesion in the left kidney	Renal infarct
3-y/o boy presents with a h/o flank mass found recently by his mother while bathing him; PE: palpable mass in left flank; abdominal CT: large mass growing out of left kidney	Wilms tumor
55-y/o with long h/o DM presents with increasing fatigue and edema; PE: ↑ BP, retinopathy, and pitting edema; W/U: severe proteinuria and glycosuria	Diabetic nephropathy (glomerulosclerosis)
21-y/o sexually active woman presents with frequency and dysuria; PE: supra-pubic tenderness; W/U: *E. coli*-positive urine cultures	Urinary tract infection (UTI)

25-y/o man presents with hemoptysis, dark urine, and fatigue; PE: bilateral crackles at lung bases; W/U: oliguria, hematuria, and anti-GBM antibodies	Goodpasture syndrome
7-y/o presents in stupor after ingesting antifreeze; PE: Kussmaul respirations and mental status changes; W/U reveals anion gap of 21 mEq/L	Metabolic acidosis (ethylene glycol toxicity)
6-y/o boy presents with hematuria and worsening vision; PE: corneal abnormalities, retinopathy, sensorineural hearing loss; W/U: hematuria with dysmorphic red cells	Alport syndrome
3-y/o boy with a h/o recent URI presents with facial edema; PE: ascitic fluid in abdomen and pedal edema; W/U reveals 4+ proteinuria and ↓ serum albumin	Minimal change disease
20-y/o otherwise healthy man presents with mild flank pain and gross hematuria 2 days after coming down with a URI; UA: hematuria with dysmorphic RBCs and RBC casts	IgA nephropathy
60-y/o woman with a long-standing h/o rheumatoid arthritis presents with several weeks of fevers, chills, flank pain, and gross hematuria; UA: hematuria, proteinuria, pyuria, and dead tissue	Renal papillary necrosis (likely 2/2 to analgesic nephropathy)

HEMATOLOGY-ONCOLOGY

50-y/o with a h/o bone marrow transplant for chronic myelogenous leukemia (CML) 3 weeks ago presents with severe pruritis, diarrhea, and jaundice; PE: violaceous rash on palms and soles; W/U: ↑ BR, ALT, and AST	Graft-versus-host disease
1-y/o Greek child presents with pallor and delayed milestones; PE: skeletal abnormalities, splenomegaly; peripheral blood smear (PBS): hypochromic microcytic RBCs, target cells, fragmented RBCs; skull XR: "hair-on-end" appearance	β-Thalassemia

10-y/o with a h/o recurrent chest pain presents with fever and bilateral leg pain; PE: febrile, multiple leg ulcers; PBS shows sickle-shaped erythrocytes; Hb electrophoresis shows HbS band	Sickle cell anemia
60-y/o presents with headache, vertigo, blurry vision, pruritus, joint pain; PE: ↑ BP, mild leukocytosis, and hyperuricemia	Polycythemia vera **plethoric splenomegaly**; W/U: Hct = 60
4-y/o boy with Down syndrome, presenting with a 1-week h/o fever, pallor, headache, and bone tenderness; PE: fever, HSM, and generalized, nontender lymphadenopathy; PBS reveals absolute lymphocytosis with abundant TdT+ lymphoblasts	Acute lymphoblastic leukemia
27-y/o presents with 2-month h/o fatigue, oropharyngeal candidiasis, pseudomonal UTI, and epistaxis; PE: numerous petechiae and ecchymoses of skin, gingival mucosal bleeding, guaiac ⊕ stools; W/U: ↑ WBC; PBS shows >30% myeloblasts with Auer rods	Acute myelocytic leukemia
17-y/o man presents with a 2-month h/o fever, night sweats, and weight loss; PE: nontender, cervical lymphadenopathy, and HSM; CBC: leukocytosis; CXR: bilateral hilar adenopathy; lymph node biopsy: Reed-Sternberg cells	Hodgkin disease
60-y/o man presents with fatigue and anorexia; PE: generalized lymphadenopathy and HSM; W/U: WBC = 250,000, positive direct Coombs test; PBS: small, round lymphocytes predominate with occasional smudge cells	Chronic lymphocytic leukemia
10-y/o African child presents with a 3-week h/o a rapidly enlarging, painless mandibular mass; CBC: mild anemia and leukopenia; cytogenetics reveal a t(8:14) translocation; excisional biopsy: "starry-sky" pattern	Burkitt lymphoma

35-y/o presents with a 3-year h/o mild weight loss, anorexia, worsening DOE; PE: splenomegaly; CBC: mild anemia, WBC = 125,000; PBS: granulocytosis with <10% myeloblasts; cytogenetics reveal a t(9:22) translocation	Chronic myelocytic leukemia
55-y/o with a recent h/o streptococcal pneumonia presents with bone pain and weight loss; W/U: mild anemia, hypercalcemia; PBS: rouleaux formation; UA: Bence-Jones proteinuria; serum electrophoresis: M spike; XR: cranial "punched-out" lesions	Multiple myeloma
18-y/o woman develops dyspnea and declining mental status 1 hour after a C-section complicated by excess blood loss; PE: mucosal bleeding, large clot in the vaginal vault; W/U: ↑ D-dimer, ↑ PT/PTT, ↓ antithrombin III, and thrombocytopenia	Disseminated intravascular coagulation
7-y/o with a h/o viral URI 1 week ago presents with epistaxis; PE: petechial hemorrhages of nasal mucosa and extremities; W/U: ↓ platelets, normal PT and PTT; bone marrow biopsy: ↑↑ megakaryocytes	Idiopathic thrombocytopenic purpura
8-y/o with a h/o vomiting and diarrhea after eating a hamburger last week presents with fatigue, periorbital edema, and oliguria; PE: purpuric rash; CBC: ↓ platelets; PBS: burr cells, helmet cells; UA: RBC casts, proteinuria, hematuria	Hemolytic uremic syndrome
8-y/o with a h/o environmental allergies presents with a painful rash on the legs, abdominal discomfort, joint pain; UA: hematuria and RBC casts; renal biopsy: glomerular mesangial IgA deposits	Henoch-Schönlein purpura
8-y/o boy presents with a swollen painful knee; FH: maternal grandfather died from hemorrhage after a cholecystectomy; PE: cutaneous ecchymoses; W/U: gross blood in swollen knee joint, ↑ PTT, normal PT and platelet count, ↑ bleeding time	Hemophilia A

2-y/o boy with a h/o recurrent epistaxis presents with the third episode of otitis media in 4 months; PE: eczematous dermatitis; W/U: thrombocytopenia, ↓ IgM, ↑ IgA

Wiskott-Aldrich syndrome

Newborn develops jaundice rapidly during the first day of life; PE: HSM; W/U: severe anemia, ⊕ indirect Coombs test in both mother and newborn

Rh incompatibility

16-y/o adolescent with a h/o menorrhagia presents with fatigue; PE: multiple cutaneous bruises; guaiac ⊕ stools; W/U: ↑ bleeding time, ↓ factor VIII, normal platelet count, PT, and PTT

von Willebrand disease

4-y/o boy brought in by parents for "behavioral problems," living in home built in the 1950s; CBC notable for mild anemia, peripheral smear showing basophilic stippling of RBCs

Lead poisoning

SKIN AND CONNECTIVE TISSUES

30-y/o man with a h/o recurrent sinusitis presents for infertility evaluation; PE: heart sounds are best heard over right side of chest

Kartagener syndrome

9-y/o with a h/o easy bruising and hyperextensible joints presents to the ER after dislocating his shoulder for the fifth time this year

Ehlers-Danlos syndrome

5-y/o presents to the ER with his sixth bone fracture in the past 2 years; PE: bluish sclera and mild kyphosis; XR: fractures with evidence of osteopenia

Osteogenesis imperfecta

8-y/o with a long h/o severe sunburns and photophobia presents to the dermatologist for evaluation of several lesions on the face that have recently changed color and size

Xeroderma pigmentosum

6-y/o boy presents to the ophthalmol-ogy clinic with sudden ↓ visual acuity; PE: unusual body habitus, long and slender fingers, pectus excavatum, and superiorly dislocated lens	Marfan syndrome
36-y/o with a h/o celiac disease pres-ents with clusters of pruritic, erythema-tous vesicular lesions over the extensor surfaces of the extremities	Dermatitis herpetiformis
5-y/o patient presents with honey-colored crusted lesions at the angle of his mouth; Gram stain of pus: gram-positive cocci in chains	Impetigo (due to *Streptococcus pyogenes*)
29-y/o HIV-positive patient presents with multiple painless pearly white umbilicated papules on the trunk and anogenital area	Molluscum contagiosum
68-y/o fair-skinned farmer presents with large, telangiectatic, and ulcerated nodule on the bridge of the nose	Basal cell carcinoma
11-y/o presents with bilateral wrist pain and a rash; PE: erythematous, reticular skin rash of the face and trunk with a "slapped-cheek appearance"	Erythema infectiosum
43-y/o woman presents with difficulty swallowing; PE: bluish discoloration of the hands and shiny, tight skin over her face and fingers	Progressive systemic sclerosis (scleroderma)
5-y/o Asian boy presents with fever and diffuse rash including the palms and soles; PE: cervical lymphade-nopathy, conjunctival injection, and desquamation of his fingertips; echo-cardiogram reveals dilation of coronary arteries	Kawasaki syndrome (mucocutaneous lymph node syndrome)
33-y/o patient presents with itchy, pur-ple plaques over her wrists, forearms, and inner thigh; PE: Wickham striae	Lichen planus
25-y/o woman with a h/o Raynaud phenomenon presents with arthralgias and myositis; W/U reveals esophageal hypomotility and ↑ anti-nRNP titers	Mixed connective tissue disease

32-y/o AA woman presents with fatigue, joint pain, and an erythematous rash on her cheeks sparing the nasolabial folds; W/U reveals +ANA and anti-dsDNA antibodies

Systemic lupus erythematosus (SLE)

45-y/o woman presents with a gradual development of weakness and difficulty performing activities of daily living over the past 3 to 4 months; skin: dusky red rash surrounding the eyelids, periungual telangiectasias; strength: 3/5 strength in hip flexion/extension, 4/5 strength in heel flexion/extension

Dermatomyositis

MUSCULOSKELETAL

25-y/o man presents with morning stiffness, heel pain, and photophobia; PE: ↓ lumbar spine extension and lateral flexion, tenderness on lumbar spinous processes and iliac crests; W/U: HLA-B27 ⊕; XR: bamboo spine

Ankylosing spondylitis

7-y/o girl presents with a limp, anorexia, and spiking fevers; PE: salmon-pink linear rash on trunk and extremities and swelling of bilateral hip, knee, elbow, and wrist joints; W/U: ↑ ESR

Juvenile rheumatoid arthritis

50-y/o woman presents with long-standing h/o morning stiffness and diffuse joint pain; PE: boutonniere and swan neck deformities of fingers, shoulder tenderness, and ↓ range of motion (ROM), symmetric and bilateral knee swelling; W/U: RF positive

Rheumatoid arthritis

25-y/o man with a h/o urethritis 2 weeks ago presents with unilateral knee pain, stiffness, and eye pain; PE: conjunctivitis, edema, and tenderness of left knee, mucoid urethral discharge; W/U: urethral swab ⊕ for *Chlamydia*

Reiter syndrome

45-y/o woman presents with dry eyes and dry mouth; PE: parotid gland enlargement, bibasilar rales; W/U: ⊕ ANA, RF, SS-A/Ro titers

Sjögren syndrome

70-y/o woman presents with pain in hands that is worse with activity; PE: Heberden and Bouchard nodes, bony enlargement at DIP and PIP joints, bilateral knee effusions; W/U: negative RF, normal ESR; hand XR: joint space narrowing, osteophytes

Osteoarthritis

72-y/o woman presents with a 6-week h/o morning stiffness in neck and shoulders; PE: low-grade fever, tenderness to palpation, and decreased ROM in neck, shoulder, hip joints; W/U: ↑ ESR and CRP, but negative RF

Polymyalgia rheumatica

50-y/o man presents with acute onset of sharp pain in the left great toe; PE: severe tenderness, swelling, and warmth of the left MTP joint; synovial fluid analysis shows negatively birefringent crystals

Gout

25-y/o woman with a 1-week h/o pain in several joints presents with swelling, redness, and pain in her right knee; PE: pustular lesions on palms, right knee shows erythema, tenderness, and ↓ ROM; W/U: gram-negative diplococci in synovial fluid

Gonococcal arthritis

28-y/o woman presents with difficulty keeping her eyelids open and holding her head up during the day; PE: weakness of facial muscles, deltoids; W/U: anti-ACh titer +; CXR: anterior mediastinal mass

Myasthenia gravis (associated with thymoma)

20-y/o black woman presents with fatigue, arthralgias, Raynaud phenomenon, and pleuritic chest pain; PE: butterfly malar facial rash; W/U: ↓ platelets, proteinuria, and ⊕ ANA, anti-dsDNA, and anti-Smith Abs

SLE

20-y/o with a h/o developmental delay presents with facial weakness; PE: cataracts, marked weakness in muscles of hand, neck, and distal leg with sustained muscle contraction; genetic testing: CTG repeat expansion within *DMPK* gene

Myotonic dystrophy

BEHAVIORAL SCIENCE

20-y/o woman presents with excessive anxiety about a variety of events for more than half of the days for the last 7 months

Generalized anxiety disorder

8-y/o boy presents with a 5-month h/o regular bedwetting episodes; PE is unremarkable and fasting glucose is WNL

Enuresis

28-y/o man who systematically checks each lock in his house every time before leaving, often causing him to be over an hour late for meetings

Obsessive-compulsive disorder

29-y/o man presents with a 9-month h/o insatiable urges to rub himself against strangers, which he has regrettably acted on several times

Frotteurism

22-y/o woman college student who is 20% below her ideal body weight complains of not having any menstrual cycles and "feeling fat"

Anorexia nervosa

26-y/o woman medical student is convinced for the past 9 months that she has SLE and despite numerous negative workups, she fears she will have to drop out of school

Hypochondriasis

17-y/o woman presents with complaints of "feeling fat" and a h/o eating dinner alone in her bedroom; PE shows normal height and weight, dental erosions, and scars on the back of her hand

Bulimia

21-y/o woman with no h/o trauma presents to the ER because she cannot feel or move her legs; W/U is WNL; detailed history reveals that her boyfriend left her this morning	Conversion disorder
43-y/o alcoholic with a h/o confabulation and amnesia presents to ER after falling down; PE shows nystagmus and ataxic gait; W/U reveals macrocytic anemia	Wernicke-Korsakoff syndrome
6-y/o presents with 8-month h/o hyperactivity, inattentiveness, and impulsivity both at school and at home; PE and W/U are WNL	Attention deficit hyperactivity disorder (ADHD)
33-y/o woman presents to your office distressed after turning down a lucrative job offer because of the requirement to speak in front of people	Social phobia
9-y/o boy with 2-year h/o involuntary tics is brought to your office because he has recently been shouting obscenities	Tourette syndrome
33-y/o woman nurse presents with recent occurrences of hypoglycemia; PE reveals multiple crossed scars on abdomen; W/U shows insulin/C-peptide ratio >1.0	Factitious disorder (Munchausen syndrome)
33-y/o is referred to you for reports of random episode of shouting and screaming during the night; he has no recollection of the event and denies having nightmares	Sleep terror disorder
16-y/o with a h/o sudden-onset daytime sleep attacks with loss of muscle tone and audiovisual hallucinations while waking and falling asleep	Narcolepsy
19-y/o with an 8-month h/o deteriorating grades and social withdrawal presents with auditory hallucinations; PE shows odd thinking patterns, tangential thoughts, and flattened effects	Schizophrenia

24-y/o with a h/o depression presents with ↓ need for sleep and auditory hallucinations; PE reveals easy distractibility and pressured speech; W/U shows normal TSH and negative toxicology screen	Bipolar disorder—type 1 (manic episode)
48-y/o woman presents with recent h/o early morning waking, ↓ appetite, feelings of guilt, and loss of interest in her usual hobbies over the past 3 months; PE and laboratory results are WNL	Major depressive disorder
68-y/o veteran presents with complaints of vivid flashbacks, hypervigilance, and difficulty falling asleep for the past several years; patient appears very anxious during the PE	Posttraumatic stress disorder
6-month-old child presents with unyielding crying; PE reveals multiple bruises in different stages of healing and bilateral retinal hemorrhages; XR shows multiple, healing fractures along posterior ribs	Shaken baby syndrome
43-y/o woman from Boston finds herself in Utah, but does not remember why she is there or how she got there; PE and W/U are WNL; detailed history reveals that her son suddenly died 1 week ago	Dissociative fugue
3-y/o boy with a h/o of poor cuddling presents with severely delayed language and social development; PE reveals below normal intelligence with unusual calculating abilities and repetitive behaviors	Autism

Index